Lippincott Williams & Wilkins'

ADMINISTRATIVE
Medical Assisting

Lippincott Williams & Wilkins'

ADMINISTRATIVE
Medical Assisting

Elizabeth A. Molle, MS, RN
Nurse Educator
Middlesex Hospital
Middletown, Connecticut

Laura Southard Durham, BS, CMA
Medical Assisting Program Coordinator
Forsyth Technical Community College
Winston-Salem, North Carolina

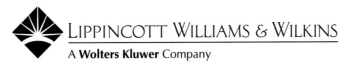

A **Wolters Kluwer** Company

Philadelphia • Baltimore • New York • London
Buenos Aires • Hong Kong • Sydney • Tokyo

Senior Acquisitions Editor: John Goucher
Managing Editor: Rebecca Keifer
Marketing Manager: Hilary Henderson
Production Editor: Bill Cady
Designer: Risa Clow
Compositor: Maryland Composition
Printer: RR Donnelley

Copyright © 2004 Lippincott Williams & Wilkins

351 West Camden Street
Baltimore, MD 21201

530 Walnut Street
Philadelphia, PA 19106

Printed in the United States of America

Library of Congress Cataloging-in-Publication Data
Molle, Elizabeth A.
  Lippincott Williams and Wilkins' administrative medical assisting / Elizabeth A. Molle, Laura Southard Durham.
      p. ; cm.
  Includes references and index.
  ISBN 0-7817-3775-3
    1. Medical assistants. 2. Medical offices—Management. I. Title: Lippincott Williams & Wilkins' administrative medical assisting. II. Title: Administrative medical assisting. III. Durham, Laura Southard. IV. Title.
    [DNLM: 1. Medical Secretaries—organization & administration. 2. Practice Management, Medical. W 80 M726L 2004]
  R728.8.M655 2004
  651'.961—dc22

                                                                                              2003054466

The publishers have made every effort to trace the copyright holders for borrowed material. If they have inadvertently overlooked any, they will be pleased to make the necessary arrangements at the first opportunity.

To purchase additional copies of this book, call our customer service department at **(800) 638-3030** or fax orders to **(301) 824-7390**. International customers should call **(301) 714-2324**.

Visit Lippincott Williams & Wilkins on the Internet: http://www.LWW.com. Lippincott Williams & Wilkins customer service representatives are available from 8:30 am to 6:00 pm, EST.

03 04 05 06 07
1 2 3 4 5 6 7 8 9 10

This book is dedicated to Ken: Thank you for your love, support, and understanding. To my friends and colleagues in the Department of Education at Middlesex Hospital, thank you for your support and encouragement.

ELIZABETH A. MOLLE

This book is dedicated to all the people who made it possible. To my daughter, Amanda, who makes me whole. To the rest of my family members who have sacrificed a great deal: Brad, Susan, Jihad, Dana, Laila, Ramsey, and Ellen. To my parents, Mamie and Joe, who taught me to work hard. They are proud of me, even from heaven. To Jenifer and Rhea for getting me through all the ups and downs of the past year. To LeRoy who loves and encourages me in everything I do. To my students who keep me centered. And especially to Gracie Ruth Melton, my granddaughter, who gives me wings.

LAURA SOUTHARD DURHAM

PREFACE

This is an exciting and challenging time to enter the field of medical assisting. You are uniquely poised to function as the most versatile professional in the medical office. As a medical assistant, you will have the opportunity to perform a variety of clinical and administrative skills. The skills you will perform and your job title will vary among offices. This book was written to help you succeed in performing a variety of administrative medical assisting procedures.

Lippincott Williams & Wilkins' Administrative Medical Assisting will define your roles and responsibilities as a professional medical assistant. The book is based on the American Association of Medical Assisting (AAMA) role delineation components for certified medical assistants and the competencies described by the American Medical Technologists (AMT) Registered Medical Assistant Competency Inventory. These roles have evolved and grown over the past decade and will continue to expand to meet the needs of the medical profession.

ORGANIZATION OF THE TEXT

As experienced medical assisting instructors, we understand the complexity of this subject matter can be overwhelming to a new student. Great care and concern were taken to organize this book into a logical and reader friendly presentation. The book is divided into three sections:

- Section I, Introduction to Medical Assisting, consists of two units. Unit 1 provides you with a brief history of the medical profession and the practice of medical assisting. Legal and ethical issues governing the medical community and your practice are also discussed. Unit 2 helps you sharpen your communication skills, and its final chapter gives you the tools to deliver effective patient education.
- Section II, The Administrative Medical Assistant, consists of two units. Unit 3 helps you master basic administrative skills. Unit 4 explores financial management of the medical office.
- Section III, Career Strategies, helps you make a smooth transition from the classroom environment to the workforce.

Lippincott Williams & Wilkins' Administrative Medical Assisting is packaged with a complimentary CD-ROM to help you prepare for examinations. The CD-ROM contains questions to help you prepare for CMA and RMA certification and four interactive case studies that place you inside actual situations you will encounter in practice.

FEATURES

Our goal is to make this textbook the most student friendly resource available in the medical assisting field. For students who use English as a second language (ESL), an ESL learning expert reviewed the entire text to ensure the language is appropriate and understandable to non-native English students. To aid these students, the ESL Glossary is provided.

A variety of key features are included to spark interest and promote comprehension. Most chapters include the following:

- A chapter outline
- Learning objectives and performance objectives
- Role delineation components as set forth by AAMA and AMT
- Key terms and key points
- Step-by-step procedure boxes
- Spanish terms and phrases
- Relevant Web addresses
- Critical thinking challenges
- Checkpoint questions
- Unique information boxes, tables, and displays
- Full color illustrations

TEACHING AND LEARNING PACKAGE

This textbook is fully supported with a robust teaching and learning package, each element of which is designed to help you and your instructor get the most out of the textbook. The resource package includes the following:

- A student study guide to enhance learning and comprehension includes competency evaluation forms for each procedure in the textbook and self-assessment exercises, such as matching, multiple-choice, skill drills, critical thinking, and patient teaching.
- A complete instructor's resource kit accompanying the textbook includes suggested classroom activities; answers to workbook questions; and questions and answers on starting a medical assisting program, gaining and maintaining accreditation, changing textbooks, setting goals and objectives for students, and general teaching guide. A CD-ROM with a test generator and PowerPoint slides is packaged with the instructor's manual.

As medical assisting instructors, we hope this books exceeds your expectations. May your career in medical assisting be challenging and fulfilling!

Elizabeth A. Molle, MS, RN
Laura Southard Durham, BS, CMA

REVIEWERS

We are grateful to the reviewers who read the proposal and drafts of all of the chapters. They provided helpful feedback that has resulted in a stronger book. We thank them all. Some of the reviewers wish to remain anonymous. We acknowledge:

Patricia Davis Christian, Program Director
Business Office Technology
Southwest Georgia Technical College
Thomasville, GA

Glenn Grady, MEd, BSMT(ASCP), CMA
Miller-Motte Technical College
Wilmington, NC

Chris Hollander, CMA, BS
Westwood College of Technology
Denver, CO

Sharon Anne Kerber, MAA
Instructor
St. Louis, MO

Debra J. Paul, AAS, CMA
Michiana College,
South Bend, Indiana

Susan Sniffin, MBA, CMA-C, LRT
Indian River Community College
Fort Pierce, Florida

PUBLISHER'S ACKNOWLEDGMENT

Lippincott Williams & Wilkins would like to thank the following medical assisting instructors for taking the time to provide valuable product and market feedback throughout the development of this text. Your input is greatly appreciated, and it has helped to shape this book.

Connie Allen
Nina Beaman
Cyndi Brassington
Becky Briggs
Beth Buchholz
Michelle Buchman
Shirley Buzbee
Theresa Cyr
Rose Dovenbarger
Kent Earley
George Fakhoury
Pamela Fleming
Dr. Eugenia Fulcher

Rena Gizicki
Robyn Gohsman
Rene Griffee
Kris Hardy
Alicia Hill
Elizabeth Hoffman
Michaelea Holten
Stacy Horn
Alexis Jenkins
Ray Johns
Linda Johnson
Marcie Jones
Kathryn Kalanick

Geri Kale-Smith
J. Kaltz
Diana Kendrick
Dorothy Kiel
Diane Klieger
Wendy Leer
Connie Lieseke
Cynthia Lundgren
Mary Marks
Tanya Mercer
Tammy Miller
Pat Moeck
Jahangir Moini, MD

Ethel Morikis
Donna Otis
Lori Rager
Deanna Rieke
Deborah Rojas
Suzette Simonson
Stacey Singer
Cathy Soto
Nina Thierer
Valeria Truitt
Debra Tymcio
Jane Vallely
Deborah Westervelt

AUTHOR'S ACKNOWLEDGMENTS

A book of this size and complexity cannot be accomplished without the hard work and dedication of many people and businesses. From the book's conception to its production, John Goucher, acquisitions editor, was there. Thank you for believing in this project and making it a reality. A special thank you to all the staff of Lippincott Williams & Wilkins for your hard work and dedication to publishing this book and other medical assisting textbooks. We thank all of the reviewers for their prompt, honest, and thorough reviews. Your reviews provided invaluable suggestions and comments for improving the quality of the book.

Thank you to Leo Hurst for helping with the Spanish translations. We also thank Karen Santiago and Neuva Esperanza for developing the ESL section. Thank you to John Briggs and Mark Lozier for lending your expertise in photography. In addition, a special thank you to the following people who served as models, coordinators, and medical experts for the pictures: Britt Butterfield, Kelli Campbell, Risa Clow, Ted Clow, Robert Homan, Ramona Hunter, Jacqui Merrell, Phillip Olive, Rob Randall, Patrick Sheridan, and Shelley Welch. We also thank Dr. Rosen and the staff of Ardmore Family Practice for their assistance on various content issues. A special thank you to Melissa Hurley for helping with the editing of numerous chapters. Thank you to my colleagues and friends with the North Carolina Society of Medical Assistants and Forsyth-Stokes-Davie chapter of Medical Assistants for being an invaluable resource to this book. Thank you to my colleagues at MICA Information Systems for supplying illustrations. Finally, a special thank you to Carol Turiello, RN, RDMS, CPC, from Upstate Medical University in Syracuse, New York, for implementing the reviews and the development editor's comments into several chapters.

USER'S GUIDE

Lippincott Williams & Wilkins' Administrative Medical Assisting is not just a textbook, it is a complete learning resource that will help you to understand important information, master skills, and become a success in your chosen field of Medical Assisting. To achieve all of this, the authors and publisher have included features and tools throughout the text to help you work through the material presented. Please take a few moments to look through this User's Guide, which will introduce you to the features that will enhance your learning experience.

Chapter Competencies
Learning objectives at the beginning of each chapter tell you the skills you must know by the end of the chapter.

Role Delineation Components
The components from the AAMA's Role Delineation Study that are covered within a chapter are listed at the beginning of each chapter. This list helps you focus on the essential information & skills covered on your certification exam.

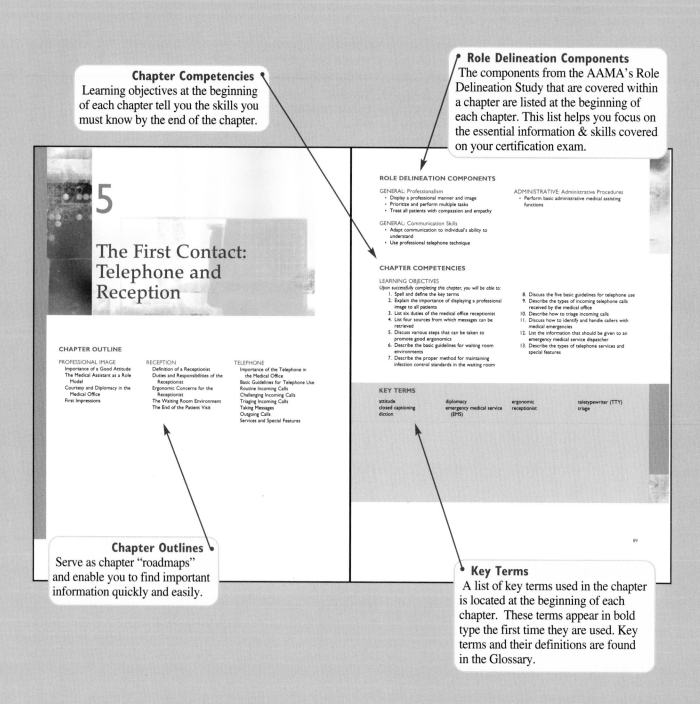

5

The First Contact: Telephone and Reception

CHAPTER OUTLINE

PROFESSIONAL IMAGE
Importance of a Good Attitude
The Medical Assistant as a Role Model
Courtesy and Diplomacy in the Medical Office
First Impressions

RECEPTION
Definition of a Receptionist
Duties and Responsibilities of the Receptionist
Ergonomic Concerns for the Receptionist
The Waiting Room Environment
The End of the Patient Visit

TELEPHONE
Importance of the Telephone in the Medical Office
Basic Guidelines for Telephone Use
Routine Incoming Calls
Challenging Incoming Calls
Triaging Incoming Calls
Taking Messages
Outgoing Calls
Services and Special Features

ROLE DELINEATION COMPONENTS

GENERAL: Professionalism
• Display a professional manner and image
• Prioritize and perform multiple tasks
• Treat all patients with compassion and empathy

GENERAL: Communication Skills
• Adapt communication to individual's ability to understand
• Use professional telephone technique

ADMINISTRATIVE: Administrative Procedures
• Perform basic administrative medical assisting functions

CHAPTER COMPETENCIES

LEARNING OBJECTIVES
Upon successfully completing this chapter, you will be able to:
1. Spell and define the key terms
2. Explain the importance of displaying a professional image to all patients
3. List six duties of the medical office receptionist
4. List four sources from which messages can be retrieved
5. Discuss various steps that can be taken to promote good ergonomics
6. Describe the basic guidelines for waiting room environments
7. Describe the proper method for maintaining infection control standards in the waiting room

8. Discuss the five basic guidelines for telephone use
9. Describe the types of incoming telephone calls received by the medical office
10. Describe how to triage incoming calls
11. Discuss how to identify and handle callers with medical emergencies
12. List the information that should be given to an emergency medical service dispatcher
13. Describe the types of telephone services and special features

KEY TERMS

attitude
closed captioning
diction

diplomacy
emergency medical service (EMS)

ergonomic
receptionist

teletypewriter (TTY)
triage

89

Chapter Outlines
Serve as chapter "roadmaps" and enable you to find important information quickly and easily.

Key Terms
A list of key terms used in the chapter is located at the beginning of each chapter. These terms appear in bold type the first time they are used. Key terms and their definitions are found in the Glossary.

CALL OUT BOXES

The most important information is emphasized throughout the text in call-out boxes. The following boxes are included:

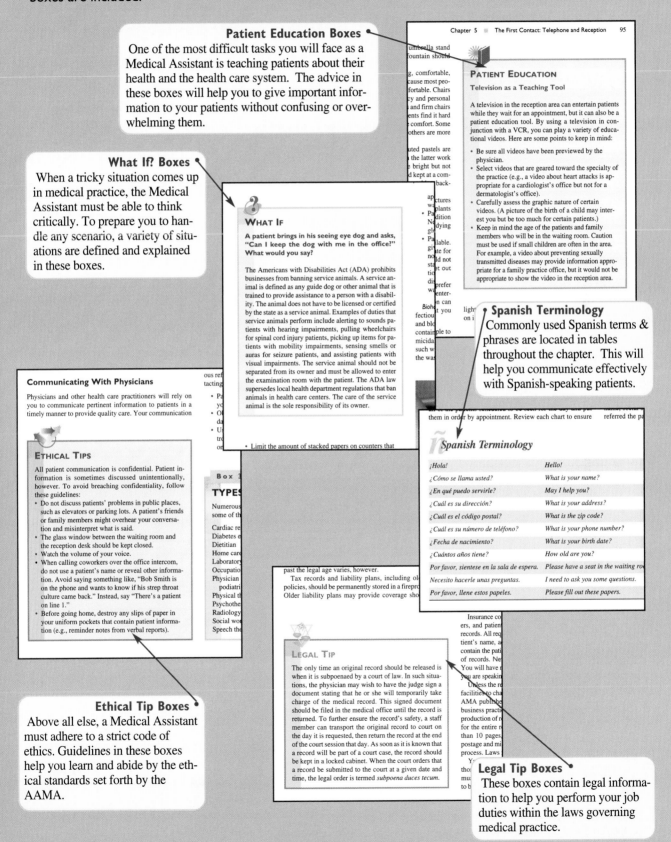

Patient Education Boxes
One of the most difficult tasks you will face as a Medical Assistant is teaching patients about their health and the health care system. The advice in these boxes will help you to give important information to your patients without confusing or overwhelming them.

What If? Boxes
When a tricky situation comes up in medical practice, the Medical Assistant must be able to think critically. To prepare you to handle any scenario, a variety of situations are defined and explained in these boxes.

Spanish Terminology
Commonly used Spanish terms & phrases are located in tables throughout the chapter. This will help you communicate effectively with Spanish-speaking patients.

Ethical Tip Boxes
Above all else, a Medical Assistant must adhere to a strict code of ethics. Guidelines in these boxes help you learn and abide by the ethical standards set forth by the AAMA.

Legal Tip Boxes
These boxes contain legal information to help you perform your job duties within the laws governing medical practice.

PATIENT EDUCATION
Television as a Teaching Tool

A television in the reception area can entertain patients while they wait for an appointment, but it can also be a patient education tool. By using a television in conjunction with a VCR, you can play a variety of educational videos. Here are some points to keep in mind:

- Be sure all videos have been previewed by the physician.
- Select videos that are geared toward the specialty of the practice (e.g., a video about heart attacks is appropriate for a cardiologist's office but not for a dermatologist's office).
- Carefully assess the graphic nature of certain videos. (A picture of the birth of a child may interest you but be too much for certain patients.)
- Keep in mind the age of the patients and family members who will be in the waiting room. Caution must be used if small children are often in the area. For example, a video about preventing sexually transmitted diseases may provide information appropriate for a family practice office, but it would not be appropriate to show the video in the reception area.

WHAT IF

A patient brings in his seeing eye dog and asks, "Can I keep the dog with me in the office?" What would you say?

The Americans with Disabilities Act (ADA) prohibits businesses from banning service animals. A service animal is defined as any guide dog or other animal that is trained to provide assistance to a person with a disability. The animal does not have to be licensed or certified by the state as a service animal. Examples of duties that service animals perform include alerting to sounds patients with hearing impairments, pulling wheelchairs for spinal cord injury patients, picking up items for patients with mobility impairments, sensing smells or auras for seizure patients, and assisting patients with visual impairments. The service animal should not be separated from its owner and must be allowed to enter the examination room with the patient. The ADA law supersedes local health department regulations that ban animals in health care centers. The care of the service animal is the sole responsibility of its owner.

Communicating With Physicians

Physicians and other health care practitioners will rely on you to communicate pertinent information to patients in a timely manner to provide quality care. Your communication

ETHICAL TIPS

All patient communication is confidential. Patient information is sometimes discussed unintentionally, however. To avoid breaching confidentiality, follow these guidelines:

- Do not discuss patients' problems in public places, such as elevators or parking lots. A patient's friends or family members might overhear your conversation and misinterpret what is said.
- The glass window between the waiting room and the reception desk should be kept closed.
- Watch the volume of your voice.
- When calling coworkers over the office intercom, do not use a patient's name or reveal other information. Avoid saying something like, "Bob Smith is on the phone and wants to know if his strep throat culture came back." Instead, say "There's a patient on line 1."
- Before going home, destroy any slips of paper in your uniform pockets that contain patient information (e.g., reminder notes from verbal reports).

Spanish Terminology

¡Hola!	Hello!
¿Cómo se llama usted?	What is your name?
¿En qué puedo servirle?	May I help you?
¿Cuál es su dirección?	What is your address?
¿Cuál es el código postal?	What is the zip code?
¿Cuál es su número de teléfono?	What is your phone number?
¿Fecha de nacimiento?	What is your birth date?
¿Cuántos años tiene?	How old are you?
Por favor, siéntese en la sala de espera.	Please have a seat in the waiting roo
Necesito hacerle unas preguntas.	I need to ask you some questions.
Por favor, llene estos papeles.	Please fill out these papers.

past the legal age varies, however.

Tax records and liability plans, including ol
policies, should be permanently stored in a firepro
Older liability plans may provide coverage sho

LEGAL TIP

The only time an original record should be released is when it is subpoenaed by a court of law. In such situations, the physician may wish to have the judge sign a document stating that he or she will temporarily take charge of the medical record. This signed document should be filed in the medical office until the record is returned. To further ensure the record's safety, a staff member can transport the original record to court on the day it is requested, then return the record at the end of the court session that day. As soon as it is known that a record will be part of a court case, the record should be kept in a locked cabinet. When the court orders that a record be submitted to the court at a given date and time, the legal order is termed *subpoena duces tecum*.

Procedure Boxes

Detailed procedures are broken down step-by-step, showing you how to properly perform essential skills. The needed equipment & supplies are listed. Purposes are given for each step to ensure greater understanding.

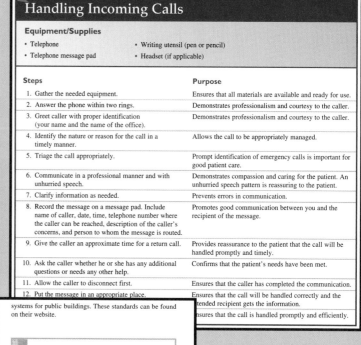

Procedure 5-1

Handling Incoming Calls

Equipment/Supplies

- Telephone
- Telephone message pad
- Writing utensil (pen or pencil)
- Headset (if applicable)

Steps	Purpose
1. Gather the needed equipment.	Ensures that all materials are available and ready for use.
2. Answer the phone within two rings.	Demonstrates professionalism and courtesy to the caller.
3. Greet caller with proper identification (your name and the name of the office).	Demonstrates professionalism and courtesy to the caller.
4. Identify the nature or reason for the call in a timely manner.	Allows the call to be appropriately managed.
5. Triage the call appropriately.	Prompt identification of emergency calls is important for good patient care.
6. Communicate in a professional manner and with unhurried speech.	Demonstrates compassion and caring for the patient. An unhurried speech pattern is reassuring to the patient.
7. Clarify information as needed.	Prevents errors in communication.
8. Record the message on a message pad. Include name of caller, date, time, telephone number where the caller can be reached, description of the caller's concerns, and person to whom the message is routed.	Promotes good communication between you and the recipient of the message.
9. Give the caller an approximate time for a return call.	Provides reassurance to the patient that the call will be handled promptly and timely.
10. Ask the caller whether he or she has any additional questions or needs any other help.	Confirms that the patient's needs have been met.
11. Allow the caller to disconnect first.	Ensures that the caller has completed the communication.
12. Put the message in an appropriate place.	Ensures that the call will be handled correctly and the intended recipient gets the information.

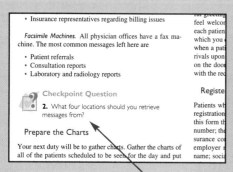

- Insurance representatives regarding billing issues

Facsimile Machines. All physician offices have a fax machine. The most common messages left here are

- Patient referrals
- Consultation reports
- Laboratory and radiology reports

Checkpoint Question

2. What four locations should you retrieve messages from?

Prepare the Charts

Your next duty will be to gather charts. Gather the charts of all of the patients scheduled to be seen for the day and put

Checkpoint Questions

Located throughout the chapter, these questions quiz you on the material covered and reinforce key points in the reading. Answers to these questions are located at the end of each chapter.

Critical Thinking Challenges

Located at the end of each chapter, these challenges encourage you to apply the knowledge gained throughout the chapter in a real-life scenario.

systems for public buildings. These standards can be found on their website.

CHAPTER SUMMARY

As the receptionist, you are the most visible and accessible representative of the medical practice. Duties and responsibilities of a receptionist vary among office settings. The key to being a good receptionist is to demonstrate tact and diplomacy in all interactions with patients. Providing a positive attitude will ease the patient's anxiety and ensure the best and most confident image of the practice is projected. Proper telephone etiquette and manners are essential for good patient care and to achieve effective communication among various health care providers. Triaging incoming calls is a skill that you must master if you are to be an effective receptionist.

Chapter Summary

Each chapter is summarized in a few paragraphs at the end of the chapter. This helps you review important topics covered in the chapter.

Critical Thinking Challenges

1. How would you calm an irate patient on the telephone? Identify some phrases that you might use to calm the caller. What phrases may make the situation worse?
2. Assume you are working in an obstetrician's office. What kinds of educational videos might be appropriate for the waiting room? What if you were working in an orthopedic office or for a surgeon?
3. Here is a triage scenario. Line 1 is a home calling the office with a patient status update

CD-ROM for Lippincott Williams & Wilkins'
ADMINISTRATIVE Medical Assisting

Back-of-Book CD-ROM

Interactive Case Studies

These computer based, interactive case studies present you with different scenarios that you will face in the medical office. The timely scenarios will encourage you to think critically and apply multiple skills that are taught in the text.

Case study topics include:
- Dealing with an emergency situation
- Patient education, health promotion and disease prevention
- Medical law & ethics and confidentiality
- Accounting & billing

Certification Exam Review Questions

These questions help you prepare for the National Certification exams. A practice exam is included, with questions that closely resemble those that are on the tests.

WWW.GO Websites

These websites can provide you with some additional information:

American Academy of Pediatrics
www.aap.org
American Heart Association
www.americanheart.org
CDC
www.cdc.gov
Federal Communications Commission
www.fcc.gov/cib/dro
Institute for Disabilities Research and Training
www.idrt.com
Online Yellow Pages
www.smartpages.com
OSHA
www.osha.gov
Telecommunications for the Deaf
www.amrad.org
U. S. Department of Justice/Americans with Disabilities Act
www.usdoj.gov/crt/ada

Websites

Listed at the end of each chapter, these online resources will help you to stay up to date in the medical field. Both medical professional sites and patient resources are given.

CONTENTS

EXPANDED CONTENTS

SECTION III

CAREER STRATEGIES, 307

Unit Five

Competing in the Job Market, 309

CHAPTER 19: Making the Transition: Student to Employee, 310

APPENDICES, 329

Section I

Introduction to Medical Assisting

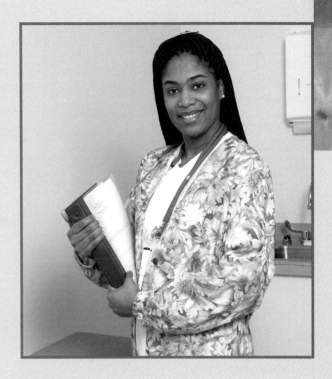

Understanding the Profession

Welcome! The world of medicine is an exciting and challenging frontier. This unit consists of two chapters that will introduce you to the field of medicine and medical assisting. In the first chapter, you will learn how medicine has evolved through the years from an era of superstition and magical cures to an age of modern technology. The second chapter introduces you to legal and ethical roles that affect medical professionals. Sometimes, the advances in medicine challenge our laws and ethics. This unit will help you to understand the bond between medicine, law, and ethics. Let the exploration begin!

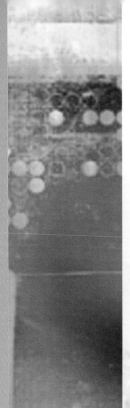

Medicine and Medical Assisting

CHAPTER OUTLINE

ROLE DELINEATION COMPONENTS

GENERAL: Professionalism
- Display a professional manner and image
- Demonstrate initiative and responsibility
- Work as a member of the health care team
- Promote the CMA credential
- Enhance skills through continuing education

GENERAL: Legal Concepts
- Perform within legal and ethical boundaries

CHAPTER COMPETENCIES

LEARNING OBJECTIVES
Upon successfully completing this chapter, you will be able to:

1. Spell and define the key terms
2. Outline a brief history of medicine
3. Identify the key founders of medical science
4. Explain the system of health care in the United States
5. Discuss the typical medical office
6. List medical specialties a medical assistant may encounter
7. List the duties of a medical assistant
8. Describe the desired characteristics of a medical assistant
9. Explain the pathways of education for medical assistants
10. Discuss the importance of program accreditation
11. Name and describe the two nationally recognized accrediting agencies for medical assisting education programs
12. Explain the benefits and avenues of certification for the medical assistant
13. List the benefits of membership in a professional organization
14. Identify members of the health care team
15. List settings in which medical assistants may be employed

KEY TERMS

accreditation	cloning	medical assistant	outpatient
administrative	continuing education units	multidisciplinary	recertification
caduceus	externship	multiskilled health	role delineation chart
certification	inpatient	professional	specialty
clinical	laboratory		

WELCOME TO THE FIELD of medicine and to the medical assisting profession! You have selected a fascinating and challenging career, one of the fastest growing specialties in the medical field. The need for the **multiskilled health professional**—an individual with versatile training in the health care field—will continue to grow within the foreseeable future, and you are now a part of this exciting career direction.

To help you understand the significance of the medical knowledge and skills you will receive during your course of study, we begin by taking a chronological look at the history of medicine and then explore the profession of medical assisting.

HISTORY OF MEDICINE

Tremendous achievements in the general health, comfort, and well-being of patients have been made just within the past 100 to 150 years, with the greatest advances occurring in the 20th century. It is difficult to imagine health care without antibiotics, x-ray machines, or anesthesia, but these developments are fairly new to medicine. For example, penicillin was not produced in large quantities until World War II, and surgery was performed without anesthesia until the mid 1800s.

Ancient Medical History

The earliest recorded evidence of medical history dates to the early Egyptians. Papyrus records of tuberculosis, pneumonia, and arteriosclerosis are still in existence from 4000 B.C. It is evident that during this time the Egyptians performed surgeries, including brain surgery. Fossil remains have shown patients with fractures (broken bones) that were splinted and subsequently healed. Although many cultures practiced primitive forms of surgery, most early practitioners used a combination of religion and superstition to heal ailments. Herbs, roots, and plants were used as medications.

Some of these early medications played a key role in the development of our modern pharmacology. Digitalis, from the common garden plant foxglove, is still in use today for its original purpose of strengthening the heart's action. Opium, from the pods of the poppy plant, is still used to induce stupor and a level of painlessness. Supplemental iron as a method of treating anemia was recognized by the Chinese as early as 2500 B.C. Medical research is constantly uncovering evidence that previously used treatment methods were based on sound theory and are being incorporated into our modern arsenal against illness.

More than 1000 years before Christ, Moses was appointed the first public health officer. He wrote rules for sanitation. He stated that all people preparing and serving public food must be neat and clean. In the days long before refrigeration, it became a religious law that only freshly slaughtered animals could be eaten. Moses also required that serving dishes and cooking utensils be washed between customers at public restaurants.

Aesculapius, Greek god of healing and the son of Apollo, had many followers who used massage and exercise to treat patients. This god is also believed to have used the magical powers of a yellow, nonpoisonous serpent to lick the wounds of surgical patients. Aesculapius was often pictured holding the serpent wrapped around his staff or wand; this staff is a symbol of medicine. Another medical symbol is the **caduceus**, the staff of the Roman god Mercury, shown as a winged staff with two serpents wrapped around it (Fig. 1-1).

Around 400 B.C., Hippocrates practiced medicine and set high behavioral standards for practicing physicians. Hippocrates, called the "Father of Medicine," turned medicine into a science and erased the element of mysticism that it once held. He wrote the Hippocratic Oath, which is still part of medical school graduation ceremonies.

The Greek physician Galen (131–201 A.D.), became known as the "Father of Experimental Physiology." He was the first physician to document a patient's pulse, although he did not know that the pulse was related to the heart. Galen identified many parts of the body. His anatomic findings were mostly incorrect, however, because they were based on the dissection of apes and swine. Postmortem human dissections were illegal and were considered sacrilegious until the Renaissance (1350–1650).

The rule of the Roman Empire, from about 200 B.C. until its dissolution several centuries later, brought great strides in public health. Water was brought from clean mountain streams by way of raised aqueducts that were regularly cleaned and maintained; sewers carried wastes away from the cities; and personal cleanliness was encouraged. One Roman physician Mar-

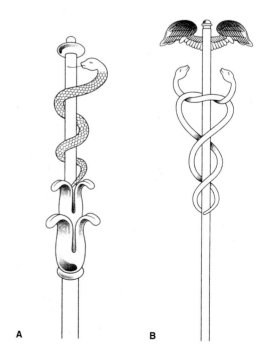

FIGURE 1-1.   (**A**) Staff of Aesculapius. (**B**) Caduceus.

cus Varro (116–21 B.C.) even suggested that there might be creatures too small to be seen that caused illness. This was 1800 years before the invention of the microscope.

During the Dark Ages (400–800 A.D.) and through the Middle Ages (800–1400 A.D.), few advances were made in the medical field. Medicine was practiced primarily in convents and monasteries and consisted of simply comforting patients rather than trying to find a cure for the illness. The population became more mobile, ranging away from traditional homelands for war, crusades, and exploration. Each venture exposed whole cultures to diseases against which they had no immunity. Cities grew larger but without the Roman technology for maintaining sanitation. Ignorance, crowding, and poor health practices led to the eruption of the bubonic plague, which twice swept through Europe and Asia, killing approximately 20 million people. This deadly disease, the greatest killer in our history, spread from rat fleas to humans, killing approximately half of the known population within a few years.

Checkpoint Question

1. Why were Galen's anatomic findings considered incorrect?

Modern Medical History

The Renaissance was a period of enlightenment in all areas of art, science, and education, and it fostered great strides in medicine. The advent of the printing press and the establishment of great universities made the practice of medicine more accessible to larger numbers of practitioners. Great minds collaborated to advance medical and scientific theories and perform experiments that led to discoveries of enormous benefit in the fight against disease.

During this period, Andreas Vesalius (1514–1564) became known as the "Father of Modern Anatomy." He corrected many of Galen's errors and wrote the first relatively correct anatomy textbook. Soon afterward, William Harvey identified the pumping action of the heart. He described circulation as a continuous circuit pumped by the heart to carry blood through the body. Harvey studied the action of the heart using dogs, not humans.

The microscope was invented in the mid 1660s by a Dutch lens maker, Anton von Leeuwenhoek. He was the first person to observe bacteria under a lens, although he had no idea of the significance of the microorganisms to human health. His instrument also allowed him to accurately describe a red blood cell.

John Hunter (1728–1793) became known as the "Father of Scientific Surgery." He developed many surgical techniques that are still used today. Hunter also developed and inserted the first artificial feeding tube into a patient in 1778 and was the first to classify teeth in a scientific manner.

In 1796, Edward Jenner, a physician in England, overheard a young milkmaid explain that she could not catch smallpox because she had already had the very mild cowpox caught while milking her cows. Several weeks later, Jenner inoculated a small boy with smallpox crusts. The boy did not contract the disease, and the prevention for smallpox was discovered. Jenner's discovery of the smallpox vaccine led to more emphasis on prevention of disease rather than on cures.

The 1800s brought the first notable records of the contributions of women to the medical field. Florence Nightingale (1820–1910) was the founder of modern nursing. She set standards for nurses and developed educational requirements for nurses (Fig. 1-2).

Also during the early 1800s, the importance of the mind as a part of the health care process was becoming a recognized field of medicine. The first extensive work and writing on mental health was published in 1812 by Benjamin Rush, entitled *Medical Inquiries and Observations upon Diseases of the Mind*. He advocated humane treatment of the mentally ill at a time when most were imprisoned, chained, starved, exhibited like animals, or simply killed. Rush's influence began the separate field of study into the working of the mind that became modern psychiatry. The mid 1880s saw a surge in the study of disease transmission. Louis Pasteur (1822–1895) became famous for his work with bacteria. Pasteur discovered that wine turned sour because of the presence of bacteria. He found that when the bacteria were eliminated, the wine lasted longer. Pasteur's discovery that bacteria in liquids could be eliminated by heat led to the process known as pasteurization. This finding led to using heat to sterilize surgical instruments. Pasteur has been called the "Father of Bacteriology" for this accomplishment. Pasteur also focused on preventing the transmission of anthrax and discovered the rabies vaccine and was honored with the title "Father of Preventive Medicine" for this work.

In the mid 1880s, Ignaz Semmelweiss, a Hungarian physician, noticed that women whose babies were born at home with a midwife in attendance had childbed fever less

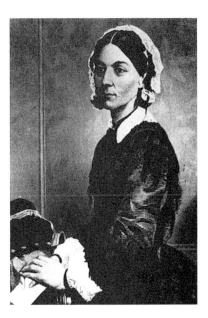

FIGURE 1-2. Florence Nightingale.

often than those who delivered in well-respected hospitals with prestigious physicians at the bedside. He was ridiculed by the medical establishment and was fired from his position when he required medical personnel to wash their hands in a solution of chlorinated lime before performing obstetric examinations. He was right, of course, and hand-washing is still the most important factor in the fight against disease transmission.

At about the same time, Joseph Lister began to apply antiseptics to wounds to prevent infection. The concept was not clearly understood, but before Lister's practices, as many patients died of infection as died of the primitive surgical techniques of the early part of the century.

Modern anesthesia was discovered in 1842 by Crawford Williamson Long. The effects of nitrous oxide were known by the mid 1700s, but Long discovered its therapeutic use by accident when he observed a group of chemistry students inhaling it for amusement. Before this time, anesthesia consisted of large doses of alcohol or opium, leather straps for patient restraint, or the unconsciousness resulting from pain. Ether and chloroform came into use at about this time.

Elizabeth Blackwell (1821–1910) became the first woman to complete medical school in the United States when she graduated from Geneva Medical College in New York. In 1869, Blackwell established her own medical school in Europe for women only, opening the door for a rapidly expanding role for women in the medical field.

Clara Barton (1821–1912) founded the American Red Cross in 1881 and was its first president. She identified the need for psychological as well as physical support for wounded soldiers in the Civil War.

X-rays were discovered in 1895 by Wilhelm Konrad Roentgen when he observed that a previously unknown ray generated by a cathode tube could pass through soft tissue and outline underlying structures. Medical diagnosis was revolutionized, earning Roentgen a Nobel Prize in 1901 for his discovery. The therapeutic uses of x-rays were recognized much later.

Marie Curie (1867–1934), a brilliant science student, married Pierre Curie, and together they discovered polonium and radium. Their discovery revolutionized the principles of energy and radioactivity. Marie and Pierre Curie shared the Nobel Prize for chemistry in 1903. Marie continued the research after his death and again won the Nobel Prize for physics in 1911.

In 1928, Sir Alexander Fleming, a bacteriologist, accidentally discovered penicillin when his assistant forgot to wash the Petri dishes Fleming had used for experiments. When he noticed the circles of nongrowth around areas of a certain mold, he was able to extract the prototype for one of our most potent weapons against disease. He won the Nobel Prize in 1945 for this accomplishment.

Jonas Edward Salk and Albert Sabin discovered the vaccines for polio in the 1950s, which led to near eradication of one of the 20th century's greatest killers.

Checkpoint Question

2. What did Louis Pasteur discover about bacteria found in liquids?

Recent Medical History

Throughout the next three decades, public health protection improved and advancements continued. Government legislation mandated clean water, and citizens reaped the benefits of preventive medicine and education about health issues.

In the 1980s, advancements in radiology gave doctors ways to see inside a patient with such accuracy that patients no longer had to have exploratory surgery. With computed tomography (CT scan) radiologists can see tumors, cysts, inflammation, and so on, with cross-sectional slices of the patient's body. Magnetic resonance imaging (MRI) uses a strong magnetic field to realign ions to form an image on a screen. MRI is used to detect internal bleeding, tumors, cysts, and so on. Positron emission tomography has further revolutionized radiology.

In July 1998, Ryuzo Yanagimachi of the University of Hawaii announced the **cloning** of mice when 7 of 22 mice were cloned from the cell of a single mouse. In December 1998, researchers from Kinki University in Nara, Japan, cloned 8 calves from a single cell.

On June 26, 2000, after 10 years of work, a team of scientists from both the public and private sectors announced the completion and availability of a rough draft of the identification and mapping of human genes. Mapping the sequence of the letters of the human genome that represent the handbook of a human being is a breakthrough that will revolutionize the practice of medicine by paving the way for new drugs and therapies. The achievement is being hailed as one of the most significant scientific landmarks of all time, comparable to the landing on the moon or splitting the atom. Already many medicines that can be tailored to an individual's genetic makeup are on the market or in development.

New discoveries will continue to expand the parameters of medicine as further research in recombinant DNA, transplantation, immunizations, diagnostic procedures, and so forth push back the boundaries of health care and make today's therapies seem as primitive as those we have just covered. You will be a part of this fascinating evolution of health care. Within the next decade expect to see immunization against or cures for many of the illnesses that continue to plague us.

Your role as a **medical assistant**, the ultimate multiskilled health care professional, will expand as the need for highly trained, versatile medical personnel keeps pace with the ever-changing practice of medicine. Today, heart bypass surgeries and organ transplants are performed routinely. Research continues to search for the cures for cancer, acquired immunodeficiency syndrome, and many other ailments. As a medical assistant, you play a key role in advancing the medical profession in the 21st century.

THE AMERICAN HEALTH CARE SYSTEM

The American health care system is complex and has seen many changes in the past few decades. Twenty years ago, a patient had medical insurance that paid a percentage of his or her medical bills. In today's world of managed care, which is discussed in the chapter on health insurance, patients are a part of a group of covered members of a HMO (health management organization). With this change came new ways of treating patients. The doctor–patient relationship was one of trust and privacy. In today's health care system, patients are treated as outlined by the insurance companies. The purpose of this change was to control health care costs. The government monitors medical finances and controls the Medicare and Medicaid systems through the Centers for Medicare & Medicaid Services (CMS). This government agency was formerly called Health Care Financing Administration (HFCA). It has been estimated that by 2013, 60% of patients being seen in the medical office will be over 65 years of age and will be covered under the Medicare system of insurance for the elderly. The need to adhere to the rules and regulations of the government drives the management practices of the **outpatient** medical facility. The allied health care arena has grown quickly. New professions have been added to the health care team, and each one is an important part of a patient's total care. As an allied health student, you have an exciting course of study ahead of you. Soon you will find yourself among a caring and conscientious group of health care professionals.

THE MEDICAL OFFICE

Today's medical office is quite different from the office of the past, where patients were treated by their family physician, insurance was filed, and reimbursement was based on a percentage of the cost. Large corporations and hospitals now own many medical clinics, and physicians are their employees. Medical practices now have the capability to maintain a patient's record without a single piece of paper. Office employees need a general understanding of the many regulations of insurance carriers. Every employee must be computer literate and should understand the legal aspects of the medical office. Although there are many medical specialties, the skills and basic functions of any medical office will be similar. Many years ago, a physician might teach a neighbor the skills needed to work with him. Those days are over. With the new technology and the need for constant monitoring of regulations and changes, the medical office employee is now expected to acquire a formal education and certification.

The typical medical office employs one or more physicians. To assist with examining and treating patients, the physician may employ physician assistants and/or nurse practitioners. These are the providers, and they need support staff. The goal of any medical practice is to provide quality care while maintaining sound financial practices within the laws and ethics of the medical profession. To achieve this goal, the physician needs a solid team. The administrative staff handles the financial aspects of the practice, and the clinical staff assists the providers with patient care. Both aspects of the office must run smoothly to reach the ultimate goal of the practice. The makeup of the team may differ among specialties. For example, a doctor who treats broken bones may have an x-ray technologist on staff, or an obstetrician may have an on-site sonographer to perform ultrasounds on mothers-to-be. Regardless of the mix of the team, the certified medical assistant is an integral part.

The day-to-day operation of a medical office requires all the skills you learn in your curriculum. The patient's health care encounter can be pleasant or unpleasant, depending on the skills and the attitude of the team.

Checkpoint Question

3. Which members of the health care team are considered providers?

MEDICAL SPECIALTIES

After completion of medical school, physicians choose a **specialty**. Some prefer treating patients of all ages and will choose family medicine or internal medicine. Others choose surgery and further specialize in fields like cosmetic surgery or vascular surgery. Table 1-1 lists the most common surgi-

Table 1–1 SURGICAL SPECIALTIES	
Surgical Specialty	**Description**
Cardiovascular	Repairs physical dysfunctions of the cardiovascular system
Cosmetic, reconstructive	Restores, repairs, or reconstructs body parts
General	Performs repairs on a variety of body parts
Maxillofacial	Repairs disorders of the face and mouth (a branch of dentistry)
Neurological	Repairs disorders of the nervous system
Orthopedic	Corrects deformities and treats disorders of the musculoskeletal system
Thoracic	Repairs organs within the rib cage
Trauma	Limited to correcting traumatic wounds
Vascular	Repairs disorders of blood vessels, usually excluding the heart

T a b l e 1 – 2 SPECIALISTS WHO EMPLOY MEDICAL ASSISTANTS	
Specialist	**Description**
Allergist	Performs tests to determine the basis of allergic reactions to eliminate or counteract the offending allergen
Anesthesiologist	Determines the most appropriate anesthesia during surgery for the patient's situation
Cardiologist	Diagnoses and treats disorders of the cardiovascular system, including the heart, arteries, and veins
Dermatologist	Diagnoses and treats skin disorders, including cosmetic treatments for the reversal of aging
Emergency care physician	Usually works in emergency or trauma centers
Endocrinologist	Diagnoses and treats disorders of the endocrine system and its hormone-secreting glands, e.g., diabetes and dwarfism
Epidemiologist	Specializes in epidemics caused by infectious agents, studies toxic agents, air pollution, and other health-related phenomena, and works with sexually transmitted disease control
Family practitioner	Serves a variety of patient age levels, seeing patients for everything from ear infections to school physicals
Gastroenterologist	Diagnoses and treats disorders of the stomach and intestine
Gerontologist	Limits practice to disorders of the aging population and its unique challenges
Gynecologist	Diagnoses and treats disorders of the female reproductive system and may also be an obstetrician or limit the practice to gynecology, including surgery
Hematologist	Diagnoses and treats disorders of the blood and blood-forming organs
Immunologist	Concentrates on the body's immune system and disease incidence, transmission, and prevention
Internist	Limits practice to diagnosis and treatment of disorders of internal organs with medical (drug therapy and lifestyle changes) rather than surgical means
Neonatologist	Limits practice to the care and treatment of infants to about 6 weeks of age
Nephrologist	Diagnoses and treats disorders of the kidneys
Obstetrician	Limits practice to care and treatment for pregnancy, the postpartum period, and fertility issues
Oncologist	Diagnoses and treats tumors, both benign (noncancerous) and malignant (cancerous)
Ophthalmologist	Diagnoses and treats disorders of the eyes, including surgery (an optometrist monitors and measures patients for corrective lenses, and an optician makes the lenses or dispenses contact lenses)
Orthopedist	Diagnoses and treats disorders of the musculoskeletal system, including surgery and care for fractures
Otorhinolaryngologist	Diagnoses and treats disorders of the ear, nose, and throat
Pathologist	Analyzes tissue samples or specimens from surgery, diagnoses abnormalities, and performs autopsies
Pediatrician	Limits practice to childhood disorders or may be further specialized to early childhood or adolescent period
Podiatrist	Diagnoses and treats disorders of the feet and provides routine care for diabetic patients, who may have poor circulation and require extra care
Proctologist	Limits practice to disorders of the colon, rectum, and anus
Psychiatrist	Diagnoses and treats mental disorders
Pulmonologist	Diagnoses and treats disorders of the respiratory system
Radiologist	Interprets x-rays and imaging studies and performs radiation therapy
Rheumatologist	Diagnoses and treats arthritis, gout, and other joint disorders
Urologist	Diagnoses and treats disorders of the urinary system, including the kidneys and bladder, and disorders of the male reproductive system

cal specialties. Table 1-2 lists specialists who may employ medical assistants.

 Checkpoint Question

4. What is the specialty that treats newborn babies?

THE MEDICAL ASSISTING PROFESSION

What Is a Medical Assistant?

A medical assistant is a multiskilled allied health professional, a member of the health care delivery team who performs administrative and clinical procedures. **Clinical** tasks generally involve direct patient care; **administrative** tasks usually focus on office procedures. Medical assistants are employed in physicians' offices and ambulatory care settings. Salaries, hours, and benefits depend on experience, size of practice or corporation, and geographic salary ranges. Working conditions for medical assistants vary greatly according to state laws regarding the medical assisting profession and the scope of the certified medical assistant (CMA), specialty of employer, and job responsibilities.

Duties of a Medical Assistant

The duties of a medical assistant are divided into two categories: administrative and clinical, which includes **laboratory** duties. The ratio of administrative to clinical duties varies with your job description. For example, if you work in a family practice office, you may do mostly clinical work; a psychiatric practice will probably require primarily administrative duties.

Administrative Duties

Performing administrative tasks correctly and in a timely manner will make the office more efficient and productive. Conversely, an office that is not managed correctly can result in loss of business, poor patient service, and loss of revenue. Following is a partial list of standard administrative duties:

- Managing and maintaining the waiting room, office, and examining rooms
- Handling telephone calls
- Using written and oral communication
- Maintaining medical records
- Bookkeeping
- Scheduling appointments
- Ensuring good public relations
- Maintaining office supplies
- Screening sales representatives
- Filing insurance forms
- Processing the payroll
- Arranging patient hospitalizations
- Sorting and filing mail
- Instructing new patients regarding office hours and procedures
- Applying computer concepts to office practices
- Implementing ICD-9 and CPT coding for insurance claims
- Completing medical transcriptions

Clinical Duties

Clinical responsibilities vary among employers. State laws regarding the scope of practice for medical assistants also differ. In some states, CMAs are not allowed to perform invasive procedures, such as injections or laboratory testing.

Most states, however, leave the responsibility for the medical assistant's actions with the physician-employer. AAMA has outlined the scope of practice for the medical assistant. Following is a partial list of clinical duties:

- Preparing patients for examinations and treatments
- Assisting other health care providers with procedures
- Preparing and sterilizing instruments
- Completing electrocardiograms
- Applying Holter monitors
- Obtaining medical histories
- Administering medications and immunizations
- Obtaining vital signs (blood pressure, pulse, temperature, respirations)
- Obtaining height and weight measurements
- Documenting in the medical record
- Performing eye and ear irrigations
- Recognizing and treating medical emergencies
- Initiating and implementing patient education

Laboratory Duties

- Low- and moderate-complexity laboratory tests as determined by the Clinical Laboratory Improvement Amendments (CLIA) of 1988
- Collecting and processing laboratory specimens

 Checkpoint Question

5. What are five administrative duties and five clinical or laboratory duties performed by a medical assistant?

CHARACTERISTICS OF A PROFESSIONAL MEDICAL ASSISTANT

Medical assistants play a key role in creating and maintaining a professional image for their employers. Medical assistants must always appear neat and well groomed. Clothing should be clean, pressed, and in good condition. Footwear should be neat, comfortable, and professional. If sneakers are approved by your supervisor, they should be all white. Only minimal makeup and jewelry should be worn. You should wear a watch with a second hand. Fingernails should be clean and at a functional length. If polish is worn, it should be pale or clear.

Medical assistants must be dependable and punctual (Fig. 1-3). Tardiness and frequent absences are not acceptable. If you are not at work, someone must fill in for you. Medical assistants must be flexible and adaptable to meet the constantly changing needs of the office. Weekend and holiday hours may be required in some specialties.

Additional characteristics vital to the profession include the following:

- Excellent written and oral communications skills. You will be required to interact with patients and other health

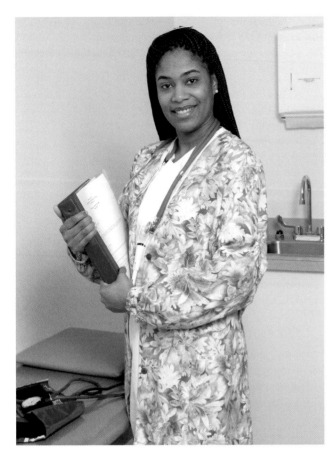

FIGURE 1–3. Medical assistants play a key role in creating and maintaining a professional image for their employers.

care workers on a professional basis. Only the best spelling and grammar skills are acceptable. (Communication skills are covered in appropriate sections of this text.)

- Maturity. Remaining calm in an emergency or during stressful situations and being able to calm others is a key skill. You must also be able to accept criticism without resentment.
- Accuracy. The physician must be able to trust you to pay close attention to detail because the health and well-being of the patients are at stake. Careless errors could cause harm to the patient and result in legal action against the physician.
- Honesty. If errors are made, they must be admitted, and corrective procedures must be initiated immediately. Covering up errors or blaming others is dishonest. So are using office property for personal business, making telephone calls during work time, and falsifying time records. Such practices can ruin your career and are to be strictly avoided.
- Ability to respect patient confidentiality. Few issues in health care can damage your career as profoundly as divulging confidential patient information.

- Empathy. The ability to care deeply for the health and welfare of your patients is the heart of medical assisting.
- Courtesy. Every patient who enters the office must be treated with respect and gracious manners.
- Good interpersonal skills. Tempers may flare in stressful situations; learn to keep yours in check and work well with all levels of interaction.
- Ability to project a positive self-image. If you are confident in your abilities as a professional, this attitude will reflect in all of your relationships.
- Ability to work as a team player. The patient's return to health is the most important objective of the office. Each staff member must work toward this goal.
- Initiative and responsibility. The entire team expects each of its members to perform assigned responsibilities.
- Tact and diplomacy. The right word at the right moment can calm and soothe anger, depression, and fear and relieve a potentially unsettling situation.
- High moral and ethical standards. Project for your profession the highest level of professionalism.

 Checkpoint Question

6. What are eight characteristics that a professional medical assistant should have?

MEMBERS OF THE HEALTH CARE TEAM

As a medical assistant, you will work with a variety of health care workers. Today's health care team must be **multidisciplinary**. A multidisciplinary team is a group of specialized professionals who are brought together to meet the needs of the patient. Some patients will need the assistance of many individuals, whereas other patients may only need one or two members of the team. The team may be broken into three groups: physicians, nurses, and allied health care providers.

Physicians

Physicians generally are the team leaders. They are responsible for diagnosing and treating the patient. Minimum education for a physician consists of a 4-year undergraduate degree, often consisting of premedical studies, 4 years of medical school, followed by a residency program usually concentrating on a certain specialty. The residency program can vary from 2 to 6 years based on the field of study. Physicians must pass a licensure examination for the state in which they wish to practice.

Physician Assistants

Physician assistants (PAs) are specially trained and usually licensed. They work closely with a physician and may perform many of the tasks traditionally done by physicians. Preliminary physical examinations and basic diagnostic and treatment procedures that do not require an intense medical background may be assigned to a physician's assistant. Their educational levels vary from several months to 2 years, depending on the program and the individual's background in medicine. National certification is available through the American Association of Physician Assistants.

Nurses

Nurses work with physicians and implement various patient care needs in the **inpatient** or hospital setting. Their job descriptions vary according to their experiences, specialties, and certifications. There are several levels of nursing education.

- Bachelor of science in nursing   4 years
  (BSN)   of education
- Associate degree in nursing   2 years
  (ADN)

- Registered nurse (RN)   2 to 3 years
- Licensed practical nurse (LPN)   1 year
- Licensed vocational nurse (LVN) 1 year
- Certified nursing assistant   4- to 6-week
  (CNN I and II)   certificate

Nurse Practitioners

Nurse practitioners (NPs) may practice medicine independently. In some states, NPs can write prescriptions, operate their own offices, and admit patients to hospitals. In other states, NPs work more closely with a physician. All NPs are experienced RNs and in most cases have a master's degree in nursing with the addition of specialized training as an NP.

Allied Health Professionals

Allied health care professionals make up a large section of the health care team. Box 1-1 lists and describes some of these

---

Box 1-1

ALLIED HEALTH CARE PROFESSIONALS

Chiropractor—Manipulates the musculoskeletal system and spine to relieve symptoms

Dental hygienist—Trained and licensed to work with a dentist by providing preventive care

Dietitian—Trained nutritionist who addresses dietary needs associated with illness

Electrocardiograph technician—Assists with the performance of diagnostic procedures for cardiac electrical activity

Electroencephalograph technician—Assists with the diagnostic procedures for brain wave activity

Emergency medical technician—Trained in techniques of administering emergency care en route to trauma centers

Histologist—Studies cells and tissues for diagnosis

Infection control officer—Identifies risks of transmission of infection and implements preventive measures

Laboratory technician—Trained in performance of laboratory diagnostic procedures

Medical assistant—Trained in administrative, clinical, and laboratory skills for the medical facility

Medical coder—Assigns appropriate codes to report medical services to third party payers for reimbursement

Medical office assistant—Trained in the administrative area of the outpatient medical facility

Medical transcriptionist—Trained in administrative skills; produces printed records of dictated medical information

Nuclear medical technician—Specializes in diagnostic procedures using radionuclides (electromagnetic radiation); works in a radiology department

Occupational therapist—Evaluates and plans programs to relieve physical and mental barriers that interfere with activities

Paramedic—Trained in advanced rescue and emergency procedures

Pharmacist—Prepares and dispenses medications by the physician's order

Phlebotomist—Collects blood specimens for laboratory procedures by performing venipuncture

Physical therapist—Plans and conducts rehabilitation to improve strength and mobility

Psychologist—Trained in methods of psychological assessment and treatment

Radiographer—Works with a radiologist or physician to operate x-ray equipment for diagnosis and treatment

Respiratory therapist—Trained to preserve or improve respiratory function

Risk manager—Identifies and corrects high-risk situations within the health care field

Social worker—Trained to evaluate and correct social, emotional, and environmental problems associated with the medical profession

Speech therapist—Treats and prevents speech and language disorders

Unit clerk—Performs the administrative duties in a hospital patient care unit

team members. The educational requirements and responsibilities vary greatly among these professionals. One thing they all have in common is the support of a professional organization. Medical assistants fall into this category.

THE HISTORY OF MEDICAL ASSISTING

Medical assisting as a separate profession dates from the 1930s. In 1934, Dr. M. Mandl recognized the need for a medical professional possessing skills required in an office environment and opened the first school for medical assistants in New York City. Although medical assistants were employed before 1934, no formal schooling was available. Office assistants were trained on the job to perform medical procedures or nurses were trained to perform administrative procedures. The need for a highly trained professional with a background in administrative and clinical skills led to the formation of an alternative field of allied health care. In 1955, the American Association of Medical Assistants (AAMA), a professional organization for medical assistants, was founded during a meeting of medical assistants in Kansas City, Kansas. The resolutions adopted by the group were accepted and commended by the American Medical Association (AMA), the professional association of licensed physicians. In 1959, Illinois recognized the AAMA as a not-for-profit educational organization. The national office was established in Chicago with state and local chapters throughout the United States. The AAMA has guided the practice of medical assisting with strong leadership and vision. With its help, the medical assistant has grown into a highly respected and versatile member of the health care team. In 1963, a certification examination for CMA was developed that would set the standards required for medical assistant education. The first AAMA examinations were given in Kansas, California, and Florida. In the next two decades, the profession grew rapidly. The AMA collaborated in the development of the curriculum and accreditation of educational programs. In 1978, the U. S. Department of Education recognized the AAMA as an official accrediting agency for medical assisting programs in public and private schools.

In 1991, the Board of Trustees of the AAMA approved the current definition of medical assisting: Medical assisting is an allied health profession whose practitioners function as members of the health care delivery team and perform administrative and clinical procedures. Medical assistants continue to be vigilant of threats to their right to practice their profession. Each state mandates the actions of allied health professionals. It is the responsibility of the medical assistant to be familiar with the laws of the state in which he or she is working. The profession has been listed as one of the fastest growing careers of the 1990s, with 74% growth predicted by the U. S. Department of Labor in its 2002 Employment Outlook. Membership in the AAMA reached 18,500, with 525 local chapters in 47 states and the District of Columbia. Today, the organization's membership exceeds 30,000 medical assistants.

Checkpoint Question

7. What prompted the establishment of a school for medical assistants?

MEDICAL ASSISTING EDUCATION

A medical assisting curriculum prepares individuals for entry into the medical assisting profession. Medical assisting programs are found in postsecondary schools, such as private business schools and technical colleges, 2-year colleges, and community colleges. Programs vary in length. Programs of 6 months to a year offer a certificate of graduation or a diploma, and 2-year programs award the graduate an associate degree. The 2-year curriculum usually includes general studies, such as English, mathematics, and computer skills, in addition to the core courses, such as medical terminology and insurance coding. The curriculum in every accredited program must include the skills determined by the accrediting agency. Specific requirements for an accredited program are discussed later.

Accredited programs must include an **externship**. An externship is an educational course offered in the last module or semester during which the student works in the field gaining hands-on experience. It varies in length from 60 to 240 hours. Students are not paid but are awarded credit toward the degree. (See Chapter 19 for more detailed information.) Some schools offer job placement services.

After you finish school, your education should not stop. You should continue to take courses on various related topics. These may include new computer programs, new clinical procedures, new laws and regulations, or pharmaceutical updates. Some employers pay for conferences. In some situations, conference costs may be listed for tax credit when filing your income tax.

Box 1-2 outlines important changes made by the House of Delegates of the AAMA.

Checkpoint Question

8. What is an externship?

Medical Assisting Program Accreditation

In 1995, the AMA House of Delegates voted to require graduation from an accredited medical assisting program for admission to the CMA examination. This change went into effect in January 1998. **Accreditation** is a nongovernmental professional peer review process that provides technical as-

AAMA HOUSE OF DELEGATE CHANGES

- In 1995, the AAMA House of Delegates approved changing the eligibility pathway for candidates of the AAMA certification examination as follows: "Any candidate for the AAMA Certification Exam must be a graduate of a CAAHEP-accredited medical assisting program." Before January 1998, medical assistants who had been employed by a physician for 1 year full-time or 2 years part-time were eligible to sit for the certification examination.
- In 2001, AAMA made the decision to grant graduates of ABHES-accredited medical assisting programs immediate eligibility to sit for the CMA examination beginning in January 2002.
- Effective January 1, 2003, all CMAs employed or seeking employment must have current certification to use the CMA credential in connection with employment.

WHAT IF

You plan to work in a state that does not require certification to work as a medical assistant in a physician's office. Why become certified?

Certification is a mark of excellence. It proves to a potential employer that you have successfully completed a program of study covering the skills you will be expected to perform. Since the physician takes legal responsibility for his employees, it is in the best interest of physician-employer to seek out trained and certified assistants.

sistance and evaluates educational programs for quality based on preestablished academic and administrative standards. Medical assisting program accreditation is based on a school's adherence to the scientifically grounded occupational analysis known as the AAMA Role Delineation Chart: Occupational Analysis of the Medical Assisting Profession. The **role delineation chart** is a list of the areas of competence expected of the graduate (see Appendix I). Role delineation components covered are listed at the beginning of each chapter of this textbook.

The Commission of Accreditation of Allied Health Education Programs

The Commission on Accreditation of Allied Health Education Programs (CAAHEP) in collaboration with the curriculum review board of the American Association of Medical Assistants' Endowment accredits medical assisting programs in both public and private postsecondary institutions throughout the United States. CAAHEP accredits many allied health education programs included in Box 1-1.

The Accrediting Bureau of Health Education Schools

The Accrediting Bureau of Health Education Schools (ABHES) accredits private postsecondary registered medical assistant (RMA) **certification** through a program review process conducted by the American Medical Technologists (AMT). This body has accredited medical technicians,

medical laboratory technicians, and dental technicians since the late 1930s but offered its first medical assisting examination in 1972.

MEDICAL ASSISTING CERTIFICATION

The AAMA and the AMT have developed certification examinations that test the knowledge of a graduate and indicate entry level competency. After passing the examination, the person can use the initials CMA (certified medical assistant) or RMA (registered medical assistant) after his or her name (Box 1-3).

CHARTING EXAMPLE USING THE CMA OR RMA DESIGNATION

Medical assistants who pass the AAMA certification examination are certified and may use the designation CMA after their name. Those who pass the AMT certification examination become registered medical assistants and may use the designation RMA after their name.

4/25/03
9:30 A.M. Patient complaining of sore throat. Throat culture taken and sent to the laboratory. Dr. Rogers in to see patient. Heather Wood, CMA
4/25/03
11:30 A.M. Amoxicillin 250 mg p.o. given to patient. Leslie Roope, RMA

Certified Medical Assistant

Graduates of medical assisting programs accredited by CAAHEP or ABHES are immediately eligible to take the CMA certification examination of the AAMA. Examinees who pass this test are designated as CMAs. The National Board of Medical Examiners, which administers several medical specialty examinations, serves as test consultant for the CMA certification examination of the AAMA.

Once you pass the examination and become a CMA, you are required to recertify every 5 years. **Recertification** may be obtained either by taking the examination again or by completing 60 **continuing education units** (CEUs) in a 5-year period. CEUs are awarded for attendance at approved local and state AAMA meetings and seminars, completion of guided study courses, and journal articles designed to submit a posttest for CEU credit.

Registered Medical Assistant

In 1972, the AMT offered the first RMA examination. Graduates from ABHES-accredited medical assisting programs are immediately eligible to take the RMA examination. Medical assistants who have been employed in the profession for a minimum of 5 years, no more than 2 of which may have been as an instructor, are also eligible. Those who pass this examination are designated as RMAs.

Although formal recertification is not required by AMT, members and nonmembers are invited to participate in the STEP program, a continuing education home study program for health care practitioners. AMT keeps a record of earned credit and issues annual reports of STEP activities to program participants.

Checkpoint Question

9. What is required to maintain current status as a CMA?

MEDICAL ASSISTING AND RELATED ALLIED HEALTH ASSOCIATIONS

Association Membership

You are not required to join a national organization to work as a medical assistant or to be eligible to take the certification examination. The associations have many benefits, however, for members. These benefits include the following:

- Access to educational seminars
- Access to continuing education units
- Subscription to the professional journals that alert you to new procedures and trends in medicine
- Access to the annual conventions
- Group insurance plans
- Networking opportunities

For further information on these organizations, visit the websites listed at the end of the chapter. Contact your local chapter or speak with your instructor for the procedure for applying for membership. You can download applications and requirements from the AAMA website (http://www.aama-ntl.org) and the AMT website (http://www.amt1.com).

American Association of Medical Assistants

The purpose of the AAMA is to promote the professional identity and stature of its members and the medical assisting profession through education and credentialing. *CMA Today*, which is published and distributed to members of the organization, includes articles of interest to the medical assistant to keep knowledge and skills current. Readers may take a posttest at the end of the article and receive CEU. Accredited continuing education opportunities are available through the national organization, and free transcripts of acquired AAMA-approved CEUs are available online with a member number. Professional benefits, such as insurance, are also made available to AAMA members. Active members are CMAs; non-CMAs, such as some medical assisting educators and those interested in medical assisting, are associate members. Students are encouraged to join and stay active in AAMA. Student members receive a reduced dues rate while in school and for a year following graduation. Figure 1-4 displays the insignia of the AAMA.

American Medical Technologists

The AMT and its governing body are set up similarly to the AAMA, with local, state, and national affiliations, opportunities for continuing education, professional benefits, and a professional journal. Members include medical technologists, medical laboratory technicians, medical assistants, dental assistants, office laboratory technicians, phlebotomy technicians, laboratory consultants, and allied health instructors. To join AMT, you need to be certified by meeting edu-

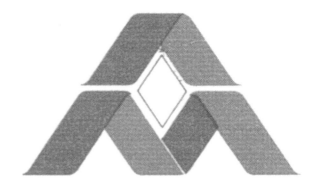

F I G U R E I – 4 .   Insignia of affiliates of the AAMA.

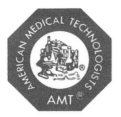

FIGURE 1-5. Insignia of AMT.

cational, professional experience, and examination requirements. Figure 1-5 displays the insignia of the AMT.

Professional Coder Associations

The American Academy of Professional Coders (AAPC) is dedicated to providing the highest standard of professional coding and billing services to employers, clients, and patients. Services to members include discounts on services and products and networking opportunities. AAPC provides a credentialing program that offers examinations to obtain the credential certified professional coder (CPC).

The American Health Information Management Association

The American Health Information Management Association (AHIMA) is a national professional organization dedicated

PATIENT EDUCATION

The Health Care System

As a medical assistant, you play a key role in teaching patients not only about their health, but also about the health care system. Some patients become confused and are overwhelmed by the number and variety of health care workers. You can help by providing the answers to these common questions:

- What is a multidisciplinary team?
- Who will conduct the examination (physician, physician's assistant, or nurse practitioner)?
- What is a medical assistant?
- What do medical assistants do?
- What kind of training is required for medical assistants?
- What does certification or registration mean for a medical assistant?
- When patients understand the health care field and know what to expect, they recover more quickly and are more comfortable asking questions about their health than they otherwise would.

to supporting the medical records or health information specialists. AHIMA administers the examination and awards the certified coding specialist (CCS) and certified coding specialists–physician-based (CCS-P) through testing at a specified time and place.

American Association of Medical Transcription

The mission of the American Association of Medical Transcriptionists (AAMT) is to represent and advance the profession of medical transcription and its practitioners. The AAMT offers a two-part examination that awards the credential certified medical transcriptionist (CMT). The written component of the examination is given at a specified testing site at the examinee's convenience. The practical examination is administered by a proctor of the examinee's choosing (approved by AAMT).

For more information, see the listing of website addresses at the end of the chapter for these organizations.

 Checkpoint Question

10. What are the two organizations that accredit medical assisting programs?

EMPLOYMENT OPPORTUNITIES

The outlook for medical assisting employment is highly promising. Health care is being restructured to be more productive and cost effective. Medical assistants are the most cost-effective employees in health care today because of the flexible, multiskilled nature of their education. Medical assistants can work in a variety of health care settings where they are under the direct supervision of a licensed health care provider. They perform many functions. Following are examples of settings where a medical assistant may work with a variety of responsibilities:

- Ambulatory care centers
- Walk-in care centers
- Physician offices
- Adult day care centers
- Research centers
- Clinics

 Checkpoint Question

11. List the settings that may employ a medical assistant.

CHAPTER SUMMARY

Medicine is a constantly changing science that grows more complex with each new medical discovery. The well-trained and certified medical assistant will be a part of the most exciting and challenging era of medical advances in the history of patient care. The health care team works together to deliver quality patient care and remain financially sound. Whatever avenue a medical assistant pursues, certification or registration gives the medical assistant increasing marketability in the health care arena. The medical office requires the skills provided by the medical assistant. By ensuring that educational levels are constantly enhanced and by continuing to grow professionally, the medical assistant graduate will prepare for the challenge of a lifelong career that is both fascinating and rewarding.

Critical Thinking Challenges

1. Review the list of characteristics for medical assistants. Which characteristics do you already have? How will you acquire the others? Are there additional characteristics that you have that will make you a good medical assistant?
2. Look at the list of physician specialties. Which type of physician would you want to work for and why? Which physician specialties would you least want to work with? Explain your response.
3. What part does a professional organization play in the career of an allied health professional?
4. How does certification or registration as a medical assistant improve your success in the profession?
5. What is the importance of continuing education?

Answers to Checkpoint Questions

1. Galen's anatomic findings were mostly incorrect because they were based on the dissection of apes and swine, not humans.
2. Pasteur discovered that bacteria in liquids could be destroyed by heating the liquid.
3. The providers in the medical office might include the physician, physician's assistant, and/or nurse practitioner.
4. The specialty that treats newborn babies is neonatology.
5. Examples of administrative duties include managing the medical office, handling telephone calls, preparing written communications, bookkeeping, scheduling, filing, and sorting mail. Examples of clinical duties include preparing patients for examinations, collecting and processing urine and blood specimens, completing electrocardiograms, and applying Holter monitors.
6. Professional characteristics include punctuality, dependability, honesty, showing respect for patient confidentiality, courtesy, diplomacy, and having high ethical and moral standards.
7. The first school for medical assistants was established because of the need for a highly trained professional with secretarial and clinical skills.
8. An externship is unpaid student work experience in a medical office. The student receives academic credit for the time worked.
9. To remain current, a CMA who takes the AAMA examination must recertify every 5 years by either taking a certification examination again or acquiring 60 continuing education units.
10. The two accrediting agencies for medical assisting are CAAHEP and ABHES.
11. Settings where medical assistants may work include physician offices, ambulatory care centers, walk-in care centers, adult day care centers, insurance companies, and research centers.

 Websites

AAPC—American Academy of Professional Coders
  http://www.aapc.com/aboutus/index.html
AAMA—American Association of Medical Assistants
  http://www.aama-ntl.org
AAMT—American Association of Medical Transcriptionists
  hhtp://www.aamt.org
ABHES—Accrediting Bureau of Health Education Schools
  http://www.abhes.org
AHIMA—American Health Information Management Association
  http://www.ahima.org
AMT—American Medical Technologists
  http://www.amt1.com
CAAHEP—Council on Accreditation of Allied Health Education Programs
  http://www.caahep.org
For information on medical specialties
  http://www.abms.org
Centers for Medicare & Medicaid Services
  http://cms.hhs.gov
For information on Vaccine Information Statement
  http://www.immunize.org

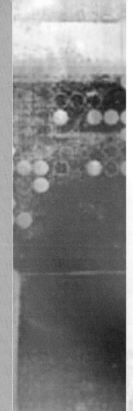

2

Law and Ethics

CHAPTER OUTLINE

ROLE DELINEATION COMPONENTS

GENERAL: Professionalism
- Demonstrate initiative and responsibility
- Treat all patients with compassion and empathy

GENERAL: Legal Concepts
- Perform within legal and ethical boundaries
- Prepare and maintain medical records

- Document accurately
- Follow employer's established policies dealing with the health care contract
- Implement and maintain federal and state health care legislation and regulations

CHAPTER COMPETENCIES

LEARNING OBJECTIVES
Upon successfully completing this chapter, you will be able to:

1. Spell and define the key terms
2. Identify the two branches of the American legal system
3. List the elements and types of contractual agreements and describe the difference in implied and express contracts
4. List four items that must be included in a contract termination or withdrawal letter
5. List six items that must be included in an informed consent form and explain who may sign consent forms
6. List five legally required disclosures that must be reported to specified authorities
7. Describe the purpose of the Self-Determination Act
8. Describe the four elements that must be proven in a medical legal suit
9. Describe four possible defenses against litigation for the medical professional
10. Explain the theory of respondeat superior, or law of agency, and how it applies to the medical assistant
11. List ways that a medical assistant can assist in the prevention of a medical malpractice suit
12. Outline the laws regarding employment and safety issues in the medical office
13. List the requirements of the Americans with Disabilities Act relating to the medical office
14. Differentiate between legal issues and ethical issues
15. List the seven American Medical Association principles of ethics
16. List the five ethical principles of ethical and moral conduct outlined by the American Association of Medical Assistants
17. List 10 opinions of the American Medical Association's Council pertaining to administrative office procedures

KEY TERMS

abandonment
advance directive
age of majority
appeal
artificial insemination
assault
battery
bench trial
bioethics
blood-borne pathogens
breach
censure
certification
civil law
coerce
common law

comparative negligence
confidentiality
consent
consideration
contract
contributory negligence
cross-examination
damages
defamation of character
defendant
depositions
direct examination
durable power of attorney
duress
emancipated minor
ethics

expert witness
expressed consent
expressed contracts
fee splitting
fraud
implied consent
implied contracts
informed consent
intentional tort
legally required disclosure
libel
licensure
litigation
locum tenens
malpractice
negligence

noncompliant
plaintiff
precedents
protocol
registered
res ipsa loquitur
res judicata
respondeat superior
slander
stare decisis
statutes
statute of limitations
tort
unintentional tort
verdict

DURING YOUR CAREER AS A medical assistant, you will be involved in many medical situations with potential legal implications. You must uphold ethical standards to ensure the patient's well-being. Ethics deals with the concept of right and wrong. Laws are written to carry out these concepts. Physicians may be sued for a variety of reasons, including significant clinical errors (e.g., removing the wrong limb, ordering a toxic dose of medication), claims of improperly touching a patient without consent, or failure to properly diagnose or treat a disease. Medicare **fraud** (concealing the truth) and falsifying medical records can also result in a lawsuit. Medical assistants and other health care workers are included in many of the suits brought to court. You may help to prevent many of these claims against your physician, and to protect yourself, by complying with medical laws, keeping abreast of medical trends, and acting in an ethical manner by maintaining a high level of professionalism at all times.

THE AMERICAN LEGAL SYSTEM

Our legal system is in place to ensure the rights of all citizens. We depend on the legal system to protect us from the wrongdoings of others. Many potential medical suits prove to be unwarranted and never make it into the court system, but even in the best physician–patient relationships, **litigation** (lawsuits) between patients and physicians may occur. Litigation may result from a single medication error or a mistake that costs a person's life. It is essential that you have a basic understanding of the American legal system to protect yourself, your patients, and your physician-employer by following the legal guidelines. You must know your legal duties and understand the legal nature of the physician–patient relationship and your role and responsibilities as the physician's agent.

Sources of Law

Laws are rules of conduct that are enforced by appointed authorities. The foundation of our legal system is our rights outlined in the Constitution and the laws established by our Founding Fathers. These traditional laws are known as **common law**.

Common law is based on the theory of **stare decisis**. This term means "the previous decision stands." Judges usually follow these **precedents** (previous court decisions) but sometimes overrule a previous decision, establishing new precedent. **Statutes** are another source of law. Federal, state, or local legislators make laws or statutes, the police enforce them, and the court system ensures justice. Statutes pertaining to Medicare, Medicaid, and the Food and Drug Administration are common examples in the medical profession.

The third type of law is administrative. These laws are passed by governmental agencies, such as the Internal Revenue Service.

Branches of the Law

The two main branches of the legal system are public law and private or **civil law**.

Public Law

Public law is the branch of law that focuses on issues between the government and its citizens. It can be divided into four subgroups:

1. Criminal law is concerned with issues of citizen welfare and safety. Examples include arson, burglary, murder, and rape. A medical assistant must stay within the boundaries of the profession. Treating patients without the physician's orders could result in a charge of practicing medicine without a license—an act covered under criminal law.
2. Constitutional law is commonly called the law of the land. The United States government has a constitution, and each state has a constitution of its own, laws, and regulations. State laws may be more restrictive than federal laws but may not be more lenient. Two examples of constitutional law are laws on abortion and civil rights.
3. Administrative law is the regulations set forth by governmental agencies. This category includes laws pertaining to the Food and Drug Administration, the Internal Revenue Service, and the Board of Medical Examiners.
4. International law pertains to treaties between countries. Related issues include trade agreements, extradition, boundaries, and international waters.

Private or Civil Law

Private or civil law is the branch of the law that focuses on issues between private citizens. The medical profession is primarily concerned with private law. The subcategories that pertain to the medical profession are contract, commercial, and tort law. Contract and commercial laws concern the rights and obligations of those who enter into contracts, as in a physician–patient relationship. **Tort** law governs the righting of wrongs or injuries suffered by someone because of another person's wrongdoing or misdeeds resulting from a **breach** of legal duty. Tort law is the basis of most lawsuits against physicians and health care workers. Other civil law branches include property, inheritance, and corporation law.

 Checkpoint Question

I. Which branch of law covers a medical assistant charged with practicing medicine without a license?

The Rise in Medical Legal Cases

Since World War II, the number of medical malpractice cases brought to court has increased significantly. **Malpractice** refers to an action by a professional health care worker that harms a patient. A rise in the amounts of settlement awards has had a negative impact on the cost and coverage of malpractice insurance. With this rise, some physicians have actually changed the scope of their practice to reduce their costs. For example, an obstetrician may choose to limit practice to the care of nonpregnant women to avoid the high cost of malpractice insurance for physicians who deliver babies. In an attempt to protect professionals, legislation designed to limit the amount a jury can award has been introduced in Congress. Legal issues involving the medical field are referred to as medicolegal, which combines the words medical and legal.

A government task force found four primary reasons for the rise in malpractice claims:

1. *Scientific advances.* As new and improved medical technology becomes available, the risks and potential for complications of these procedures escalate, making physicians more vulnerable to litigation.
2. *Unrealistic expectations.* Some patients expect miracle cures and file lawsuits because recovery was not as they hoped or expected, even if the physician is not at fault.
3. *Economic factors.* Some patients view lawsuits as a means to obtain quick cash. (In fact, the number of lawsuits filed has increased during economic recessions.)
4. *Poor communication.* Studies show that when patients do not feel a bond with their physician, they are more likely to sue. Attention to customer service helps develop a good rapport between patients, the provider, and the staff.

PHYSICIAN–PATIENT RELATIONSHIP

Rights and Responsibilities of the Patient and Physician

In any contractual relationship, both parties have certain rights and responsibilities. The rights of the patient include the ability to choose a physician. This right may be limited to a list of participating providers under a patient's insurance plan. Patients have the right to determine whether to begin medical treatment and to set limits on that treatment. The patient also has the right to know in advance what the treatment will consist of, what effect it may have, and what dangers are to be expected. The concept of informed consent is discussed later in the chapter.

Physicians have the right to limit their practice to a certain specialty or a certain location. For example, patients may not expect a physician to treat them at home. Physicians also have the right to refuse service to new patients or existing patients with new problems unless they are on emergency room call, in which case they must continue to treat patients seen during this time. The subject of abandonment is discussed later. Doctors have the right to change their policies or availability as long as they give patients reasonable notice of the change. This can be done through a local newspaper advertisement and/or a letter to each patient. Box 2-1 lists the patient's and physician's responsibilities.

Contracts

A **contract** is an agreement between two or more parties with certain factors agreed on among all parties. The physician–patient relationship is reinforced by the formation of a contract. All contractual agreements have three components:

1. Offer (contract initiation)
2. Acceptance (both parties agree to the terms)
3. **Consideration** (the exchange of fees for service)

A contract is not valid unless all three elements are present. A contract offer is made when a patient calls the office to request an appointment. The offer is accepted when you make an appointment for the patient. You have formed a contract that implies that for a fee, the physician will do all in his or her power to address the health concerns of the patient.

Certain individuals, such as children and those who are mentally incompetent or temporarily incapacitated, are not legally able to enter contracts. Patients in this category do not have the capacity to enter into a contract, and therefore decisions about health care should be made by a competent party acting as a health care decision maker for the minor or incompetent person.

The two types of contracts between physicians and patients are implied and expressed.

Implied Contracts

Implied contracts, the most common kind of contract between physicians and patients, are not written but are assumed by the actions of the parties. For example, a patient calls the office and requests to see Dr. Smith for an earache. The patient arrives for the appointment, is seen by the physician, and receives a prescription. It is *implied* that because the patient came on his own and requested care that he wants this physician to care for him. The physician's action of accepting the patient for care *implies* that he acknowledges responsibility for his part of the contract. The patient *implies* by accepting the services that he will render payment even if the price was not discussed.

Expressed Contracts

Expressed contracts, either written or oral, consist of specified details. A mutual sharing of responsibilities is always stated in an expressed contract. The agreement you have

Box 2-1

RESPONSIBILITIES OF THE PATIENT AND THE PHYSICIAN

Responsibilities of the Patient	Responsibilities of the Physician
Provide the physician with accurate data about the duration and nature of symptoms	Respect the patient's confidential information
Provide a complete and accurate medical history to the physician	Provide reasonable skill, experience, and knowledge in treating the patient
Follow the physician's instructions for diet, exercise, medications, and appointments	Continue treating the patient until the contract has been withdrawn or as long as the condition requires treatment
Compensate the physician for services rendered	Inform patients of their condition, treatments, and prognosis
	Give complete and accurate information
	Provide competent coverage during time away from practice
	Obtain informed consent before performing procedures (informed consent is a statement of approval from the patient for the physician to perform a given procedure after the patient has been educated about the risks and benefits of the procedure)
	Caution against unneeded or undesirable treatment or surgery

with your creditors is an expressed contract. These kinds of contracts are not used as often in the medical setting as implied contracts.

Checkpoint Question

2. An orthopedic surgeon decides to make a change in his services. He wants to limit his practice to nonsurgical patients. What action should the physician take?

Termination or Withdrawal of the Contract

A contract is ideally resolved when the patient is satisfactorily cured of the illness and the physician has been paid for the services. The patient may end the contract at any time, but the physician must follow legal **protocol** to dissolve the contract if the patient still seeks treatment and the physician wishes to end the relationship.

Patient-Initiated Termination. A patient who chooses to terminate the relationship should notify the physician and give the reasons. You must keep this letter in the medical record. After the receipt of this letter, the physician should then send a letter to the patient stating the following:

- The physician accepts the termination.
- Medical records are available on written request.
- Medical referrals are available if needed.

If the patient verbally asks to end this relationship, the physician should send a letter to the patient documenting the conversation and again offering referrals and access to the medical records. Clear documentation is essential.

Physician-Initiated Termination. The physician may find it necessary to end the relationship. A physician may terminate the contract if the patient is **noncompliant** or does not keep appointments or for personal reasons. The physician must send a letter of withdrawal that includes:

- A statement of intent to terminate the relationship
- The reasons for this action
- The termination date at least 30 days from the date of receipt of the letter
- A statement that the medical records will be transferred to another physician at the patient's request
- A strong recommendation that the patient seek additional medical care as warranted

The letter must be sent by certified mail with a return receipt requested. A copy of the termination letter and the return receipt are placed in the patient's record. Figure 2-1

Amy Fine, MD
Charlotte Family Practice
220 NW 3rd Avenue
Charlotte, NC 25673

August 22, 2003

Regina Dodson
Jones Hill Road
Charlotte, NC 25673

Dear Ms. Dodson:

Due to the fact that you have persistently refused to follow my medical advice and treatment of your diabetes, I will no longer be able to provide medical care to you. Since your condition requires ongoing medical care, you must find another physician as soon as possible. I will be available to you until that time, but no longer than 30 days.

To assist you in continuing to receive care, we will make records available to your new physician as soon as you authorize us to send them.

Sincerely,

Amy Fine, MD

FIGURE 2–1. Letter of intent to terminate physician–patient relationship.

shows a sample letter of intent to terminate a physician–patient relationship.

Abandonment. If a contract is not properly terminated, the physician can be sued for abandonment. **Abandonment** may be charged if the physician withdraws from the contractual relationship without proper notification while the patient still needs treatment. Physicians must always arrange coverage when absent from the office for vacations, conferences, and so on. Patients may sue for abandonment in any instance that a suitable substitute is not available for care. Coverage may be provided by a **locum tenens**, a substitute physician.

Other examples of abandonment:

- The physician abruptly and without reasonable notice stops treating a patient whose condition requires additional or continued care.
- The physician fails to see a patient as often as the condition requires or incorrectly advises the patient that further treatment is not needed.

Checkpoint Question

3. What five elements must be in a physician's termination intent letter?

Consent

The law requires that patients must **consent** or agree to being touched, examined, or treated by the physician or agents of the physician involved in the contractual agreement. No treatment may be made without a consent given orally, nonverbally by behavior, or clearly in writing. Patients have the right to appoint a health care surrogate or health care power of attorney who may make health care decisions when the patient is unable to make them. A health care surrogate may be a spouse, a friend, a pastor, or an attorney. A **durable power of attorney** for health care gives the patient's representative the ability to make health care decisions as the health care surrogate. A patient's physician should be aware of the power of attorney agreement, and a copy of the legal documentation should be kept in the office medical record.

Implied Consent

In the typical visit to the physician's office, the patient's actions represent an informal agreement for care to be given. A patient who raises a sleeve to receive an injection implies agreement to the treatment. **Implied consent** also occurs in an emergency. If a patient is in a life-threatening situation and is unable to give verbal permission for treatment, it is implied that the patient would consent to treatment if possible. As soon as possible, informed consent should be signed by either the patient or a family member in this type of situation. When there is no emergency, implied consent should be used only if the procedure poses no significant risk to the patient.

Informed or Expressed Consent

The physician is responsible for obtaining the patient's **informed consent** whenever the treatment involves an invasive procedure such as surgery, use of experimental drugs, potentially dangerous procedures such as stress tests, or any treatment that poses a significant risk to the patient. A federal law discussed later requires that health care providers who administer certain vaccines give the patient a current vaccine information statement (VIS). A VIS provides a standardized way to give objective information about vaccine benefits and adverse events (side effects) to patients. The VIS is available online through the Centers for Disease Control and Prevention (CDC) in 26 languages. Informed consent is also referred to as **expressed consent**.

Informed consent is based on the patient's right to know every possible benefit, risk, or alternative to the suggested treatment and the possible outcome if no treatment is initiated. The patient must voluntarily give permission and must understand the implications of consenting to the treatment. This requires that the physician and patient communicate in a manner understandable to the patient. Patients can be more active in personal health care decisions when they are educated about and understand their treatment and care.

A consent form must include the following information:

1. Name of the procedure to be performed
2. Name of the physician who will perform the procedure
3. Name of the person administering the anesthesia (if applicable)
4. Any potential risks from the procedure
5. Anticipated result or benefit from the procedure
6. Alternatives to the procedure and their risks
7. Probable effect on the patient's condition if the procedure is not performed
8. Any exclusions that the patient requests
9. Statement indicating that all of the patient's questions or concerns regarding the procedure have been answered
10. Patient's and witnesses' signatures and the date

As the medical assistant, you will frequently be required to witness consent signatures. A sample consent form is seen in Figure 2-2.

The informed consent form supplied for the patient's signature must be in the language that the patient speaks. Most physicians who treat multicultural patients have consent

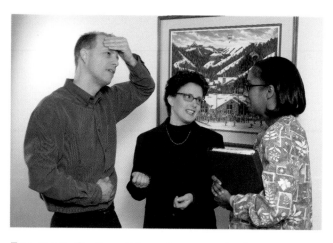

FIGURE 2–3.   Using an interpreter, the CMA helps this patient understand the procedure.

forms available in a variety of languages. Never ask a patient to sign a consent form if he or she:

- Does not understand the procedure
- Has unanswered questions regarding the procedure
- Is unable to read the consent form

Never **coerce** (force or compel against his or her wishes) a patient into signing a consent form. Figure 2-3 shows a deaf patient, a signing interpreter, and a certified medical assistant (CMA) with a consent form.

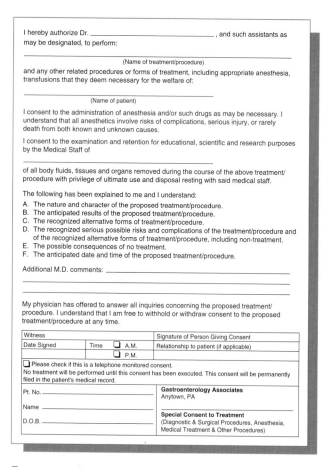

I hereby authorize Dr. _____ , and such assistants as may be designated, to perform:

_____
(Name of treatment/procedure)

and any other related procedures or forms of treatment, including appropriate anesthesia, transfusions that they deem necessary for the welfare of:

_____
(Name of patient)

I consent to the administration of anesthesia and/or such drugs as may be necessary. I understand that all anesthetics involve risks of complications, serious injury, or rarely death from both known and unknown causes.

I consent to the examination and retention for educational, scientific and research purposes by the Medical Staff of

_____

of all body fluids, tissues and organs removed during the course of the above treatment/ procedure with privilege of ultimate use and disposal resting with said medical staff.

The following has been explained to me and I understand:

A. The nature and character of the proposed treatment/procedure.
B. The anticipated results of the proposed treatment/procedure.
C. The recognized alternative forms of treatment/procedure.
D. The recognized serious possible risks and complications of the treatment/procedure and of the recognized alternative forms of treatment/procedure, including non-treatment.
E. The possible consequences of no treatment.
F. The anticipated date and time of the proposed treatment/procedure.

Additional M.D. comments: _____

_____

_____

My physician has offered to answer all inquiries concerning the proposed treatment/ procedure. I understand that I am free to withhold or withdraw consent to the proposed treatment/procedure at any time.

Witness	Signature of Person Giving Consent
Date Signed	Time □ A.M. □ P.M.	Relationship to patient (if applicable)

□ Please check if this is a telephone monitored consent.
No treatment will be performed until this consent has been executed. This consent will be permanently filed in the patient's medical record.

Pt. No. _____	Gastroenterology Associates Anytown, PA
Name _____	
D.O.B. _____	Special Consent to Treatment (Diagnostic & Surgical Procedures, Anesthesia, Medical Treatment & Other Procedures)

FIGURE 2–2.   Sample consent form.

WHAT IF

A well-meaning family member asks for information about her mother's condition. What should you say?

Tell the family member that you are not allowed to discuss the patient without his or her permission. No information should be released to anyone—friends, family, media, or insurance companies—without prior written approval from the patient.

At the first visit, you should establish the patient's wishes about giving information to family members and friends. If there is a particular family member who brings the patient to the office, the patient may sign a release form giving that person the right to receive information. Many physicians provide the patient with a short progress report including the patient's test results, diagnosis, treatment, and next appointment. A form could be designed for this purpose. This gives the patient the opportunity to share complete and accurate information if they choose.

Who May Sign a Consent Form?. An adult (usually someone over age 18) who is mentally competent and not under the influence of medication or other substances may sign a consent form. A minor may sign a consent form if he or she is:

- In the armed services
- Requesting treatment for communicable diseases (including sexually transmitted diseases)
- Pregnant
- Requesting information regarding birth control, abortion, or drug or alcohol abuse counseling
- Emancipated

An **emancipated minor** is under the **age of majority** but is either married or self-supporting and is responsible for his or her debts. The age of majority varies from state to state and ranges from 18 to 21. Minors may give consent if any one of the above-listed criteria is present.

Legal guardians may also sign consent forms. A legal guardian is appointed by a judge when the court has ruled an individual to be mentally incompetent. Health care surrogates may also sign consent forms. Health care surrogates are discussed later in the chapter.

Checkpoint Question

4. Under what circumstances should a patient never be asked to sign a consent form?

Refusal of Consent

Patients may refuse treatment for any reason. Sometimes, patients make treatment choices based on religious or personal beliefs and preferences. For instance, a Jehovah's Witness may refuse a blood transfusion on religious grounds, or an elderly person may not want to undergo serious surgery because the potential complications may limit future lifestyle options. In this situation, the patient must sign a refusal of consent form indicating that the patient was instructed regarding the potential risks and benefits of the procedure as well as the risks if the procedure is not allowed. If the patient is a minor, the courts may become involved at the request of the physician or hospital and may award consent for the child. In this situation, the physician should follow legal counsel and document the incident carefully. In any instance that the patient refuses treatment, documentation must be made to protect the physician. The physician has a legal right to refuse to perform elective surgery on a patient who refuses to receive blood if needed.

Releasing Medical Information

The medical record is a legal document. Although the medical record itself belongs to the physician, the information belongs to the patient. Patients have the right to their medical information, and they have the right to deny the sharing of this information.

Requests for medical records are common. Other health care facilities, insurance companies, and patients themselves may need information from the medical chart. Staying within the law when releasing medical information is covered in Chapter 8.

Legally Required Disclosures

Even though patients have the right to limit access to their medical records, health care facilities have a responsibility to report certain events to governmental agencies without the patient's consent, which are referred to as **legally required disclosures**. You and other health care providers must report to the department of public health the situations described in the following sections.

Vital Statistics

All states maintain records of births, deaths, marriages, and divorces. These records include the following:

- Birth certificates.
- Stillbirth reports. Some states have separate stillbirth forms; other states use a regular death certificate.
- Death certificates. These must be signed by a physician. The cause and time of death must be included.

You may assist the physician in completing a death certificate and filing the finished report in the patient's chart.

Medical Examiner's Reports

Each state has laws pertaining to which deaths must be reported to the medical examiner's office. Generally, these include the following:

- Death from an unknown cause
- Death from a suspected criminal or violent act
- Death of a person not attended by a physician at the time of death or for a reasonable period preceding the death
- Death within 24 hours of hospital admission

Infectious or Communicable Diseases

These reports are made to the local health department. The information is used for statistical purposes and for preventing or tracking the spread of these diseases. Although state guidelines vary, there are usually three categories of reports:

- Telephone reports are required for diphtheria, cholera, meningococcal meningitis, and plague, usually within 24 hours of the diagnosis. Telephone reports must always be followed by written reports.
- Written reports are required for hepatitis, leprosy, malaria, rubeola, polio, rheumatic fever, tetanus, and tuberculosis. Sexually transmitted diseases must also

PATIENT EDUCATION

Legally Required Disclosures

Patient's who have conditions that require legal disclosure should be informed about the applicable law. Patients should be assured that all steps to ensure their confidentiality will be followed. Patients should be educated about why the disclosure is necessary, who receives the information, what particular forms will be completed, and any anticipated follow-up from the organization. For example, you are required to report to the local health department the name, address, and condition of a patient with sexually transmitted disease. It is the responsibility of the health department to contact the patient to acquire the names of the patient's sexual contacts. These contacts are notified and counseled by the health department official. Patients who are educated about these legally required disclosures will be more understanding and accepting of the need to file official reports.

be reported. Notification is usually required within 3 days of the date of discovery.

- Trend reports are made when your office notes an unusually high occurrence of influenza, streptococcal infections, or any other infectious diseases. Box 2-2 is a sample of reportable diseases and their time frames.

The CDC keeps a watchful eye on the public health. When necessary, the CDC establishes directives for the protection of the public. For example, when the public appeared to be at risk for contracting anthrax in 2001, the CDC mandated that documented anthrax cases be reported immediately. Fax machines and e-mail help facilitate such urgent public health communication.

National Childhood Vaccine Injury Act of 1986

Health care providers who administer certain vaccines and toxoids must report to the U. S. Department of Health & Human Services (DHHS) the occurrence of any side effects listed in the manufacturer's package insert. In addition, health care providers must record in the patient's record the following information:

1. Date the vaccine was administered
2. Lot number and manufacturer of vaccine
3. Any adverse reactions to the vaccine
4. Name, title, and address of the person who administered the vaccine

Box 2-2

REPORTABLE CONDITIONS

Chapter 19—Health: Epidemiology
Subchapter 19a—Communicable Disease Control
Section .0100—Reporting of Communicable Diseases
.0101 Reportable Diseases and Conditions
(a) The following named diseases and conditions are declared to be dangerous to the public health and are hereby made reportable within the time period specified after the disease or condition is reasonably suspected to exist:

acquired immune deficiency syndrome (AIDS)— 7 days
amebiasis—7 days
anthrax—24 hours
blastomycosis—7 days
botulism—24 hours
brucellosis—7 days
Campylobacter infection—24 hours
chancroid—24 hours
chlamydial infection (laboratory confirmed)—7 days
cholera—24 hours
dengue—7 days
diphtheria—24 hours
E. coli infection—24 hours
encephalitis—7 days
food-borne disease, including but not limited to
Clostridium perfringens, staphylococcal, and *Bacillus cereus*—24 hours
gonorrhea—24 hours
granuloma inguinale—24 hours
Haemophilus influenzae, invasive disease—24 hours
hepatitis A—24 hours
hepatitis B—24 hours
hepatitis B carriage—7 days
hepatitis non-A, non-B—7 days
human immunodeficiency virus infection (HIV) confirmed—7 days
legionellosis—7 days
leprosy—7 days
leptospirosis—7 days
Lyme disease—7 days
lymphogranuloma venereum—7 days
malaria—7 days
measles (rubeola)—24 hours
meningitis, pneumococcal—7 days
meningitis, viral (aseptic)—7 days
meningococcal disease—24 hours
mucocutaneous lymph node syndrome (Kawasaki syndrome)—7 days
mumps—7 days

Excerpt from the North Carolina Administrative Code Regarding Reporting of Communicable Diseases

VACCINATIONS REQUIRING VACCINE INFORMATION STATEMENTS

Anthrax
Chickenpox
Diphtheria, tetanus, and pertussis
Hib
Hepatitis A
Hepatitis B
Influenza
Lyme disease
Measles, mumps, and rubella
Meningococcal
Pneumococcal polysaccharide
Pneumococcal conjugate
Polio

Box 2-3 lists the vaccines and toxoids covered by the National Childhood Vaccine Injury Act.

Abuse, Neglect, or Maltreatment

Abuse, neglect, or maltreatment of any person who is incapable of self-protection usually falls under this category and may include the elderly or the mentally incompetent. Each state has its own regulations regarding what must be reported. Patient confidentiality rights are waived when the law requires you to report certain conditions.

Abuse is thought to be the second most common cause of death in children under age 5. The Federal Child Abuse Prevention and Treatment Act mandates that threats to a child's physical and mental welfare be reported. Health care workers, teachers, and social workers who report suspected abuse are not identified to the parents and are protected against liability. State laws vary regarding the procedure for reporting abuse. Local regulations should be outlined in the policies and procedures manuals at any outpatient facility. If you suspect a child is being abused, relay your suspicions to the physician. The physician will make the formal report. When authorities receive a report from a health care provider, they follow up by investigating the situation. For assistance in reporting suspected child abuse, you may call the national 24-hour hotline at 800-4 A CHILD (800-422-4453).

Spousal abuse is on the rise in this country. Many women and children are trapped in a cycle of abuse. Mothers who are financially dependent on their abusers may see no way out. You should record any information gathered in the patient interview or anything observed in the course of dealing with the patient that may indicate abuse. Report these observations to the physician. Most communities have anonymous safe places for victims of domestic abuse, and you should be familiar with these services. With proper referrals, you may be able to help break the cycle of domestic abuse.

This country is also undergoing a rise in elderly parents being cared for by their adult children who also have the responsibility of raising young children. This phenomenon can cause great stress among caregivers. Abuse of the elderly can be in the form of mistreatment or neglect (not providing appropriate care). You should pay attention to observations and information provided by your elderly patients. If mistreatment is suspected, alert the physician. Support groups for those caring for the elderly are useful in dealing with the challenges of caring for others.

Violent Injuries

Health care providers have the legal duty to report suspected criminal acts. Injuries resulting from weapons, assault, attempted suicide, and rape must be reported to local authorities.

Other Reports

A diagnosis of cancer must be reported to assist in tracking malignancies and identifying environmental carcinogens. Just as the CDC keeps track of all communicable diseases reported, a database of treated tumors is kept in hospitals through a tumor registry. Some states also require that epilepsy (a seizure condition) be reported to local motor vehicle departments. The testing of newborns for phenylketonuria (PKU), which can cause mental retardation, is required in all states. Some states require positive PKU results to be reported to the health department so that close observation and follow-up care are ensured to prevent serious complications for the infant. Infantile hypothyroidism is also a reportable condition in some states.

 Checkpoint Question

5. What are six situations and conditions you are legally required to report?

SPECIFIC LAWS AND STATUTES THAT APPLY TO HEALTH PROFESSIONALS

Medical Practice Acts

Although each state has its own medical practice act, the following elements are usually included:

- Definition of the practice of medicine.
- Requirements that the physician must have graduated from an accredited medical school and residency program and have passed the state medical examination.
- Description of the procedure for **licensure**.

- Description of the conditions for which a license can be suspended or revoked.
- Description of the renewal process for licensure. Most states require the physician to have attended a certain number of continuing education hours.
- Personal requirements necessary to become a licensed physician. Generally, a licensed physician must be a state resident, of good moral character, a U. S. citizen, and 21 years of age or older.

A physician may have his or her license revoked or suspended by the board of medical examiners in most states for a variety of reasons, including certain criminal offenses, unprofessional conduct, fraud, or professional or personal incompetence. Criminal offenses include but are not limited to murder, manslaughter, robbery, and rape. Examples of unprofessional conduct may include invasion of a patient's privacy, excessive use of alcohol or use of illegal drugs, and **fee splitting** (sharing fees for the referral of patients to certain colleagues). Fraud is a common reason for revoking a license. Fraud may include filing false Medicare or Medicaid claims, falsifying medical records, or professional misrepresentation. Examples of misrepresentation or fraud include advertising a medical cure that does not exist, guaranteeing 100% success of a treatment, or falsifying medical credentials. Incompetence is often a hard charge to prove. The three most common examples are insanity, senility, and other documented mental incompetence.

As a medical assistant, it is your responsibility to report illegal or unethical behavior or signs of incompetence in the medical office. See Box 2-11 and think about how would you handle this difficult situation. (We will discuss ethics later in this chapter.)

Licensure, Certification, and Registration

Medical professionals can be licensed, certified, or **registered**. Licensure is regulated by laws, such as medical practice acts and nursing practice acts. If a particular profession is a licensed one, it is mandatory that one maintain a license in each state where he or she works. Each state determines the qualifications and requirements for licensure of a particular profession. A state agency will be responsible for issuing and renewing licenses. Most professionals are licensed to practice their profession according to certain guidelines and are limited to specific duties. For example, nurses are licensed. In North Carolina, the nursing practice act specifically prohibits a nurse from delegating professional authority to unlicensed personnel.

The term *registered* indicates that a professional has met basic requirements, usually for education, has passed standard testing, and has been approved by a governing body to perform given tasks within a state. X-ray technologists are registered as registered radiologic technologists. A national registry is available to verify a potential employee's status.

Certification is a voluntary process regulated through a professional organization. Standards for certification are set by the organization issuing the certificate. The CMA and registered medical assistant (RMA) credentials are nationally recognized and do not require any action when moving from one state to another. Remember, you must adhere to the laws regarding the CMA or RMA in the state where you work.

As a medical assistant, you are not licensed and therefore not limited to certain duties. The physician-employer has the sole responsibility of setting any limits on the duties of a medical assistant. Although most states do not require certification for employment, employers seek the CMA or RMA because certification indicates the achievement of certain standards of competence. A few states require that you take a test or short course before performing certain clinical duties.

Controlled Substances Act

The Controlled Substances Act of 1970 is a federal law enforced by the Drug Enforcement Agency (DEA). The act regulates the manufacture, distribution, and dispensing of narcotics and nonnarcotic drugs considered to have a high potential for abuse. This act was designed to decrease the illegal use of controlled substances and to prevent substance abuse by medical professionals. The law requires that any physician who dispenses, administers, or prescribes narcotics or other controlled substances be registered with the DEA.

Physicians who maintain a stock of controlled substances in the office for dispensing or administration must use a special triplicate order form available through the DEA. A record of each transaction must be kept and retained for 2 to 3 years. The record must be available for inspection by the DEA at any time. The act requires that all controlled substances be kept in a locked cabinet out of the patients' view and that the keys be kept secure. Theft should be reported immediately to the local police and the nearest DEA office. Prescription pads used for prescribing controlled substances must remain in a safe place at all times. Box 2-4 lists steps you can take to keep these prescription pads safe.

This act also requires a physician to return all registration certificates and any unused order forms to the DEA if the practice is closed or sold. Violation of this act is a criminal offense. Penalties range from fines to imprisonment. Table 2-1 outlines the classification of controlled substances.

Good Samaritan Act

As the number of lawsuits against physicians began to rise, physicians feared that giving emergency care to strangers outside the office could lead to malpractice suits. To combat that fear, all states now have Good Samaritan acts. Good Samaritan acts ensure that caregivers are immune from liability suits as long as they give care in good faith and in a manner that a reasonable and prudent person would in a

Box 2-4

PRESCRIPTION PAD SAFETY TIPS

- Keep only one prescription pad in a locked cabinet in the examining room. All other pads should be locked away elsewhere. Do not leave prescription pads unattended.
- Keep a limited supply of pads. It is better to reorder on a regular basis than to overstock.
- Keep track of the number of pads in the office. If a burglary occurs, you will be able to advise the police regarding the number of missing pads.
- Report any prescription pad theft to the police and alert local pharmacies of the theft. If the theft involves the loss of narcotic pads, the Drug Enforcement Agency must be notified.

similar situation. Each state has specific guidelines. Some even set standards for various professional levels, such as one set of standards for a physician and another set of standards for emergency medical technicians. Your state's Good Samaritan Act will not protect you if you are grossly negligent or willfully perform negligent acts.

You are not covered by the Good Samaritan Act while you are working as a medical assistant, nor does it cover physicians in the performance of their duties. Liability and malpractice insurance policies are available to protect you in those situations. If you render emergency care and accept compensation for that care, the act does not apply.

The provisions only cover acts outside of the formal practice of the profession.

BASIS OF MEDICAL LAW

Tort Law

A tort is a wrongful act that results in harm for which restitution must be made. The two forms of torts are intentional and unintentional. An allegation of an **unintentional tort** means that the accuser (the **plaintiff**) believes a mistake has been made; however, the plaintiff believes the caregiver or accused party (the **defendant**) was operating in good faith and did not intend the mistake to occur. Consider this scenario as an example of an unintentional tort: A medical assistant giving a patient a heat treatment for muscle aches inadvertently burns the arm of a patient because the equipment is faulty. This act was not intentional or malicious, but it caused damage to the patient. About 90% of suits against physicians fall into this category.

Schedule	Description	Examples
Table 2-1 CONTROLLED SUBSTANCES		
I	These drugs have the highest potential for abuse and have no currently accepted medical use in the United States. There are no accepted safety standards for use of these drugs or substances even under medical supervision, although some are used experimentally in carefully controlled research projects.	Opium Marijuana Lysergic acid diethylamide (LSD) Peyote Mescaline
II	These drugs have a high potential for abuse. They have accepted medicinal use in the United States but with severe restrictions. Abuse of these drugs can lead to dependence, either psychological or physiological. Schedule II drugs require a written prescription and cannot be refilled or called in to the pharmacy by the medical office. Only in extreme emergencies may the physician call in the prescription. A handwritten prescription must be presented to the pharmacist within 72 hours.	Morphine Codeine Seconal Cocaine Amphetamine Dilaudid Ritalin
III	These drugs have a limited potential for psychological or physiological dependence. The prescription may be called in to the pharmacist by the physician and refilled up to 5 times in a 6-month period.	Paregoric Tylenol with codeine Fiorinal
IV	These drugs have a lower potential for abuse than those in Schedules II and III. They can be called in to the pharmacist by a medical office employee and may be refilled up to 5 times in a 6-month period.	Librium Valium Darvon Phenobarbital
V	These drugs have a lower potential for abuse than those in Schedules I, II, III, and IV.	Lomotil Dimetane expectorant DC Robitussin-DAC

Negligence and Malpractice (Unintentional Torts)

Most unintentional torts involve negligence. These are the most common forms of medical malpractice suits.

Negligence is performing an act that a reasonable health care worker or provider would not have done or the omission of an act that a reasonable professional or provider would have done. Failure to take reasonable precautions to prevent harm to a patient is termed **negligence**. If a physician is involved, the term usually used is malpractice. Malpractice is said to have occurred when the patient is harmed by the professional's actions. There are three types of malpractice:

- Malfeasance—incorrect treatment
- Misfeasance—treatment performed incorrectly
- Nonfeasance—treatment delayed or not attempted

In a legal situation, the standard of care determines what a reasonable professional would have done. Standards of care are written by various professional agencies to clarify what the reasonable and prudent physician or health care worker would do in a given situation. For example, a patient comes to an orthopedist's office after falling from a horse and complains of arm pain. The standard of care for orthopedists would require an x-ray of the injured extremity after trauma. Standards of care vary with the level of the professional. A registered nurse is not held to the same standards of care as a physician, nor is the medical assistant expected to perform by the same standards as the registered nurse. Each must practice within the scope of their training. The representing attorney may seek an **expert witness** to state under oath the standards of care for a specific situation. Expert witnesses may be physicians, nurses, physical therapists, or other specialized practitioners who have excellent reputations in their field.

Expert witnesses are always used in malpractice cases, except when the doctrine of **res ipsa loquitur** is tried. This doctrine means "the thing speaks for itself." In other words, it is obvious that the physician's actions or negligence caused the injury. A judge must preapprove the use of this theory in pretrial hearings. An example of a case tried under this doctrine might be a fracture that occurred when the patient fell from an examining table.

For negligence to be proved, the plaintiff's attorney must prove four elements were present: duty, dereliction of duty, direct cause, and damage. The courts place the burden of proof on the plaintiff; the physician is assumed to have given proper care until proven otherwise.

Duty

Duty is present when the patient and the physician have formed a contract. This is usually straightforward and the easiest of the elements to prove.

Dereliction of Duty

The patient must prove that the physician did not meet the standard of care guidelines, either by performing an act inappropriately or by omitting an act.

Direct Cause

The plaintiff must prove that the derelict act directly caused the patient's injury. This can be difficult to prove if the patient has an extensive medical history that may have contributed to the injury.

Damage

The plaintiff must prove that an injury or **damages** occurred. Documentation must be available to prove a diagnosis of an injury or illness.

Jury Awards

There are three types of awards for damages:

1. *Nominal.* Minimal injuries or damages occurred and compensation is small.
2. *Actual (compensatory).* Money is awarded for the injury, disability, mental suffering, loss of income, or the anticipated future earning loss. This payment is moderate to significant.
3. *Punitive.* Money is awarded to punish the practitioner for reckless or malicious wrongdoing. Punitive damages are the most costly. (Note: A physician may have committed a medical error, but if the patient suffered no injuries or damages, he or she cannot win the suit. Also, if the outcome was not as expected but the physician cannot be shown to be at fault, the patient will not be compensated.)

 Checkpoint Question

6. What four elements must be proved in a negligence suit?

Intentional Torts

An **intentional tort** is an act that takes place with malice and with the intent of causing harm. Intentional torts are the deliberate violation of another person's legal rights. Examples of intentional torts are assault and battery, use of duress, invasion of privacy, defamation of character, fraud, tort of outrage, and undue influence. These are described next.

Assault and Battery

Assault is the unauthorized attempt or threat to touch another person without consent. **Battery** is the actual physical touching of a patient without consent; this includes beating and physical abuse. By law, a conscious adult has the right to refuse medical care. An example of battery might be suturing a laceration against the patient's expressed wish.

Duress

If a patient is coerced into an act, the patient can possibly sue for the tort of **duress**. Following is an example in which a patient may be able to sue successfully for assault, battery, and duress: A 22-year-old woman arrives at a pregnancy center. She is receiving public assistance and has five children. Her pregnancy test is positive. The staff persuades her to have an abortion. She signs the consent form, and the abortion is performed. Later she sues, stating that she was verbally coerced into signing the consent form (duress) and that the abortion was performed against her wishes (assault and battery).

Invasion of Privacy

Patients have the right to privacy. Most offices have patients sign an authorization to release information to their insurance company on their first visit. This covers each return visit unless the insurance carrier changes. Written permission must be obtained from the patient to:

- Release medical records or personal data
- Publish case histories in medical journals
- Make photographs of the patient (exception: suspected cases of abuse or maltreatment)
- Allow observers in examination rooms

For example, a 57-year-old woman is seen in your office for a skin biopsy. Her insurance company calls asking for information regarding the bill and asks for the biopsy report. You give the requested information and then find that the patient never signed a release form. She has a valid case for invasion of privacy.

Defamation of Character

Making malicious or false statements about a person's character or reputation is **defamation of character**. **Libel** refers to written statements and **slander** refers to oral statements. For example, a patient asks for a referral to another physician. She states that she has heard "Dr. Rogers is a good surgeon." You have heard that he has a history of alcoholism. You tell the patient that he is probably not a good choice because of his drinking. That is defamation of his character, and you could be sued for saying it.

Fraud

Fraud is any deceitful act with the intention to conceal the truth, such as:

- Intentionally raising false expectations regarding recovery

- Not properly instructing the patient regarding possible side effects of a procedure
- Filing false insurance claims

Tort of Outrage

Tort of outrage is the intentional infliction of emotional distress. For this tort to be proved, the plaintiff's attorney must show that the physician:

- Intended to inflict emotional distress
- Acted in a manner that is not morally or ethically acceptable
- Caused severe emotional distress

Undue Influence

Improperly persuading another to act in a way contrary to that person's free will is termed undue influence. For instance, preying on the elderly or the mentally incompetent is a common type of undue influence. Unethical practitioners who gain the trust of these persons and persuade them to submit to expensive and unnecessary medical procedures are practicing undue influence.

Checkpoint Question

7. What is the difference between assault and battery?

THE LITIGATION PROCESS

The litigation process begins when a patient consults an attorney because he or she believes a health care provider has done wrong or becomes aware of a possible prior injury. The patient's attorney obtains the medical records, which are reviewed by medicolegal consultants. (Such consultants may be nurses or physicians who are considered experts in their field.) Then the plaintiff's attorney files a complaint, a written statement that lists the claim against the physician and the remedy desired, usually monetary compensation.

The defendant and his or her attorney answer the complaint. The discovery phase begins with interrogatories and **depositions**. During this phase, attorneys for both parties gather relevant information.

Next, the trial phase begins. A jury is selected unless the parties agree to a **bench trial**. In a bench trial, the judge hears the case without a jury and renders a **verdict** (decision or judgment). Opening statements are given, first by the plaintiff's attorney, then by the defendant's attorney. The plaintiff's attorney presents the case. Expert witnesses are called, and the evidence is shown. Examination of the witnesses begins. **Direct examination** involves questioning by one's own attorney; **cross-examination** is questioning by the opposing attorney. When the plaintiff's attorney is finished, the defense presents the opposing arguments and evidence. The plaintiff's attorney may cross-examine the defendant's witnesses. Closing arguments are heard. Finally, a verdict is made.

If the defendant is found guilty, damages are awarded. If the defendant is found not guilty, the charges are dismissed. The decision may be appealed to a higher court. An **appeal** is a process by which the higher court reviews the decision of the lower court.

DEFENSES TO PROFESSIONAL LIABILITY SUITS

The objective of all court proceedings is to uncover the truth. Many defenses are available to a health care worker who is being sued. These include the medical record, statute of limitations, assumption of risk, res judicata, contributory negligence, and comparative negligence, discussed next.

Medical Records

The best and most solid defense the caregiver has is the medical record. Every item in the record is considered to be a part of a legal document. Juries may believe a medical record regardless of testimony. Juries tend to believe these records because they are tangible items from the actual time the injury occurred. There is a common saying in the medicolegal world: "If it's not in the chart, it did not happen." This means that even negative findings should be listed. For example, instead of saying that the patient's neurological history is negative, the documentation might say the patient reports no headaches, seizures, one-sided weakness, and so on. Entries in the medical record refresh the memory of the defendant and provide documentation of care. As a medical assistant, you must make sure that all of your documentation is timely, accurate, and legible. (See Chapter 8 for specific information regarding charting practices.)

Statute of Limitations

Each state has a statute that defines the length of time during which a patient may file a suit against a caregiver. When the **statute of limitations** expires, the patient loses the right to file a claim. Generally, the limits vary from 1 to 3 years following the alleged occurrence. Other states use a combination rule. Some states allow 1 to 3 years following the patient's discovery of the occurrence. States vary greatly when an alleged injury involves a minor. The statute may not take effect until the minor reaches the age of majority and then may extend 2 to 3 years past this time. Some states have longer claim periods in wrongful death suits.

Assumption of Risk

In the assumption of risk defense, the physician will claim that the patient was aware of the risks involved before the procedure and fully accepted the potential for damages. For example, a patient is instructed regarding the adverse effects of chemotherapy. The patient fully understands these risks, receives the chemotherapy, and wants to sue for alopecia (hair loss). Alopecia is a given risk with certain forms of chemotherapy. A signed consent form indicating that the patient was informed of all of the risks of a procedure proves this point.

Res Judicata

The doctrine of **res judicata** means "the thing has been decided." Once the suit has been brought against the physician or patient and a settlement has been reached, the losing party may not countersue. If, for instance, the physician sues a patient for not paying bills and the court orders the patient to pay, the patient cannot sue the physician for malpractice. The opposite may occur as well. If the physician is sued for malpractice and loses, he cannot countersue for defamation of character.

Contributory Negligence

With the **contributory negligence** defense, the physician usually admits that negligence has occurred; he or she will claim, however, that the patient aggravated the injury or assisted in making the injury worse. For example, the patient's laceration is stitched with only 3 sutures when 10 were needed. The physician instructs the patient to limit movement of the arm. The patient plays baseball; the laceration reopens, causing infection; and subsequently, extensive scar tissue forms. Both the patient and the physician contributed to the postoperative damages. Most states do not grant damage awards for contributory negligence. If an award is granted, the courts assess **comparative negligence**.

Comparative Negligence

In comparative negligence, the award of damages is based on a percentage of the contribution to the negligence. If the patient contributed 30% to the damage, the damage award is 30% less than what was granted. In the example in the previous paragraph, the courts may decide that the negligence is shared at 50%. Therefore, if the court assessed damages of $20,000, the physician would be responsible for $10,000.

In the past, contributory negligence, such as a patient not returning for appointments, was seen as absolute defense for the physician. Since the 1970s, however, the trend has been toward using the defense of comparative negligence, with the responsibility shared between the physician and the patient.

Immunity

The Federal Tort Claim Act of 1946 prohibits suits against any U. S. governmental facility, such as veterans hospitals or military bases. This provides immunity to all of their employees for ordinary negligence but not for intentional torts.

DEFENSE FOR THE MEDICAL ASSISTANT

Respondeat Superior or Law of Agency

The doctrine of **respondeat superior** literally means "let the master answer." This may also be called law of agency. This doctrine implies that physicians are liable for the actions of their employees. The physician is responsible for your actions as a medical assistant as long as your actions are within your scope of practice. Figure 2-4 features a scope-of-practice decision tree designed to help you make such decisions.

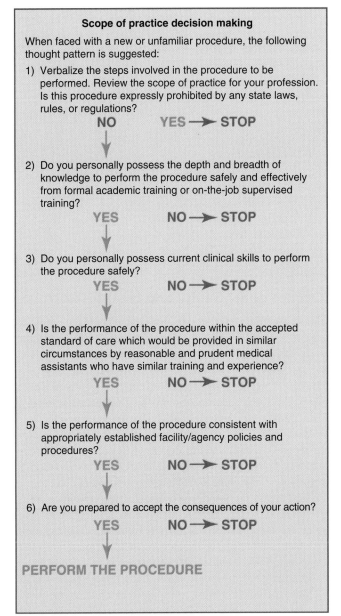

Scope of practice decision making

When faced with a new or unfamiliar procedure, the following thought pattern is suggested:

1) Verbalize the steps involved in the procedure to be performed. Review the scope of practice for your profession. Is this procedure expressly prohibited by any state laws, rules, or regulations?
   NO   YES → STOP

2) Do you personally possess the depth and breadth of knowledge to perform the procedure safely and effectively from formal academic training or on-the-job supervised training?
   YES   NO → STOP

3) Do you personally possess current clinical skills to perform the procedure safely?
   YES   NO → STOP

4) Is the performance of the procedure within the accepted standard of care which would be provided in similar circumstances by reasonable and prudent medical assistants who have similar training and experience?
   YES   NO → STOP

5) Is the performance of the procedure consistent with appropriately established facility/agency policies and procedures?
   YES   NO → STOP

6) Are you prepared to accept the consequences of your action?
   YES   NO → STOP

PERFORM THE PROCEDURE

FIGURE 2–4. Scope of practice decision-making tree. (Adapted from the Washington State Department of Health, Nursing Care Quality Assurance Commission, "Scope of Practice Decision Tree.")

As a new medical assistant, you can use this tool to guard against overconfidence. If your actions exceed your abilities or training, the physician is not generally responsible for any error that you make. You must understand that you can be sued in this instance and that respondeat superior does not guarantee immunity for your actions.

For example, Mrs. Smith is a chronic complainer, calling your office frequently with minor concerns. Today, she calls complaining of tingling in her arms. The physician has left for the day, so you tell Mrs. Smith, "Don't worry about this; take your medication and call us tomorrow." During the night a blood vessel in Mrs. Smith's brain bursts. She has a cerebral hemorrhage (bleeding inside the brain) and dies. The family sues. The physician claims that you were instructed not to give advice over the telephone. You are not covered by respondeat superior because you acted outside of your scope of practice.

To protect yourself from situations such as this, have your job description in written form and always practice within its guidelines. Do not perform tasks that you have not been trained to do. Never hesitate to seek clarification from a physician. If you are not sure about something, such as a medication order, ask!

Malpractice insurance is available to allied health care professionals for further protection. Malpractice premiums are inexpensive and afford protection against losing any personal assets if sued. The insurance company would pay damages as assessed by a jury. Of course, as with any insurance policy, there will be conditions of coverage and maximum amounts the company will pay. Box 2-5 provides some additional tips for preventing lawsuits.

Box 2-5

YOU CAN AVOID LITIGATION

- Keep medical records neat and organized. Always document and sign legibly.
- Stay abreast of new laws and medical technology.
- Become a certified or registered medical assistant (CMA or RMA).
- Keep your CPR and first aid certification current.
- Never give any information over the telephone unless you are sure of the caller's identity and you have patient consent.
- Keep the office neat and clean. Make sure that children's toys are clean and in good condition to avoid injuries. Perform safety checks frequently.
- Limit waiting time for patients. If an emergency arises, causing a long wait, explain to the patients in a timely and professional manner.
- Practice good public relations. Always be polite, smile, and show genuine concern for your patients and their families.

Checkpoint Question

8. What is the law of agency, and how does it apply to the medical assistant?

EMPLOYMENT AND SAFETY LAWS

Civil Rights Act of 1964, Title VII

Title VII of the Civil Rights Act of 1964 protects employees from discrimination in the workplace. The Equal Employment Opportunity Commission (EEOC) enforces the provisions of the act and investigates any possible infractions. Employers may not refuse to hire, limit, segregate or classify, fire, compensate, or provide working conditions and privileges on the basis of race, color, sex, religion, or national origin. This act determines the questions that may be asked in a job interview. For example, a potential employee cannot be asked questions that would reveal age, marital status, religious affiliation, height, weight, or arrest record. It is acceptable, however, to ask if an applicant has ever been convicted of a crime. In the health care setting, employers can require a criminal records check and even drug screening to ensure the safety of the patients. The American Association of Medical Assistants (AAMA) has made recent changes to prohibit convicted felons from taking the CMA examination.

Sexual Harassment

In recent years, Title VII has been expanded to include sexual harassment. Sexual harassment is defined by the EEOC as unwelcome sexual advances or requests for sexual favors in the workplace. The definition includes other verbal or physical conduct of a sexual nature when such conduct is made a condition of an individual's employment, is used as a basis for hiring or promotion, or has the purpose or effect of unreasonably interfering with an individual's work performance. If such behavior creates an intimidating, hostile, or offensive working environment, it is considered sexual harassment. In the past two decades court decisions have confirmed that this form of harassment is a cause for both criminal prosecution and civil litigation.

In the medical office setting, the office manager must be alert for signs of harassment and should have in place a policy for handling complaints.

Americans with Disabilities Act

Title VII also includes the Americans with Disabilities Act (ADA), which prohibits discrimination against people with substantial disabilities in all employment practices, including job application procedures, hiring, firing, advancement, compensation, training, benefits, and all other privileges of employment. The ADA applies to all employers with 15 or more employees. The law covers those with impairments that limit their major life activities. The statute also protects those with AIDS or HIV-positive status and individuals with a history of mental illness or cancer. ADA also requires that employers provide basic accommodations for disabled employees. Those basic accommodations include extra-wide parking spaces close to the door, ramps or elevators, electric or easily opened doors, bathroom facilities designed for the disabled, an accessible break room, and a work area with counters low enough for a person in a wheelchair.

The ADA also takes safety into consideration. Employers are permitted to establish qualification standards that will exclude individuals who pose a direct threat to others if that risk cannot be lowered to an acceptable level by reasonable accommodations. In the medical field, technical standards are established that outline physical requirements of a certain job. For example, a medical assistant needs adequate vision to see the dials on laboratory equipment. If a particular job requires reaching a certain height, it is unreasonable to expect an employer to hire a person who is too short. The law is designed to protect employees, not to require unreasonable accommodations.

The ADA also requires that all public buildings be accessible to physically challenged people. Following is a partial list of ways the medical office can comply with this act:

- Entrance ramps
- Widened rest rooms to be wheelchair accessible
- Elevated toilet bowls for easier transferring from wheelchairs
- Easy-to-reach elevator buttons
- Braille signs
- Access to special telephone services to communicate with hearing-impaired patients

Occupational Safety and Health Act

Employers must provide safe environments for their employees. In accordance with the Occupational Safety and Health Act of 1970, the Occupational Safety and Health Administration (OSHA) controls and monitors safety for workers. Specific OSHA rules and regulations protect the clinical worker from exposure to **blood-borne pathogens**. Blood-borne pathogens are organisms that can be spread through direct contact with blood or body fluids from an infected person. Universal precautions are designed to protect health care workers from blood and body fluids contaminated with HIV, hepatitis, or any contagious "bugs" by requiring that those in direct contact with patients use protective equipment (e.g., gloves, gowns, face mask). In days past, health care workers felt that they needed protection only from patients with known risk factors (sharing needles, having unprotected sexual intercourse). OSHA's regulations ensure protection from contracting a contagious disease from *any* body fluids handled.

Your medical assisting training will include an extensive study of safety issues and protection against accidental exposure to blood-borne pathogens. Box 2-6 outlines OSHA rules governing all free-standing health care providers. Box 2-7 outlines the laws governing employer and employee rights and responsibilities.

OCCUPATIONAL SAFETY AND HEALTH ACT OF 1970 RULES GOVERNING HEALTH CARE PROVIDERS

OSHA defines body fluids as semen, blood, amniotic fluids, vaginal secretions, synovial fluid (from joint spaces), pleural fluid (from the lungs), pericardial fluid (from the heart), cerebrospinal fluid (from the spinal cord), and saliva. OSHA employs inspectors who may conduct inspections and issue citations for violations and recommend penalties. Under specific rules, OSHA requires that health care facilities provide:

- A list of all employees who might be exposed to blood-borne diseases on either a regular or an occasional basis.
- A written exposure control plan that outlines steps to be taken in the event of an employee's accidental exposure to blood-borne pathogens.
- One employee who is responsible for OSHA compliance.
- Availability of protective clothing that fits properly.
- An employee training program in writing and records of sessions and participants.
- Warning labels and signs denoting biohazards (potentially dangerous materials).
- Written guidelines for identifying, containing, and disposing of medical waste, including housecleaning and laundry decontamination.
- Written guidelines and procedures to follow if any employee is exposed to blood or other potentially infectious materials, as well as a policy for reporting incidents of exposure and maintaining records.
- Postexposure evaluation procedures, including follow-up testing of the exposed employee.
- Material safety data sheets (MSDS) listing each ingredient in a product used in the office Manufacturers provide an MSDS for every product they sell Information included in the sheets includes any hazards involved or necessary precautions that must be taken when handling materials.
- Hepatitis B vaccine free of charge to employees working with body fluids.

Other Legal Considerations

The Clinical Laboratory Improvement Amendments (CLIA) of 1988 contain specific rules and regulations regarding laboratory safety.

The Joint Commission on Accreditation of Healthcare Organizations (JCAHO) is a private organization that sets stan-dards for health care administration. Each state also has specific laws regarding patient care, insurance billing, collections, and such matters.

Checkpoint Question

9. What are blood-borne pathogens? Which government agency governs their control in the medical office?

LAWS GOVERNING EMPLOYER AND EMPLOYMENT RIGHTS AND RESPONSIBILITIES

Fair Labor Standards Act of 1939
- Regulates wages and working conditions including
- Federal minimum wage, overtime compensation, equal pay requirements, child labor, hours, requirements for record keeping.

Civil Rights Act of 1964, Title VII
- Applies to employers with 15 or more employees for at least 20 weeks of the year.
- Federal regulation forbids discrimination on the basis of race, color, sex, religion, or national origin. Some state laws also prohibit discrimination for sexual orientation, personal appearance, mental health, mental retardation, marital status, parenthood, and political affiliation.

Americans with Disabilities Act of 1990
- Applies to employers with 15 or more employees.
- Prohibits discrimination against individuals with substantial impairments in all employment practices.

Age Discrimination in Employment Act of 1967
- Applies to employers with 15 or more employees.
- Regulates discrimination against workers on the basis of age. Protects those 40–65.

Family and Medical Leave Act of 1993
- Employees are covered after 1 year or 1,250 hours of employment over the past 12 months.
- Provides up to 12 weeks per year of unpaid, job-protected leave to eligible employees for certain family and medical reasons.

Immigration Reform and Control Act of 1986
- Applies to employers with four or more employees.
- Prohibits employment of illegal aliens and protects legal aliens from discrimination based on national origin or citizenship.

MEDICAL ETHICS

Medical **ethics** are principles of ethical and moral conduct that govern the behavior and conduct of health professionals. These principles define proper medical etiquette, customs, and professional courtesy. Ethics are guidelines specifying right or wrong and are enforced by peer review and professional organizations. Laws are regulations and rules that are enforced by the government. **Bioethics** are issues and problems that affect a patient's life; many bioethical issues have arisen from the advances of modern medicine.

American Medical Association (AMA) Code of Ethics

A code of ethics is a "collective statement from a professional organization that depicts the behavioral expectations for its members. Additionally, a code of ethics allows the organization to set standards by which it may discipline its members." The AMA Code of Ethics states that physicians must recognize and accept their responsibilities for both patients and society. It also states that these are "not laws but standards of conduct by which a physician's professional behavior will be assessed." Box 2-8 outlines the AMA Code of Ethics.

Box 2-8

AMA CODE OF ETHICS

Seven principles in the AMA Code of Ethics state that the physician shall:

1. Practice competent medical care with compassion while respecting human dignity.
2. Remain honest in dealings with patients and colleagues; expose colleagues with character deficiencies or who are incompetent or who engage in fraud or deception.
3. Adhere to all laws, and when needed, be a voice to lawmakers in the best interest of patient care.
4. Respect the rights of patients and other health care professionals; safeguard patient confidentiality (privacy) except within the provisions of the law.
5. Continue appropriate education to remain current; request consultation and obtain the knowledge and skills of other health professionals when needed.
6. Be free to select whom to treat, where to establish a practice, and whom to associate with except in emergency situations.
7. Participate in activities to enhance the community.

Violations of these AMA principles may result in censure, suspension, or expulsion by the state medical board. **Censure**, the least punitive action, is a verbal or written reprimand from the association indicating negative findings regarding a specific incident. Suspension is the temporary removal of privileges and association with the organization. Expulsion is a formal discharge from the professional organization and is the maximum punishment. Many of these issues, however, deal with laws and the patient's rights as established by law. When violations of laws are involved, physicians may lose their license to practice, may be fined, or may be imprisoned. Serious consequences can arise from a breach of this code of ethics.

Medical Assistant's Role in Ethics

As an agent of the physician in the medical office, you are also governed by ethical standards and are responsible for:

- Protecting patient confidentiality
- Following all state and federal laws
- Being honest in all your actions

As a medical assistant, you must apply ethical standards as you perform your duties. You must realize that your personal feelings of right and wrong should be kept separate if they differ from the ethics of your profession. For example, a medical assistant who has a strong opinion against abortion would not be happy working in a medical facility that performs abortions. The care you give patients must be objective, and personal opinions about options must not be shared.

Patient Advocacy

Your primary responsibility as a medical assistant is to be a patient advocate at all times. Advocacy requires that you consider the best interests of the patient above all other concerns. This often means setting aside your own personal beliefs, values, and biases and looking at a given situation in an objective manner. You should never, however, be asked or forced to compromise your own value system.

Patient Confidentiality

Confidentiality of patient information is one of the most important ethical principles to be observed by the medical assistant. As discussed earlier, information obtained in the care of the patient may not be revealed without the permission of the patient unless required by law. Whatever you say to, hear from, or do to a patient is confidential. Patients will reveal some of their innermost thoughts, feelings, and fears. This information is not for public knowledge. Family members, friends, pastors, or others may call the physician's office to inquire about a patient's condition. Many of these calls are made with good intentions; NO INFORMATION, however, should be released to anyone—friends, family, media, or in-

WHAT IF

A patient is hearing impaired, and you cannot communicate with him. What should you do?

If the patient does not understand the procedure, he or she is not *informed*. Legally, you have not met your responsibilities to obtain informed consent if the patient does not understand the information you are trying to convey. If the patient cannot provide his or her own assistance, it is the legal responsibility of the physician and his agents to provide the means for effective communication.

Most community colleges offer courses in sign language. The Internet offers a site for the deaf community that will direct you to resources in your area. Handspeak is a site that provides a visual language dictionary. These websites are listed at the end of this chapter.

surance companies—without prior written approval from the patient (see Chapter 8).

Honesty

One of the most important character traits for medical assistants is honesty. We all make mistakes at times; how we handle our mistakes is the indication of our ethical standards. If you make a mistake (e.g., giving the wrong medication) you must immediately report the error to your supervisor and the attending physician. The mark of a true professional is the ability to admit mistakes and take full responsibility for all actions. When speaking to patients concerning medical issues, be honest; give the facts in a straightforward manner. Never offer false expectations or hope. Never minimize or exaggerate the risks or benefits of a procedure. If you do not know the answer to a question, say, "I don't know, but I will find out for you," or refer the question to the physician. Treating the patient with dignity, respect, and honesty in all interactions will build trust in you and your professional abilities.

Checkpoint Question

10. What are the three ethical standards a CMA, as an agent of the physician, should follow?

American Association of Medical Assistants (AAMA) Code of Ethics

Principles

The AAMA has published a set of five principles of ethical and moral conduct that all medical assistants must follow in the practice of the profession. They state that the medical assistant must always strive to:

MEDICAL ASSISTANTS' CREED

The AAMA also has a written creed for medical assistants. It is generally recited as a group during graduation or pinning services. The creed of the AAMA is:

I believe in the principles and purposes of the profession.
I endeavor to be more effective.
I aspire to render greater service.
I protect the confidence entrusted to me.
I am dedicated to the care and well-being of all patients.
I am loyal to my physician-employer.
I am true to the ethics of my profession.
I am strengthened by compassion, courage, and faith.

1. Render services with respect for human dignity
2. Respect patient confidentiality, except when information is required by the law
3. Uphold the honor and high principles set forth by the AAMA
4. Continually improve knowledge and skills for the benefit of patients and the health care team
5. Participate in community services that promote good health and welfare to the general public

These principles are outlined in the AAMA creed seen in the Medical Assistants' Creed.

In 1999, the AAMA adopted *AAMA's Disciplinary Standards & Procedures for CMAs*. For the first time, a policy was established for sanctions against CMAs who violate the disciplinary standards. Possible sanctions include denial of eligibility for the certification examination, probation, reprimand, temporary revocation of the CMA credential, and permanent revocation of the CMA credential. For more information, see the AAMA website.

BIOETHICS

Bioethics deals specifically with the moral issues and problems that affect human life. As a result of advances in medicine and research, many situations require moral decisions for which there are no clear answers. Abortion and genetic engineering are examples. The goal is to make the right decision in each specific instance as it applies to an individual's specific circumstances. What may be right for one patient may be wrong for another; that is the foundation of bioethics.

American Medical Association (AMA) Council on Ethical and Judicial Affairs

Because of the broad scope of medical ethics and bioethical issues, the AMA formed a subcommittee to review AMA principles and to interpret them as they apply to everyday clinical situations. This subcommittee is called the Council on Ethical and Judicial Affairs. The council has formulated a series of opinions on various medical and bioethical issues that are intended to provide the physician with guidelines for professional conduct and responsibilities. These opinions, most recently revised in 1992, are divided into four general categories:

- Social policy issues
- Relations with colleagues and hospitals
- Administrative office procedures
- Professional rights and responsibilities

The following discussion provides a summary of these opinions along with questions designed to promote your ability to use reasoning to examine difficult ethical issues. Your workbook provides some situations for you to consider. These issues are not within the scope of decisions for medical assistants, but you will be faced with their consequences at some time in your career.

Social Policy Issues

The social policy section deals with various issues of societal importance and provides guidelines to aid the physician in making ethical choices. Five common societal topics and the opinion statements from the AMA Council on Ethical and Judicial Affairs follow.

Allocation of Resources

The term *allocate* means set aside or designate for a purpose. Allocation of resources in the medical profession may refer to many health needs:

- *Organs for transplantation.* Who gets this heart, the college professor or the young recovering addict whose heart was damaged by his lifestyle? Should lifestyle or perceived worth be considered in the decision?
- *Funds for research.* Which disease should receive more funding for research, cancer or AIDS?
- *Funds for health care.* Where should the money be spent, for keeping alive extremely premature infants or making preventive health care available for a greater number of poor children?
- *Hospital beds and professional care.* With hospital care at a premium, who will pay for the indigent? How is it decided which patient is entitled to the last bed in the intensive care unit?

Box 2-9 outlines the judicial council's viewpoints on allocation of limited resources.

Box 2-9

AMA COUNCIL ON ETHICAL AND JUDICIAL AFFAIRS VIEWPOINT STATES:

- When resources are limited, decisions for allocating health care materials should be based on fair and socially acceptable criteria. Economic or social position should not be a factor in the decision.
- Priority care is given to the person or persons who are more likely to receive the greatest long-term benefit from the treatment. Patients with other disease processes or who are not good candidates for treatment for whatever reason will be less likely to receive treatment than otherwise healthy patients. For instance, a patient with cancer in other sites would not be considered for a liver transplant, whereas a patient whose liver was damaged by trauma but who has no other involvement would probably be a good candidate.
- An individual's societal worth must not be a deciding factor during the decision process. A socially or politically prominent patient should not be considered a better recipient of treatment options than a young mother on welfare.
- Age must not be considered in the decision process. If the age of the patient is not a contraindication for the treatment, all ages should be considered on an even basis for most medical resources.

Clinical Investigations and Research

Physicians are frequently involved in studying the effectiveness of new procedures and medications, often called clinical investigations or research. New drugs and treatments are tested on animals first and then considered safe for human testing. The council's viewpoint on research investigation of new drugs and procedures states:

- *A physician may participate in clinical research as long as the project is part of a systematic program with controls for patient evaluation during all phases of the research. At all stages of the testing and at the completion of the study, a protocol must be in place to evaluate the immediate and the long-term effects of the study.*
- *The goal of the research must be to obtain scientifically valid data. The objectives of the study must be available to the physician and the patient, results must be provided to all participants on request, and the testing must serve a medically sound purpose to provide better patient care.*
- *Utmost care and respect must be given to patients involved in clinical research. They are entitled to be treated just as any other patient receiving health care.*

- *Physicians must obtain the patient's permission or consent before enrolling the patient in a research project.*
- *The patient's decision to participate in the program must be completely voluntary.*
- *The patient must be advised of any potential risks, side effects, and benefits of participating in the project.*
- *The patient must be advised that this procedure or drug is experimental. Patients must be made aware that research is not complete, that this is the purpose of the trials, and that risks and benefits are not fully known at this time.*
- *The physician and the institution must have a check and balance system in place to ensure that quality care is always given and ethical standards are followed. Documentation of patient education and instruction for following testing guidelines and patient response to the treatment must be ongoing and thorough.*

Obstetric Dilemmas

Advances in technology have created legal and ethical situations that have polarized opinions and are difficult to bring to consensus. Issues such as the beginning of life, genetic testing and engineering, sex determination, the rights of the fetus, ownership of the fertilized egg, and so forth will not be easily answered. The council formulated an opinion regarding obstetric issues as fairly as possible that states the following:

ABORTION. *As the law now stands, a physician may perform an abortion as long as state and federal laws are followed regarding the trimester in which an abortion may be performed. A physician who does not want to perform abortions cannot be forced to perform the procedure; that physician, however, should refer the patient to other health care professionals who can assist the patient.*

GENETIC TESTING. *If amniocentesis is performed on a mother and a genetic defect is found, both parents must be told. The parents may request or refuse to have the pregnancy terminated. (Amniocentesis is a procedure in which a needle is inserted in a pregnant woman's abdomen to remove and test amniotic fluid. Many abnormalities and disorders can be diagnosed early in pregnancy by this procedure.)*

ARTIFICIAL INSEMINATION. **Artificial insemination** *involves the insertion of sperm into a woman's vagina for the purpose of conception. The donor may be the husband (artificial insemination by husband [AIH]) or an anonymous donor (artificial insemination by donor [AID]). The council states that both the husband and wife must consent to this procedure. If a donor is used, the sperm must be tested for infectious and genetic disorders. Complete confidentiality for the donor and recipient must be maintained.*

Organ Transplantation

Organ transplantation became a medical option in the mid 1950s, although at that time there were many problems with rejection of the organs by the recipient's immune system. When this postoperative complication was corrected by antirejection drugs, the practice became more common. Organs are viable (able to support life) for varying lengths of time, but most can be used successfully if transplanted within 24 to 48 hours. An organization in Richmond, Virginia, the United Network of Organ Sharing, coordinates local organ procurement teams that will fly to areas where organs are to be harvested to assist with the surgery if needed and to ensure the integrity of the organ. There are far fewer organs available than are needed, and every year thousands of patients die who could have lived if an organ had been available. The scarcity of organs has caused many Third World countries to become sources of organs as poor people sell parts of their bodies to meet their basic needs.

The use of organs from a baby born without a brain (anencephaly) raises serious ethical issues. The council states that everything must be done for the infant until the determination of death can be made. For infant organs to be transplanted, both parents must consent.

The council's views on transplantation state:

- *The rights of the donor and organ recipient must be treated equally. The imminent death of the donor does not release the medical personnel from observing all rights that every patient is due.*
- *Organ donors must be given every medical opportunity for life. Life support is not removed until the patient is determined to have no brain activity and could not live without artificial support.*
- *Death of the donor must be determined by a physician who is not on the transplant team to avoid a charge of conflict of interest.*
- *Consent (permission) must be received from both the donor, if possible, and recipient before the transplant. Family members may give consent if the donor is unable to do so.*
- *Transplants can be performed only by surgeons who are qualified to perform this complex surgery and who are affiliated with institutions that have adequate facilities for the surgery and postoperative care. Box 2-10 highlights the Uniform Anatomical Gift Act.*

Withholding or Withdrawing Treatment

Physicians have a professional and ethical obligation to promote quality of life, which means sustaining life and relieving suffering. Sometimes, these obligations conflict with a patient's wishes. Patients have the right to refuse medical treatment and to request that life support or life-sustaining treatments be withheld or withdrawn. Withholding treatment means that certain medical treatments may not be initiated.

Box 2-10

UNIFORM ANATOMICAL GIFT ACT

Approximately 60 American citizens die each day waiting for an organ transplant. Many organs can be transplanted, including the liver, kidney, cornea, heart, lung, and skin. To meet the growing need for organs and to allay the concern over donor standards, the National Conference of Commissioners for Uniform State Laws passed legislation known as the Uniform Anatomical Gift Act.

All acts include the following clauses:

- Any mentally competent person over age 18 may donate all or part of his or her body for transplantation or research.
- The donor's wishes supersede any other wishes except when state laws require an autopsy.
- Physicians accepting donor organs in good faith are immune from lawsuits against harvesting organs.
- Death of the donor must be determined by a physician not involved with the transplant team.
- Financial compensation may not be given to the donor or survivors.
- Persons wishing to donate organs can revoke permission or change their minds at any time.

In most states the Department of Motor Vehicles asks applicants for a driver's license about organ donation and indicates their wishes on their license. In addition, an individual may declare the wish to donate all or parts of the body in a will or any legal document, including a Uniform Donor Card. Organ donors should make their families aware of their wishes to ensure they will be carried out.

Withdrawing treatment is terminating a treatment that has already begun. In 1991, congress passed the Self-Determination Act, which gave all hospitalized patients the right to make health care decisions on admission to the hospital. These decisions may be referred to as advance directives. Today, everyone is encouraged to participate in his or her own end-of-life decisions. We can go online and complete an advance directive. An **advance directive** is a statement of a person's wishes for medical decisions prior to a critical event. Advance directives may include specific wishes, such as whether a ventilator can be used, whether cardiopulmonary resuscitation (CPR) should be initiated, and whether a feeding tube should be inserted. Just completing an advance directive does not ensure that the patient's wishes will be carried out. It is important to make family members aware of these wishes. The patient's next of kin should keep a copy of the advance directive, and one should be placed in the medical office chart with special notation. Figure 2-5 is a sample of an advance directive.

Checkpoint Question

11. What is an advance directive? How can a patient be sure his or her wishes will be followed?

PROFESSIONAL AND ETHICAL CONDUCT AND BEHAVIOR

The council states that all health care professionals are responsible for reporting unethical practices to the appropriate agencies. No health care professional should engage in any act that he or she feels is ethically or morally wrong. Additionally, the council states:

- *A physician must never assist or allow an unlicensed person to practice medicine.*
- *Hospitals and physicians must work together for the best care for patients. Hospitals should allow physicians staff privileges based on the ability of the physician, educational background, and the needs of the community. (Staff privileges allow physicians to admit their patients to a given hospital.) Issues of a personal nature must never be considered when accepting or declining a physician's application for privileges.*
- *It is unethical for physicians to admit patients to the hospital or to order excessive treatments for the sole purpose of financial rewards.*

ETHICAL ISSUES IN OFFICE MANAGEMENT

As a medical assistant, you are directly involved in some of the council's guidelines regarding administrative issues. In relation to fees, the council states:

- *Financial interests must never come above patient care. Ordering the most expensive tests or not ordering needed tests based on the patient's ability to pay is not acceptable.*
- *If a physician's office routinely charges patients for canceling appointments within 24 hours of the actual scheduled appointment, a warning must be posted to advise patients of this charge.*
- *The medical record must never be held against non-payment of a bill.*
- *Fees cannot be excessive. They must be based on fair and standard charges for all patients. Guidelines for charges should consider the difficulty and unique nature of the services involved and the use of medical equipment.*
- *Interest on past due accounts can be charged in accordance with state laws and with prior notification to the patient.*

FIGURE 2-5. Sample advance directive.

ADVANCE DIRECTIVE

UNIFORM ADVANCE DIRECTIVE OF [list name of declarant]

To my family, physician, attorney, and anyone else who may become responsible for my health, welfare, or affairs, I make this declaration while I am of sound mind.

If I should ever become in a terminal state and there is no reasonable expectation of my recovery, I direct that I be allowed to die a natural death and that my life not be prolonged by extraordinary measures. I do, however, ask that medication be mercifully administered to me to alleviate suffering, even though this may shorten my remaining life.

This statement is made after full reflection and is in accordance with my full desires. I want the above provisions carried out to the extent permitted by law. Insofar as they are not legally enforceable, I wish that those to whom this will is addressed will regard themselves as morally bound by this instrument.

If permissible in the jurisdiction in which I may be hospitalized I direct that in the event of a terminal diagnosis, the physicians supervising my care discontinue feeding should the continuation of feeding be judged to result in unduly prolonging a natural death.

If permissible in the jurisdiction in which I may be hospitalized I direct that in the event of a terminal diagnosis, the physicians supervising my care discontinue hydration (water) should the continuation of hydration be judged to result in unduly prolonging a natural death.

I herewith authorize my spouse, if any, or any relative who is related to me within the third degree to effectuate my transfer from any hospital or other health care facility in which I may be receiving care should that facility decline or refuse to effectuate the instructions given herein.

I herewith release any and all hospitals, physicians, and others for myself and for my estate from any liability for complying with this instrument.

Signed:

_____
  [list name of declarant]

City of residence: _____
                  [city of residence]

County of residence: _____
                  [county of residence]

State of residence: _____
                  [state of residence]

Social Security Number: _____
                  [social security number]

Date: _____

_____
Witness

_____
Witness

STATE OF _____

COUNTY OF _____

This day personally appeared before me, the undersigned authority, a Notary Public in and for _____County, _____ State,

_____   _____ (Witnesses)

who, being first duly sworn, say that they are the subscribing witnesses to the declaration of [list name of declarant], the declarant, signed, sealed, and published and declared the same as and for his declaration, in the presence of both these affiants; and that these affiants, at the request of said declarant, in the presence of each other, and in the presence of said declarant, all present at the same time, signed their names as attesting witnesses to said declaration.

Affiants further say that this affidavit is made at the request of [list name of declarant], declarant, and in his presence, and that [list name of declarant] at the time the declaration was executed, in the opinion of the affiants, of sound mind and memory, and over the age of eighteen years.

Taken, subscribed and sworn to before me by _____(witness) and

_____ (witness) this _____ day of_____, 20_____.

My commission expires:_____

_____ Notary Public

Box 2-11

ETHICAL DILEMMA

Here is a hypothetical situation that could occur in a medical office. How would you handle it?

You are the office manager for a well-respected family physician in a small town. He is 70 years old and is starting to show signs of senility. He is forgetful and has even been disoriented and confused a few times. No one else seems to have noticed. Should you report your concerns? If so, to whom?

The AMA Principles of Medical Ethics require that physicians, and medical assistants through the law of agency, report unethical behavior among colleagues. The medical profession is also governed by the patient's right to safety and quality care. It is your ethical responsibility to report the doctor's condition to the administration of the hospital where the physician has privileges or to the state board of medicine. The physician's family should be involved in the situation.

- No fees can be charged for physician referrals or for admitting a patient to the hospital.
- A fee should not be charged to the patient for completing or filing a simple insurance form. If the form is extensive, a minimal fee may be charged.
- Caution must be used with computers to maintain patient confidentiality. If patient data are sent via fax machine, utmost care must be used to ensure that the material is received by only the correct recipient.
- If the physician advertises his or her practice, it must be done with the utmost honesty. Misrepresentation of information is never appropriate.
- If a physician closes the practice or dies, all patients must be notified that the office is closing and must be given instructions for retrieving their medical records. Generally, copies of medical records are transferred to another local physician. The originals are stored as directed by state law. Box 2-11 describes an ethical issue that might occur in a medical office. Read it carefully. If you were the physician, how would you handle the problem?

Checkpoint Question

12. What steps should be taken when a physician closes his or her practice?

CHAPTER SUMMARY

The fields of medicine and law are linked in common concern for the patient's health and rights. Increasingly, health care professionals are the object of malpractice lawsuits. You must keep abreast of medicolegal issues to protect yourself and other health care professionals from legal action. You can help prevent medical malpractice by acting professionally, maintaining clinical competency, and properly documenting in the medical record. Promoting good public relations between the patient and the health care team can avoid frivolous or unfounded suits and direct attention and energy toward optimum health care.

Medical ethics and bioethics involve complex issues and controversial topics. There will be no easy or clear-cut answers to questions raised by these issues. As a medical assistant, your first priority must be to act as your patients' advocate with their best interests and concerns foremost in your actions and interactions. You must always maintain ethical standards and report the unethical behaviors of others.

Many acts and regulations affect health care organizations and their operations. A medical office must keep current on all legal updates. Most states publish a monthly bulletin that reports on new legislation. Every state has a website that will link you to legislative action. Read these on a regular basis. Each office should have legal counsel who can assist in interpreting legal issues.

Critical Thinking Challenges

1. An acquaintance who knows you work in the medical field asks you to diagnose her rash. What do you say?
2. A patient owes a big bill at your office. She requests copies of her records. What do you do?
3. You suspect that a new employee in the office is misusing narcotics. What do you do?

Spanish Terminology

¿Usted entiende la información que acaba de recibir?	Do you understand the information I have given?
¿Usted nos autoriza a llevar a cabo este procedimiento médico?	Do you give us permission to perform this procedure?
Firme aquí, por favor.	Please sign here.

4. Mrs. Rodriguez has bone cancer. Her doctor has estimated she has 6 months to live. Mrs. Rodriguez wants the physician to withhold all medical treatments. She does not want chemotherapy or any life-sustaining measures. Her family disagrees. Should her family have any input into her health care decisions?

Answers to Checkpoint Questions

1. Criminal law deals with the act of practicing medicine without a license.

2. When a physician changes the scope of his practice, patients should be given advance notice. A letter should be sent to each active patient or an ad may be placed in a local newspaper.

3. The following elements must be in a physician's termination intent letter: statement of intent, explanation of reasons, termination date, availability of medical records, and a recommendation that the patient seek medical help as needed.

4. Never ask a patient to sign a consent form if the patient does not understand the procedure, has questions about the procedure, or is unable to read the consent form.

5. The six situations or conditions legally requiring disclosure are vital statistics, medical examiner reports, infectious diseases, abuse or maltreatment, violent injuries, and others according to state laws.

6. The four elements that must be proved in a negligence suit are duty, dereliction of duty, direct cause, and damages.

7. Assault is the attempt or threat to touch another person without permission; battery is the actual touching.

8. The law of agency implies that physicians are liable for the actions of their employees. The physician is responsible for your actions as a medical assistant, as long as your actions are within your scope of practice and you practice the standard of care required for your assigned duties and responsibilities

9. Blood-borne pathogens are organisms that can be spread through direct contact with blood or body fluids from an infected person. OSHA governs their control in the medical office.

10. The three ethical standards the CMA must follow are protecting patient confidentiality, following laws, and being honest.

11. An advance directive is a statement of a person's wishes for medical decisions prior to a critical event. Letting family know of these wishes and keeping a copy in the medical office chart will help ensure that these wishes are carried out.

12. If a physician closes the practice (or dies), all patients must be notified that the office is closing and must be given instructions for retrieving their medical records. Generally, copies of medical records are transferred to another local physician. The originals are stored as directed by state law.

 Websites

To keep abreast of changes in the medical field:

- Go to your state's home page and click on the link to the state legislature to view pending state legislation
- Go to The Library of Congress to view federal legislation to be considered in the coming week via the website http://Thomas.loc.gov

Equal Employment Opportunity Commission
www.eeoc.gov

For a complete text of Title VII of the Civil Rights Act
www.eeoc.gov/laws/vii.html

U. S. Department of Labor, Bureau of Labor Statistics
http://stats.bls.gov

To complete an advance directive
www.LegalZoom.com

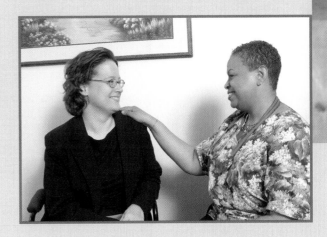

Communicating With Patients

There are two fundamental tasks that you will perform every day when working as a medical assistant. These two tasks are communication and teaching. This unit will introduce you to the skills needed to perform these tasks. Communication is the sharing of ideas between two people. Successful communication ensures that the medical office will run effectively and smoothly. Teaching occurs in all areas of the medical office and is a responsibility shared among all medical professionals. Teaching patients various skills or information helps to ensure that they have received the most comprehensive medical care possible. You will be able to master these skills after completing the next two chapters.

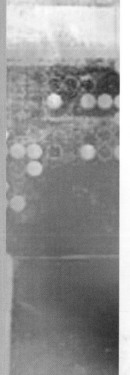

3

Fundamental Communication Skills

CHAPTER OUTLINE

ROLE DELINEATION COMPONENTS

GENERAL: Professionalism
- Display a professional manner and image
- Treat all patients with compassion and empathy

GENERAL: Communication Skills
- Recognize and respect cultural diversity
- Adapt communications to individual's ability to understand

- Use professional telephone technique
- Recognize and respond effectively to verbal, nonverbal, and written communications

ADMINISTRATIVE: Administrative Procedures
- Perform basic administrative medical assisting functions

CHAPTER COMPETENCIES

LEARNING OBJECTIVES
Upon successfully completing this chapter, you will be able to:

1. Spell and define the key terms
2. List two major forms of communication
3. Explain how various components of communication can affect the meaning of verbal messages
4. Define active listening
5. List and describe the six interviewing techniques
6. Give an example of how cultural differences may affect communication
7. Discuss how to handle communication problems caused by language barriers
8. List two methods that you can use to promote communication among hearing-, sight-, and speech-impaired patients
9. List five actions that you can take to improve communication with a child
10. Discuss how to handle an angry or distressed patient
11. Discuss your role in communicating with a grieving patient or family member
12. Discuss the key elements of interdisciplinary communication

KEY TERMS

anacusis	discrimination	messages	presbyacusis
bias	dysphasia	mourning	reflecting
clarification	dysphonia	nonlanguage	stereotyping
cultures	feedback	paralanguage	summarizing
demeanor	grief	paraphrasing	therapeutic

COMMUNICATION IS SENDING and receiving **messages** (information), verbally or otherwise. The ability to communicate effectively is a crucial skill for medical assistants. In your role, you must accurately and appropriately share information with physicians, other professional staff members, and patients. When communicating with patients you must be able to receive messages correctly, interpret them, and respond to the sender appropriately. The medical assistant is usually the first person the patient meets in the medical office. Thus, your positive attitude, pleasant presentation, and use of good communication skills will set the tone for future interactions.

BASIC COMMUNICATION FLOW

Communication requires the following elements:

- A message to be sent
- A person to send the message
- A person to receive the message

During the act of communicating, two or more people will alternate roles as sender and receiver as they seek **feedback** (responses) and **clarification** (understanding) regarding the message. The process of message exchange is a swing moving back and forth between two people. Figure 3-1 illustrates the flow of communication and its common components.

As a medical assistant, you will primarily be communicating in a therapeutic manner. This means that your com-

munication will focus on conversations regarding pertinent topics relating to office procedures, policies, and patient care. Your other responsibilities for ensuring good communication include the following:

- Clarifying confusing messages
- Validating (confirming) the patient's perceptions
- Adapting messages to the patient's level of understanding
- Asking for feedback to ensure that the messages you sent were received by the patient or other persons as intended

Checkpoint Question

1. What three elements must be present for communication to occur?

FORMS OF COMMUNICATION

Verbal Communication

Verbal communication involves an exchange of messages using words or language; it is the most commonly used form and is usually the initial form of communication. You need good verbal communication skills when performing such tasks as making appointments, providing patient education, making referrals, and sharing information with the physician.

Oral communication is sending or receiving messages using spoken language. As a professional, you should use a pleasant and polite manner of speaking. Use proper English and grammar at all times; lapsing into slang and colloquialisms projects an unprofessional image.

Gear your conversation to the patient's educational level. A well-educated patient may resent your using other than the correct terms, yet a less educated patient may be confused and intimidated by the same phrases. Avoid using elaborate medical terminology if you think it might confuse or frighten a patient. Will this patient understand "myocardial infarction," or should you say heart attack? Do not talk down to the patient, but do phrase your communication appropriately.

Be aware, too, that the meaning of spoken messages may be affected by other components of oral communication, including paralanguage and nonlanguage sounds. The cliché that it's not what you say but how you say it is true. Research shows that the primary message is transmitted more by the way it is said than by the words that are used. This refers to paralanguage. **Paralanguage** includes voice tone, quality, volume, pitch, and range. Nonlanguage sounds include laughing, sobbing, sighing, grunting, and so on. Other **nonlanguage** clues to understanding can be found in a speaker's grammatical structure, pronunciation, and general articulation, which can indicate regional or cultural background and level of education. Knowing this information can help you adapt responses and explanations to the patient's level of understanding.

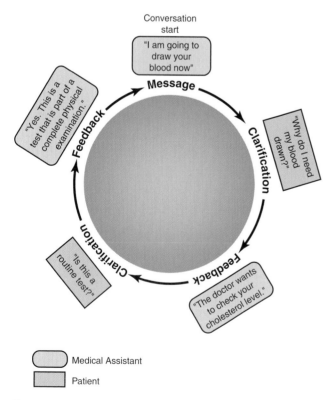

FIGURE 3–1. Flow of communication.

EXAMPLE OF WRITTEN DISCHARGE INSTRUCTIONS

Main Street Pediatric Group
343 Main Street, Suite 609
Philadelphia, PA 19106

Discharge Instructions for Otitis Media

Your child has an ear infection. It is easily treated with antibiotics. Get the prescription filled immediately. The first dose should be given as soon as you arrive home. Read the attached information on the antibiotic.

Here are some other important things to remember:
- Ear infections are not contagious.
- Symptoms usually resolve within 24 hours of beginning antibiotics. It is very important to make sure your child takes all of the prescription.
- If the pain persists for more than 48 hours, call the office.
- If you see any blood in the ear canal, call the office.

Make an appointment for a follow-up visit in 2 weeks.

_____   _____
Patient's signature   Physician's signature

Written communication uses written language to exchange messages. The ability to write clearly, concisely, and accurately is important in the health care profession (see Chapter 7). Typically, patients receive oral instructions first, as you or the physician explain key points of concern. These verbal instructions are then reinforced with written instructions (Box 3-1).

If the instructions, oral or written, are not clear, the patient may misinterpret them. This misunderstanding can hinder treatment and recovery and possibly even require the patient to be admitted to the hospital. Here is an example of unclear instruction: "Return to the office if you don't feel better." This provides the patient with no details. Clearer instructions would state, "If your fever and sore throat are not better in 24 hours, call the office to schedule a revisit." Even the most clearly outlined instructions can be misunderstood, particularly by those with deficient hearing or reading abilities. As a medical assistant, you are responsible for asking questions to verify that the patient has correctly understood the information. To verify that the patient understood these instructions, a good question to ask would be, "When should you call the office if you don't feel better?"

Checkpoint Question

2. List five examples of paralanguage.

Nonverbal Communication

Nonverbal communication—exchanging messages without using words—is sometimes called body language. Body language includes several types of behaviors, such as kinesics, proxemics, and the use of touch. Kinesics refers to body movements, including facial expressions, gestures, and eye movements. A patient's face can sometimes reveal inner feelings, such as sadness, happiness, fear, or anger, that may not be mentioned explicitly during a conversation (Fig. 3-2). Gestures also carry various meanings. For instance, shrug-

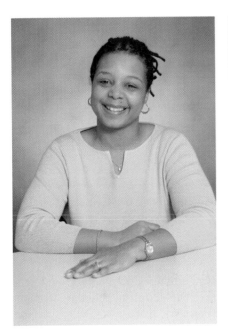
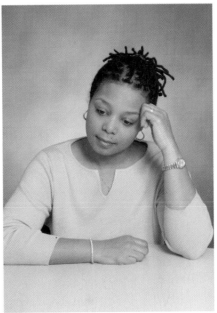
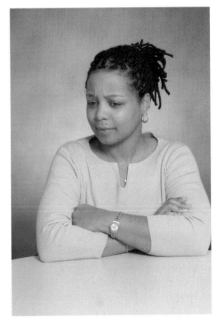

FIGURE 3-2. Different facial expressions convey different messages.

ging the shoulders can mean simple lack of interest or hopeless resignation. Eyes can often hint at what a person may be thinking or feeling. For example, a patient whose eyes wander away from you while you are talking may be impatient, lack interest, or not understand what you are saying.

Nonverbal communication may more accurately reflect a person's true feelings and attitude than verbal communication. In other words, people may say one thing but show a completely different response with their body language. For example, if the patient says, "The pain in my foot is not too bad," but the patient's face shows pain with each step, the nonverbal clues demonstrate an inconsistent message. Many patients mask their feelings, so you must learn to read their actions and nonverbal clues in addition to what they tell you. Be aware that patients are also acutely attuned to your facial and nonverbal reactions. Responding with an expression of disgust or shaking your head in a negative way can jeopardize communication and rapport between you and the patient.

How and where individuals physically place themselves in relation to others can affect communication as well. Proxemics refers to spatial relationships or physical proximity tolerated by humans. Generally, the area within a 3-foot radius around a person is considered personal space and is not to be invaded by strangers, although this area varies among individuals and people of various **cultures** (societies). To deliver care to a patient, physicians and medical assistants must enter a patient's personal space. After a patient task is completed, it is appropriate to take a few steps back and allow for more space between you and the patient. Because some individuals become uncomfortable when their space is invaded, it is essential to approach the patient in a professional manner and explain what you plan to do. Explanations help ease patient anxiety about what will happen.

Related to proxemics is the use of touch, which can be **therapeutic** (beneficial) for some patients. It can indicate emotional support and convey concern and feeling. For some patients, however, being touched by a stranger is an uncomfortable or even a negative experience. Many patients perceive touch in a medical setting as a prelude to something unpleasant, such as an injection. To change this negative perception, try offering a comforting touch when nothing invasive or painful is imminent (Fig. 3-3). Before comforting a patient by touching, assess the patient's **demeanor** (expressions and behavior) for clues indicating that touch would be acceptable.

ACTIVE LISTENING

Active listening is important to ensure that messages are correctly received and interpreted. Failure to do so can result in poor patient care. To listen actively, you must give your full attention to the patient with whom you are speaking. Interruptions should be kept to a minimum. You need to focus not only on what is being said but also on what is being conveyed through paralanguage, body language, and other aspects of communication. Occasionally, a patient's verbal messages may seem to conflict with the nonverbal messages. For example, a patient who is wringing his hands while telling you that everything is fine is sending conflicting signals that require further exploration. If a patient's verbal response does not correspond to your observations, convey your concern to the physician.

Active listening is a skill that develops with practice. To test your listening ability, try this exercise: Ask another student to speak continuously for 1 to 2 minutes while you listen. (The student should discuss a topic with which you are unfamiliar.) When he or she finishes, wait silently for the same amount of time. Then try to repeat the message. If you have trouble doing this exercise, you need to practice listening.

INTERVIEW TECHNIQUES

As a medical assistant, you are typically responsible for gathering initial information and updating existing information about the patients. This task is accomplished by interviewing the patient. The interview will consist of you asking certain questions and then interpreting the patient's responses. The initial interview includes many areas. The key areas are the patient's medical and family history, a brief review of the body systems, and a social history. Table 3-1 has sample questions that you may ask in each of these areas. The main goal is to obtain accurate and pertinent information. The interview for an established patient, however, is much different. First, you should review the chart to look at the patient's health problems. Make a list of questions regarding the pertinent medical problems. Reconfirm medication usage and any specific treatments the patient is supposed to be doing.

To conduct either type of interview, you must use effective techniques: listen actively, ask the appropriate questions, and record the answers. During the interview, you must demonstrate professionalism. Begin by introducing yourself. Always conduct the interview in a private area.

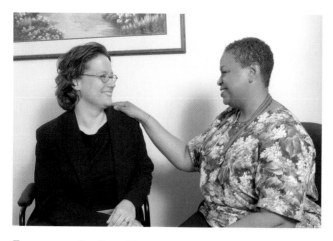

FIGURE 3–3. Therapeutic touch conveys caring and concern.

Table 3–1   INITIAL PATIENT INTERVIEW COMPONENTS

Area	Sample Questions
Past medical history	Any previous hospitalizations? If so, when?
	Any previous surgeries? If so, when?
	Any chronic problems (e.g., asthma, diabetes, heart condition)?
	Any past pregnancies? Any complications?
	Any miscarriages, stillbirths, or abortions?
Family history	Age and health of parents?
	If deceased, what was the cause and at what age did they die?
	Age and health of siblings?
	Are there any genetic disorders?
Body system review	General questions regarding all body systems: cardiovascular, pulmonary, integumentary, musculoskeletal, neurological, sensory, gastrointestinal, endocrine, immune, urological, and reproductive
Social history	Alcohol use?
	Smoking?
	Drug use?
	Hobbies?
	Education?
	Employment?
Medications	What do you take? When? How much?
	Any vitamins or herbal supplements?

Know what questions you need to ask and in what order to ask them before you begin the interview. Be organized. It is also helpful to have an extra pen. And most important, do not answer phone calls or attend to other distractions until you have finished the interview. Last, when you leave the room, let patients know who will be in to see them and the approximate time, for example, "Dr. Sanchez will be in to see you in about 10 minutes."

The six interviewing techniques are reflecting, paraphrasing, clarification, asking open-ended questions, summarizing, and allowing silences.

Reflecting

Reflecting is repeating what you have heard the patient say, using open-ended statements. With this technique, you do not complete a sentence, but leave it up to the patient to do so. For example, you might say, "Mrs. Rivera, you were saying that when your back hurts you. . . ." Reflection encourages the patient to make further comments. It also can help bring the patient back to the subject if the conversation begins to drift. (Reflecting is a useful tool, but be careful not to overuse it, because some patients find it annoying to have their words constantly parroted back.)

Paraphrasing or Restatement

Paraphrasing or restatement means repeating what you have heard, using your own words or phrases. Paraphrasing can help verify that you have accurately understood what was said. It also allows patients the opportunity to clarify their thoughts or statements. Typically, a paraphrased statement begins with "You are saying that . . . ," or "It sounds as if . . . ," followed by the rephrased content.

Asking for Examples or Clarification

If you are confused about some of the information you have received, ask the patient to give an example of the situation being described. For instance, "Can you describe one of these dizzy spells?" The patient's example should help you better understand what the patient is saying. It also may give you an insight into how the patient perceives the situation.

Asking Open-Ended Questions

The best way to obtain specific information is to ask open-ended questions that require the patient to formulate an answer and elaborate on the response. Open-ended questions usually begin with what, when, or how. For example, "What medications did you take this morning?" "When did you stop taking your medication?" "How did you get that large bruise on your arm?" Be careful about asking "why" questions, because they can often sound judgmental or accusing. For example, asking "Why did you do that?" or "Why didn't you follow directions?" may imply to patients that you have already made a negative value judgment about their behavior, and they could become defensive and uncooperative. Instead you might ask, "What part of the instructions did you not understand?" or "How can we help you follow these instructions?"

Avoid closed-ended questions that allow the patient to answer with one word, such as yes or no. For example, suppose you ask the patient, "Are you taking your medications?" The patient can easily say yes but may not be taking all of them. However, suppose you ask, "What medications do you take every day?" The patient's answer will give you a clearer understanding of whether the patient is taking the correct medications.

Summarizing

Briefly reviewing the information you have obtained, or **summarizing**, gives the patient another chance to clarify statements or correct misinformation. This technique can also help you organize complex information or events in sequential order. For example, if the patient has been feeling dizzy and stumbling a lot, you might summarize by saying, "You told me that you have been feeling dizzy for the past 3 days and that you frequently stumble as you are walking."

Allowing Silences

Periods of silence sometimes occur during the interview. These can be beneficial. Some people are uncomfortable with prolonged silences and feel a need to break the silence with words in an effort to jump-start a stalled conversation. Silences are natural parts of conversations and can give patients time to formulate their thoughts, reconstruct events, evaluate their feelings, or assess what has already been said. During moments of silence, gather your thoughts and formulate any additional questions that you may have.

 Checkpoint Question

3. What are the six interviewing techniques?

FACTORS AFFECTING COMMUNICATION

Sometimes, despite your best efforts, others may not receive your message accurately. A common occurrence that causes messages to be misinterpreted is the use of a cliché. For example, suppose you are teaching a patient to use crutches and she is having difficulty managing them. A cliché comment may be, "Don't worry. Rome wasn't built in a day. This takes time." The cliché is innocent and not meant to be demeaning, but the patient may misinterpret it to mean that she is slow, ancient. A more positive message would be, "I can see that you are making progress. Let's try walking down the hallway."

Here are some reasons for miscommunication:

1. The message may have been unclear or inappropriate to the situation. For example, "I have scheduled you for a PET scan in radiology tomorrow at 8 A.M." Keep in mind that most of your patients do not understand medical abbreviations and terms. Since positron emission tomography (PET) is newer technology, they may confuse it with computed tomography (CT). Also, where is radiology? A better message would be, "The doctor wants you to have a test done tomorrow. It is called a PET scan; here is a brochure that explains it. Go to the second floor of the outpatient center on Main Street. Do you know how to get there?"
2. The person receiving the message may have been distracted, anxious, or confused. A common cause of distraction is pain. For example, teaching a patient how to use crutches cannot be done if the patient's ankle or knee still hurts. The concentration will be on the pain, not on what you are saying. Patients who have just received positive news can also be anxious to contact loved ones. This is commonly seen with patients who have just been told that they are pregnant. The patient's focus is on calling family members and not on your conversation.
3. Environmental elements, such as noise or interruptions, may also distort messages. Environmental noises from staff lounges or break rooms can easily be overheard. Keep the doors to these areas closed. Cleaning staff should not be vacuuming or emptying trash while patients are present.

In addition to these three items, other factors may affect communication. They are discussed next.

Cultural Differences

The way a person perceives situations and other people is greatly influenced by cultural, social, and religious beliefs or firmly held convictions. Personal values (principles or ideals) are commonly developed from these same beliefs. As a medical assistant, you will interact with people from varied ethnic backgrounds and cultural origins who bring with them beliefs and values that may differ from your own. Understanding those differences can aid communication and thereby improve patient care (Table 3-2). It is very important that you not form preconceived ideas about a given culture. Remember that each patient is unique and that their health care needs differ.

Some cultures may be offended by the types of intensely personal questions necessary for a medical history and may

Table 3–2 CULTURAL FACTORS THAT AFFECT PATIENT CARE[a]			
Cultural Group	**Family**	**Folk and Traditional Health Care**	**Common Health Problems**
White	Nuclear family is highly valued Elderly family members may live in a nursing home when they can no longer care for themselves	Self-diagnosis of illnesses Use of over-the-counter drugs, especially vitamins and analgesics Dieting, especially fad diets Extensive use of exercise and exercise facilities	Cardiovascular disease Gastrointestinal disease Some forms of cancer Motor vehicle accidents Suicide Mental illness Substance abuse
African American	Close and supportive extended-family relationships Strong kinship ties with nonblood relatives from church or organizational and social groups Family unity, loyalty, and cooperation are important. Frequently matriarchal	Varies extensively and may include spiritualists, herb doctors, root doctors, conjurers, skilled elder family members, voodoo, faith healing	Hypertension Sickle cell anemia Skin disorders; inflammation of hair follicles, various types of dermatitis and excessive growth of scar tissue (keloids) Lactose enzyme deficiency resulting in poor toleration of milk products High rate of tuberculosis Diabetes mellitus Higher infant mortality rate than in the white population
Asian	Welfare of the family is valued above the individual person Extended families are common A person's lineage (ancestors) is respected Sharing among family members is expected	Theoretical basis in Taoism, which seeks balance in all things Good health is achieved through proper balance between yin (feminine, negative, dark, cold) and yang (masculine, positive, light, warm) An imbalance in energy is caused by an improper diet or strong emotions Diseases and food are classified as hot or cold, and a proper balance between them will promote wellness (e.g., treat a cold disease with hot foods) Many Asian health care systems use herbs, diet, and application of hot or cold therapy Many Asians believe some points on the body are on the meridians, or energy pathways; if the energy flow is out of balance, treatment of the pathways may be necessary to restore the energy equilibrium *Acumassage*: Manipulation of points along the energy pathways *Acupressure*: Technique for compressing the energy pathway points *Acupuncture*: Insertion of fine needles into the body at energy pathway points	Tuberculosis Communicable diseases Malnutrition Suicide Various forms of mental illness Lactose enzyme deficiency

(continued)

Table 3–2 CULTURAL FACTORS THAT AFFECT PATIENT CARE[a] *(Continued)*

Cultural Group	Family	Folk and Traditional Health Care	Common Health Problems
Hispanic, Mexican American	Familial role is important *Compadrazgo*: special bond between a child's parents and grandparents Family is the primary unit of society	*Curanderas(os)*: Folk healers who base treatments on humoral pathology: basic functions of the body are controlled by four body fluids, or humors—blood, hot and wet; yellow bile, hot and dry; black bile, cold and dry; and phlegm, cold and wet The secret of good health is to balance hot and cold within the body; therefore, most foods, beverages, herbs, and medications are classified as hot (*caliente*) or cold (*fresco, frio*); a cold disease will be cured with a hot treatment	Diabetes mellitus and its complications Problems of poverty, such as poor nutrition, inadequate medical care, and poor prenatal care Lactose enzyme deficiency
Hispanic, Puerto Rican	*Compadrazgo*: similar to Mexican American culture	Similar to that of other Spanish-speaking cultures	Parasitic diseases, such as dysentery, malaria, filariasis, hookworms Lactose enzyme deficiency
Native American	Families large and extended Grandparents are official and symbolic leaders and decision makers A child's namesake may assume equal parenting authority with biological parents	Medicine men (shamans) are frequently consulted Heavy use of herbs and psychological treatments, ceremonies, fasting, meditation, heat, and massage	Alcoholism Suicide Tuberculosis Malnutrition Communicable diseases Higher maternal and infant mortality rates than in most of the population Diabetes mellitus Hypertension Gallbladder disease

Reprinted with permission from Taylor C, Lillis C, LeMone P. Fundamentals of Nursing, 2nd ed. Philadelphia: Lippincott-Raven, 1996:122–125.

[a] The beliefs and practices vary within each group, and no assumptions should be based on a patient's cultural background alone. The factors in this table are merely a guide to some commonly observed and documented cultural factors.

perceive them as an inexcusable invasion of privacy. If this occurs, your physician may be required to intervene to allay the patient's concerns.

Looking someone else directly in the eyes, or eye contact, is also perceived differently by people of various backgrounds. Eye contact occurs more often among friends and family members than among acquaintances or strangers. In the United States, someone who maintains good eye contact is usually perceived as being honest, believable, and concerned. In contrast, in some Asian and Mideastern cultures, direct eye contact is perceived as sexually suggestive or disrespectful. In other cultures, lack of eye contact or casting the eyes downward is a sign of respect.

In addition to cultural differences in values, many differences occur among individuals. Some people are just more reserved or shy than others and may feel less comfortable in medical settings. To help avoid miscommunication and offending patients, you must be sensitive to these differences in all of your patient interactions.

Stereotyping and Biased Opinions

Medical assisting deals with people of differing ages, races, and sexual orientation. Sometimes, your values may be in stark contrast to those held by a patient, but you should not let your personal values or **bias** (opinions) affect your communication or treatment of a patient. All patients must be treated fairly, respectfully, and with dignity, regardless of their cultural, social, or personal values. To treat them in any other fashion is **discrimination**.

Stereotyping is holding an opinion of all members of a particular culture, race, religion, age group, or other group based on oversimplified or negative characterizations. It is a form of prejudice. Examples of negative stereotypes include

"All old people are frail and senile" and "Those people are always dirty and never bathe." Stereotyping and prejudice are deterrents to establishing therapeutic relationships because they do not allow for patients' individuality and can prevent quality care from being given to everyone on an equal basis.

As a health care professional, you are expected to treat all patients impartially, to guard against discriminatory practices, remain nonjudgmental, avoid stereotypes, and have a professional demeanor. By doing so, you communicate to patients that you accept human differences and that quality health care will be provided to all those who seek it.

Let's suppose Ms. Henry arrives with her 3-year-old daughter for a checkup. The mother says, "I think she has gotten head lice from someone at the shelter." Which response would be most appropriate? "Don't worry about it. The shelter is full of people with lice. Do you know anyone with lice?" or "I will mention to the doctor that you are concerned that she may have lice. Is anyone else in your family being treated for lice?" The latter response demonstrates appropriate caring and concern. It also begins the dialogue for determining additional people who may need to be checked, which is key to preventing community outbreaks. The first response communicates stereotyping of a particular lifestyle and prevents collection of additional data.

Language Barriers

Effective communication depends on the use of language, but some patients cannot speak or understand English well enough for good communication. Because it is crucial for you to give and receive accurate information, you will need to use an interpreter to help bridge any language barriers. A staff person might serve as the interpreter, or an English-speaking member of the patient's family may be able to help. In either case, be sure the interpreter fully understands what you are saying. In the absence of a reliable interpreter, a phrase book of common medical questions with lists of possible answers may be of help. If your area has a large population of non–English-speaking patients, your office should be equipped with an appropriate phrase book (See Appendix II for a list of key health care phrases in English and Spanish).

When choosing an interpreter, try to find someone of the same sex as the patient, because certain cultures prohibit members of the opposite sex (even family members) from discussing personal issues about the body. Some cultures follow religious guidelines dictating how members of the opposite sex should interact with each other.

Use the following suggestions for communicating with non–English-speaking patients:

1. Do not shout. Raising your voice will not increase their understanding.
2. Demonstrate or pantomime as needed. Gestures are usually relatively universal.
3. If you are using an interpreter, speak directly to the patient, with the interpreter in your line of vision, so that the patient can read your facial expressions.
4. Speak slowly with simple sentences and phrases that require simple answers. The patient may comprehend some simple English.
5. Avoid slang; it may not translate well.
6. Avoid distractions and provide a relaxed, quiet interview space.
7. Learn some basic phrases of the most common language used in your area. Patients appreciate your effort.

Ñ Spanish Terminology

Hable despacio, por favor.	Please speak slowly.
Sí, hablo español un poco.	Yes, I speak Spanish a little.
No, no comprendo.	No, I don't understand.
¿Comprende?	Do you understand?
¿Cuándo?	When?
¿Qué clase?	What kind?
¿Porqué?	Why?
¿Cuántos?	How many?
¿Qué, Qué tal?	What?
¿En qué puedo ayudarlo?	What can I help you with?
¿Dígame porque esta aquí?	Tell me why you are here?
¿Cómo?	How?

SPECIAL COMMUNICATION CHALLENGES

Many situations present special communication challenges. For instance, hearing- or sight-impaired patients, young children, patients with limited understanding, those who are too ill or sedated to comprehend, and those who are frightened or anxious require particular attention. In each instance, you will need to assess the situation and the patient's ability to comprehend. In some cases, a responsible family member will be with the patient and can be included in the communication process. Never exclude the patient from the exchange, but do ensure that all needed information is communicated, whether you obtain the information through questions about the patient's condition or you give instructions for further care. Patients must feel that they are part of the process even if their condition requires involvement by family members or other caregivers.

Hearing-Impaired Patients

There are many forms of hearing impairments. Impairments can vary from a partial loss to **anacusis**, complete hearing loss. The two types of impairments are conductive and sensorineural. Conductive hearing loss is caused by interference with sound in the external canal or the middle or inner ear. Sensorineural hearing loss is caused by lesions or problems with either nerves or the cochlea. The cochlea is a coiled tubular structure that turns vibrations into sounds. Most patients with anacusis are adept with communicating through sign language, interpreters, or other tools. However, patients with **presbyacusis**, a common hearing impairment in older patients, often have a more difficult time communicating and tend to be in denial about their hearing abilities. Patients with presbyacusis benefit from hearing aids and other amplification devices.

To communicate with patients who cannot hear what you are saying, you need tact, diplomacy, and patience. These suggestions may help.

1. Touch the patient gently to gain his or her attention.
2. Talk directly face-to-face with the patient, not at an angle and certainly not with your back turned.
3. Turn to the most prominent light so that your face is illuminated.
4. Lower the pitch of your voice, since higher pitches are frequently lost with nerve impairment, but speak distinctly and with force. In most instances, shouting does not help and will only distort what might be heard.
5. Use note pads or demonstration as needed.
6. Pictograms are very helpful and should be readily available. A pictogram is a flash card that shows basic medical terms.
7. Use short sentences with short words. Enunciate clearly but do not exaggerate your facial movements.

WHAT IF

You need to call a hearing-impaired patient. What should you do?

Hearing-impaired patients can make and receive calls using a special telephone with a service called converse communication center, which uses a system called telecommunication device for the deaf (TDD) or a text telephone (TTY). If your office has either of these types of phones, you call the patient and type in your message. The patient reads your message and types a response. If your office does not have one of these phones, your local telephone company can communicate with TDD/TTY users and nonusers. Check your telephone directory for more information. Most hospitals have TDD/TTY phones available.

8. Eliminate all distractions. Extraneous noises may confuse the patient.

Checkpoint Question

4. What is the term for complete hearing loss?

Sight-Impaired Patients

Sight impairments range from complete blindness to blurred vision. The changes in vision tend to be slow and progressive. Box 3-2 has a list of conditions that can cause visual im-

---

Box 3-2

MEDICAL CONDITIONS THAT CAN CAUSE VISUAL IMPAIRMENT

Below are some common medical conditions that can cause visual impairment:

Cataract
Hyperopia (farsightedness)
Glaucoma
Macular degeneration
Myopia (nearsightedness)
Nyctalopia (night blindness)
Presbyopia
Retinal detachment
Retinopathy
Strabismus

pairment. Patients who can't see lose valuable information from nonverbal communication. To improve communication with a sight impaired patient, try these suggestions.

1. Identify yourself by name each time the patient comes into the office.
2. Do not raise your voice; the patient is not hearing impaired.
3. Let the patient know exactly what you will be doing at all times and alert him or her before touching.
4. Orient the patient spatially by having him or her touch the table, the chair, the counter, and so forth.
5. Assist the patient by offering your arm and escorting him or her to the interview room.
6. Tell the patient when you are leaving the room and knock before entering.
7. Explain the sounds of machines to be used in the examination (e.g., buzzing, whirring) and what each machine will do.

Speech Impairments

Speech impairments can come from a variety of medical conditions. The medical term for difficulty with speech is **dysphasia**. Dysphasia is usually the result of a neurological problem. A common neurological condition can result in dysphasia is a stroke. **Dysphonia** is a voice impairment that is caused by a physical condition, such as oral surgery, cancer of the tongue or voice box, or cleft palate. Stuttering is another medical condition that can impair the patient's ability to communicate.

Here are some suggestions to help you communicate with a patient who has a speech impediment:

- Allow such patients time to gather their thoughts.
- Allow plenty of time for them to communicate.
- Do not rush conversations.
- Offer a note pad to write questions.
- Discuss with the physician the potential benefits for getting a speech therapist referral for the patient.

Checkpoint Question

5. What is the medical term for difficulty with speech? What does dysphonia mean?

Mental Health Illnesses

Many mental illnesses and psychiatric disorders can impair a patient's ability to communicate. These illnesses produce a broad range of communication challenges. Some illnesses can lead the patient to have uncontrollable outbursts, while others can cause a mute condition in which the patient will not communicate at all. Patients may hear voices that direct their communication to a given topic, while others may see objects that do not exist and will want confirmation from you

that you see the objects. Communicating with patients with moderate to severe psychiatric disorders requires in-depth training. It is important to stress that not all patients with mental illnesses will be challenges. Most mental illnesses can be controlled and treated with medications and other therapies. Here are a few suggestions for communicating with patients who have mental illnesses:

- Tell the patient what to expect and when things will happen.
- Keep conversations focused and professional.
- Do not force or demand answers from patients who are withdrawn or mute.
- If you feel unsafe communicating with a given patient, speak to either your supervisor or the physician regarding your concerns.
- Do not confirm hearing voices or seeing nonexistent objects.
- Orient the patient to reality as appropriate.

Patients with a history of substance abuse, alcoholism, and other addictions can also present a communication challenge. Patients may have euphoria and communicate with a flight of ideas. Or they may demonstrate aggression and agitation while they are withdrawing from the addiction. Your responsibility in communicating with patients who have any of these conditions is to identify the reasons for today's visit and follow your regular assessment duties. It is not the role of the medical assistant to recommend treatments or counseling for these patients. Your communication should be professional, nonjudgmental, and encouraging when appropriate.

Angry or Distressed Patients

Patients' emotions can run the spectrum from polite and cordial to angry and upset. There are numerous reasons for the latter. Prolonged waiting times, financial issues, and illness can spark untoward emotions. At some time in our lives we all have had a cold, felt terrible, and have snapped angrily at an innocent bystander. The key to communicating with upset patients is to prevent an escalation of the problem. Keep your patients informed about waiting times, billing and insurance changes, and other office policies that might trigger untoward emotions.

It is understandable that patients will become upset on hearing sad or unfortunate news about their health. Most patients take sad news in a calm manner. It is important to offer assistance as needed. Provide written instructions and information for the patient to read later. This material should consist of information on the diagnosis, causes of the illness, treatment options, and phone numbers that the patient may call for additional information.

Here are some suggestions that will help you communicate with an angry or distressed patient:

- Be supportive.
- Be open and honest in all communication.

- Do not provide false reassurances.
- Do not belittle the problem or concern.
- Ensure your own safety if the angry patient becomes aggressive or threatening.

Children

Levels of comprehension vary greatly during childhood, and therefore communication needs must be tailored to the specific child's needs. The following suggestions will help facilitate communication:

1. Children are responsive to eye-level contact. Either raise them to your height or lower yourself to theirs.
2. Keep your voice low-pitched and gentle.
3. Make your movements slow and keep them visible. Tell children when you need to touch them.
4. Rephrase your questions until you are sure that the child understands.
5. Be prepared for the child to return to a lower developmental level for comfort during an illness. For example, a child may revert to thumb sucking during a stressful event.
6. Use play to phrase your questions and to gain the child's cooperation. (For example, if the child appears shy and does not want to talk, start by asking the child how a stuffed animal feels today. " How does Teddy feel today?" Follow up on the child's answer with "And how do you feel?" Offering to take the teddy's temperature first may lessen any fear of thermometers.
7. Allow the child to express fear, to cry, and so on.
8. Many adolescents resent authority. During the interview, some teenagers may not want a parent in the room. Assess the situation before including the parent.
9. Never show shock or judgment when dealing with adolescents; this will immediately close communication.

Communicating With a Grieving Patient or Family Member

Occasionally, you will need to support patients who are in **grief** or great sadness caused by a loss. Grieving starts when a person has a significant loss, such as the loss of a loved one through death or the loss of a relationship, a body part, or personal health. Grief includes such emotional responses as anger, sadness, and depression, and each emotion may trigger certain behaviors. For example, anger may result in outbursts, sadness may cause crying, and depression may lead to unusual quietness or isolation.

Grieving occurs in stages: denial, anger, bargaining, depression, and acceptance. Here are some examples of what a patient in denial may say: "The doctor must have read the test wrong." "I don't have cancer; I feel fine." Anger may be voiced by, "I hate the doctor." "This is a terrible place." Bargaining is a stage in which the patient or family member tries to trade off the sad news, for example, "God, I will be the

best person I can be if you take away this disease." Depression is often expressed through quiet, withdrawn behaviors. The patient may state, "I don't care if I live anymore." Acceptance is the last stage. The patient may state, "I understand that I have terminal disease and am going to die." It is very important to stress that each person grieves in his or her own way and at his or her own pace. These stages may spread over months or years. It is possible to go through stages more than once. Sometimes, the collective signs of grief are referred to as **mourning**.

In medical settings, expect to see grief displayed in many ways. Know, too, that several factors can influence how a patient demonstrates grief and that different cultures and individuals demonstrate their grief in a variety of ways ranging from stoic, impassive responses to loud, prolonged wailing and fainting. Other responses may reflect religious beliefs about the meaning of death. Grieving is a unique and personal process. There is no set time period for grieving, and there is no "right" way to grieve.

Grieving patients may want to talk about their feelings and review events. Terminally ill patients may want to discuss their fears of dying and concerns for surviving loved ones. To support grieving patients, allow time for them to express themselves and actively listen to what they say. When appropriate, consider using touch to convey your understanding. If patients' concerns stem from a lack of understanding about their condition, provide pertinent education for them and for their caregivers (if appropriate). You should also become familiar with available community resources, such as grief or other counseling services and hospice care, so you can suggest these services when necessary.

It is normal for you to feel sad when a patient dies. It is important that your communication focus on empathy, not sympathy. Many psychologists describe sympathy as feeling *for* someone and empathy as feeling *with* someone. In the health care setting, empathy means trying to understand what patients are feeling so you can help them. Empathy can help you recognize a patient's fear and discomfort so you can do everything possible to provide support and reassurance. Sympathy, or pitying your patient, may compromise your professional distance and cause you to become personally involved. Box 3-3 offers suggestions for helping grieving patients.

 Checkpoint Question

6. What are the five stages of grieving?

ESTABLISHING POSITIVE PATIENT RELATIONSHIPS

Your approach to patients conveys a message about who you are and how you feel about yourself and your profession. Medical assistants can be role models, earning the trust and admiration of patients. To establish and maintain positive relationships with patients, speak respectfully and exhibit an appropriate demeanor during all interactions.

COMMUNICATING WITH A GRIEVING FAMILY MEMBER OR PATIENT

Patients and families faced with great loss can be helped through a variety of community resources. Hospice is national program that offers support to patients and family members dealing with a loss. Hospice deals with all types of medical conditions and with people of all ages. The earlier the patient is introduced to a hospice program, the more beneficial. Hospice does have a palliative component. Hospice staff and volunteer grief counselors are trained to answer the questions, acknowledge the fears and anger, ease the transition, and offer respite for caregivers. A patient must never be forced to join hospice or other community resources. Grieving is an individual experience. Your local hospital may also have grief counselors or social workers who can help your patients. Other community resources may be available. The knowledgeable medical assistant will, with the physician's permission, direct the patient and the family to the proper organization.

Proper Form of Address

The way you address patients provides clues about your attitude and how you will likely provide care. When greeting patients, use a proper form of address, for example, "Good morning, Mr. Jones!" or "How are you feeling, Mrs. Smith?" This type of address shows respect and sets a professional tone. In contrast, calling patients by pet names, such as sweetie, granny, gramps, or honey, can offend the person. These terms denigrate the individual's dignity and put the interaction on a personal, not professional, level.

Other inappropriate forms of address include referring to the patient as a medical condition, such as "the gallbladder in room 2" or "the broken arm in the waiting room." Patients often come to the medical office feeling anxious, so they may be particularly sensitive to everything they see and hear (or overhear). Referring to the patient as a medical condition sends the message that the staff values the patient as nothing more than an illness, which can lead to heightened anxiety.

Professional Distance

How people interact with each other is influenced by the level of emotional involvement between them. For instance, communication between a husband and wife is more intimate than the personal level of communication between friends or the social level of communication between acquaintances. In the health care setting, you must establish an appropriate level of communication to deliver direct patient care, make objective assessments, and provide quality patient teaching. You should not become too personally involved with patients because doing so may jeopardize your ability to make objective assessments. It is easy to become overattached, especially to elderly patients who are lonely. For example, do not offer to drive patients to appointments, pick up prescriptions, or do their grocery shopping. Keeping a professional distance allows you to deal objectively with patients while creating a therapeutic environment. To keep this distance, avoid revealing intimate information about yourself (e.g., marital woes, financial troubles, family conflict) that might shift the dynamics of the relationship to a more personal level. Often, in an attempt to help a patient, we might say, "My grandmother was diagnosed with cancer too, but she is fine; it's not a big deal. You will be okay too." Every situation is different. The patient may misinterpret this to mean that you don't think that his or her diagnosis of cancer is a big deal. But at that moment it is a very big deal to the patient!

TEACHING PATIENTS

One of the fundamental communication skills you will need is the ability to teach patients about their medical conditions. Teaching patients might involve something as relatively simple as explaining how often they should take a medication or instructing a newly diagnosed diabetic patient about self-injection. The guidelines listed below incorporate such key communication skills as interviewing and active listening. Follow these to provide effective patient education. (See Chapter 4.)

1. Be knowledgeable about current medical issues, discoveries, and trends.
2. Be aware of special services available in your area.
3. Have pertinent handouts or information sheets available.
4. Allow enough teaching time so that you are not interrupted or rushed.
5. Find a quiet room away from the main office flow if at all possible.
6. Give information in a clear, concise, sequential manner; provide written instructions as a follow-up.
7. Allow the patient time to assimilate this new information.
8. Encourage the patient to ask questions.
9. Ask questions in a way that will allow you to know whether the patient understands the material.
10. Invite the patient to call the office with additional questions that may arise.

PROFESSIONAL COMMUNICATION

Communicating With Peers

Communication among your peers must remain professional and appropriate throughout the workday. Discussions of non–work-related topics should be kept to a minimum and occur only during designated break times. It is not appropriate to discuss last night's TV shows, arguments with boyfriends, shopping lists, and so on in front of patients. Excessive laughing, high-pitched voice tones, and whispering can produce an unprofessional atmosphere.

During your career, you may come across a situation that requires communication with your supervisor about another peer's actions. Your communication must always be honest and accurate when reporting facts to a supervisor. Embellishing or hiding information can result in termination of your employment.

An excellent way to promote communication among your peers is to become active in your local professional organization. Your involvement at the local level can spread to national exposure. Involvement in local community organizations and support groups is also beneficial to promoting you and your profession.

Communicating With Physicians

Physicians and other health care practitioners will rely on you to communicate pertinent information to patients in a timely manner to provide quality care. Your communication must always be professional. The physician should always be addressed as doctor unless he specifies otherwise. The use of inappropriate terms is never acceptable. When possible, the correct medical terminology should be used. If you are unsure of the correct medical term, however, explain the condition rather than use a term that you do not understand. For example, if a patient comes into the office with a chief complaint of difficulty urinating, simply say, "Mr. Aramark is complaining of trouble urinating." Never use a slang expression, such as "He is having trouble peeing."

Do not feel intimidated when speaking to a physician. Speak slowly and confidently and you will develop a professional rapport. Be honest. It is better to say, "I am not sure what to do with this specimen" then to assume and make a mistake.

Remember, there is a time and place for everything. The physician may be the biggest jokester or sports fan in the office, but it is not appropriate to draw on these topics in front of patients or family members.

Communicating With Other Facilities

The medical administrative staff often makes referrals to other facilities or physicians. Box 3-4 has examples of various referrals you might make. No matter whom you are contacting, follow these key points:

- Patient confidentiality is always foremost. Make sure you have appropriate patient consent.
- Observe all legal requirements for dispensing patient data.
- Use caution with fax machines, E-mail, and other electronic devices. Make sure the intended receiver is the one who gets the communication.

ETHICAL TIPS

All patient communication is confidential. Patient information is sometimes discussed unintentionally, however. To avoid breaching confidentiality, follow these guidelines:

- Do not discuss patients' problems in public places, such as elevators or parking lots. A patient's friends or family members might overhear your conversation and misinterpret what is said.
- The glass window between the waiting room and the reception desk should be kept closed.
- Watch the volume of your voice.
- When calling coworkers over the office intercom, do not use a patient's name or reveal other information. Avoid saying something like, "Bob Smith is on the phone and wants to know if his strep throat culture came back." Instead, say "There's a patient on line 1."
- Before going home, destroy any slips of paper in your uniform pockets that contain patient information (e.g., reminder notes from verbal reports).

Box 3-4

TYPES OF REFERRALS

Numerous types of referrals can be made. Here are some of the most common examples:

Cardiac rehabilitation
Diabetes education
Dietitian
Home care services
Laboratory studies
Occupational therapy
Physician specialties (cardiologist, pulmonologist, podiatrist)
Physical therapy
Psychotherapy
Radiology
Social worker
Speech therapy

- Provide only the facts. Do not relay suspicions or assumptions.
- Always be nonjudgmental.
- Confirm that the message was received and that the referral will be handled.

CHAPTER SUMMARY

Communication is a complex and dynamic process involving the sending and receiving of messages. It includes verbal and nonverbal forms of expression and is influenced by personal and societal values, individual beliefs, and cultural orientation. In the medical practice, important aspects of patient communication are interviewing and active listening. You will need to overcome many communication challenges to communicate with all patients. These challenges include patients with hearing, sight, and speech impairments. Children, or angry or distressed patients, and patients with mental illnesses can also present a challenge to communication. To communicate effectively, you must understand the various factors that can affect the exchange of messages and use the communication techniques that are most appropriate for each individual situation.

Critical Thinking Challenges

1. Dr. Rogers has just told a patient she has breast cancer. The words breast cancer can spark many emotions and fears. Write three sample questions that you could ask the patient to promote open communication about her feelings. Suppose the diagnosis made was AIDS. What questions would you ask?
2. Dr. Blanda has just discharged a patient with specific instructions for wound care. How would you determine the patient's understanding of these instructions? Can nonverbal clues help you determine whether the patient is confused?
3. A mother brings in her 3-year-old child for a checkup. The child refuses to have her temperature taken. How would you go about communicating the importance of this? What if the child was 6 years old?
4. List five common clichés. Then select one and draw a picture illustrating how it may be misinterpreted.

5. A patient arrives in your office demanding to see the physician immediately. He is yelling and obviously very angry. The doctor is with another patient. Write three statements that you could say that might help the situation. Write three statements that would escalate the situation.
6. List five local resources that can assist a grieving patient or family member. Include the name of the agency, type of help that it offers, any special information, and its phone number.

Answers to Checkpoint Questions

1. For communication to occur, these three elements must be present: a message to be sent, a person to send the message, and a person to receive the message.
2. Voice tone, quality, volume, pitch, and range are five examples of paralanguage.
3. When interviewing patients, you can use six different techniques. These include reflecting, paraphrasing or restatement, asking for examples or clarification, asking open-ended questions, summarizing, and allowing silences.
4. The medical term for complete hearing loss is anacusis.
5. The medical term for difficulty with speech is dysphasia. Dysphonia is a voice impairment.
6. The five stages of grieving are denial, anger, bargaining, depression, and acceptance.

 Websites

Here are some websites that can give you some additional information:

National Institute of Deafness and Other Communication Disorders
www.nidcd.nih.gov
American Speech-Language-Hearing Association
www.asha.org
Hearing, Speech and Deafness Center
www.hsdc.org
National Hospice and Palliative Care Organization
www.nhpco.org

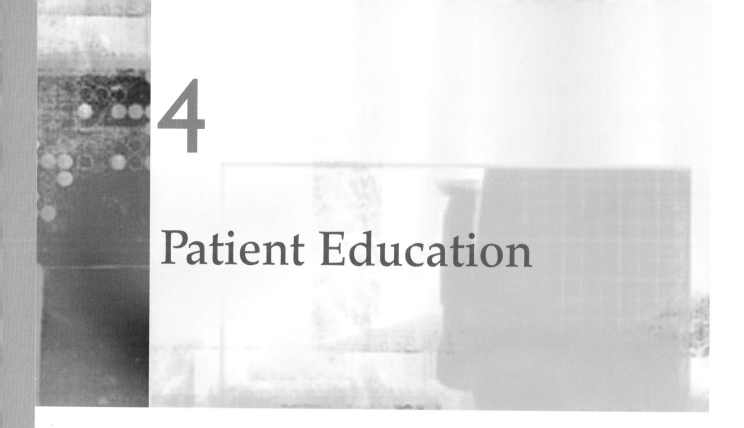

4

Patient Education

CHAPTER OUTLINE

ROLE DELINEATION COMPONENTS

GENERAL: Instruction
- Instruct individuals according to their needs
- Explain office policies and procedures
- Teach methods of health promotion and disease prevention
- Locate community resources and disseminate information
  - Develop educational materials
  - Conduct continuing education activities

GENERAL: Communication Skills
- Recognize and respect cultural diversity
- Adapt communications to individual's ability to understand
- Recognize and respond effectively to verbal, nonverbal, and written communications
- Use medical terminology appropriately

GENERAL: Legal Concepts
- Perform within legal and ethical boundaries
- Document accurately

CHAPTER COMPETENCIES

LEARNING OBJECTIVES

Upon successfully completing this chapter, you will be able to:

1. Spell and define the key terms
2. Explain the medical assistant's role in patient education
3. Define the five steps in the patient education process
4. Identify five conditions that are needed for patient education to occur
5. Explain Maslow's hierarchy of human needs
6. List five factors that may hinder patient education and at least two methods to compensate for each of these factors
7. Discuss five preventive medicine guidelines that you should teach your patients
8. Explain the kinds of information that should be included in patient teaching about medication therapy
9. Identify the components of a healthy diet, and explain how to use a food guide pyramid
10. Explain the importance of teaching range-of-motion exercises to patients
11. Explain your role in teaching patients about alternative medicine therapies
12. List and explain relaxation techniques that you can teach patients to help with stress management
13. List three national organizations that can help patients with smoking cessation
14. Identify a national organization that can assist patients with treating alcoholism
15. Describe how to prepare a teaching plan
16. List potential sources of patient education materials

KEY TERMS

alternative	detoxification	learning objectives	planning
assessment	documentation	noncompliance	psychomotor
carbohydrates	evaluation	nutrition	range-of-motion
coping mechanisms	implementation	placebo	stress

IN THE CURRENT HEALTH care climate of short hospital stays, patients seen in the medical office typically have acute conditions requiring intensive and extensive education from their health care provider. This will be one of your most challenging and rewarding roles as a medical assistant. Of course, you will not be responsible for teaching patients everything they need to know about health care. Patient education is performed under the direction of the physician. The amount and types of education that you will be expected to do will vary greatly from office to office. This chapter will give you the foundation needed for providing patient education.

THE PATIENT EDUCATION PROCESS

Patient education involves more than telling patients which medications they need to take or which lifestyle behaviors they need to change and expecting them to follow these instructions blindly. To educate patients effectively, you need to help them accept their illness, involve them in the process of gaining knowledge, and provide positive reinforcement. Ultimately, that knowledge should lead to a change in behavior or attitudes.

The process of patient education involves five major steps:

- Assessment
- Planning
- Implementation
- Evaluation
- Documentation

These five steps collectively produce the teaching plan. The plan may be formally written as the process is occurring or may be documented after the event. You must follow all these steps to achieve effective patient education.

Assessment

Before you begin to teach, you must assess your feelings and attitudes about the patient and the topic to be taught. Sometime in your career as a medical assistant, you may encounter situations or patients that make you feel uncomfortable. Your role as an educator, however, requires that you set aside your own personal feelings and life experiences to instruct the patient objectively and to the best of your ability. Always consider how your responses and actions will affect the patient and be sure to treat each patient impartially.

Assessment requires gathering information about the patient's present health care needs and abilities. In addition to knowing the present health care needs, you must also look at these other areas:

- Past medical and surgical conditions
- Current understanding and acceptance of health problems
- Needs for additional information

- Feelings about their health care status
- Factors that may hinder learning (covered in detail later in the chapter)

You may obtain this information from a number of sources. The most comprehensive source will be the medical record. The patient's medical record consists of all information regarding current diagnoses, treatments, medications, past medical history, and a variety of other documentation. Most medical records have a problem list on the inside cover. This will provide you with a snapshot of the patient and save you time from reading the entire document. Other sources of information will be the physician, family members, significant others, and other members of the health care team. When you have collected all of the assessment data, you are ready to start the next step of the education process: planning.

   Checkpoint Question

1. What is the purpose of the assessment step during patient education?

Planning

Planning involves using the information you have gathered during the assessment phase to determine how you will approach the patient's learning needs. If possible, involve the patient in this part of the process. Learning goals and objectives that are established with input from the patient are most meaningful. A patient's learning goal is what the patient and educator want to be the outcome of the program. The patient's **learning objectives** include procedures or tasks that will be discussed or performed at various points in the program to help achieve the goal. Make certain the objectives

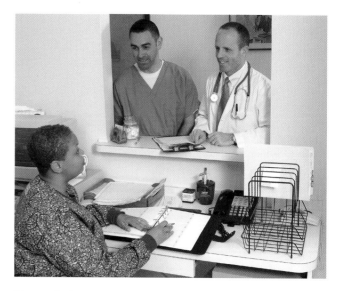

The medical assistant may obtain information regarding the patient's condition from the physician and other members of the health care team.

you establish are specific for each individual patient and are measurable in some manner. If the objectives are measurable, you will be able to evaluate when or whether the patient successfully completed them.

For example, consider a patient who needs to limit his fluid intake. Which of the following objectives is more specific and would allow you to evaluate the patient's progress: (1) the patient understands why he should limit his fluid intake, or (2) the patient is able to prepare a schedule for daily fluid intake and explain why it is important that he limits his fluids? The second objective is more specific and not only evaluates the patient's understanding but also requires the patient to demonstrate understanding. Having patients prepare their own schedule gets them involved in their health care. It allows them to customize the schedule to fit their lifestyle, which is likely to increase compliance.

Implementation

After you establish the need for patient teaching and agree on the goals and objectives, you begin implementation. **Implementation is the process used to perform the actual teaching.** The teaching usually is carried out in several steps. Box 4-1 presents some commonly used teaching strategies.

Box 4-1

IMPLEMENTATION STRATEGIES

Implementing the learning process should be individualized to the patient's best method of comprehension and retention. These may include:

1. *Lecture and demonstration.* This method presents the information in the most basic form but requires no patient participation for reinforcement and retention.
2. *Role playing and demonstration.* The patient watches you perform a medical procedure, then performs it to ensure understanding. Information is more likely to be recalled if the patient actively participates in the process.
3. *Discussion.* This two-way exchange of information and ideas works well for lifestyle changes (e.g., making dietary changes to lower cholesterol) rather than for medical procedures.
4. *Audiovisual material.* Audiocassettes or videos can often be taken home and reviewed by the patient and family members as needed. This allows for reinforcement of teachings and provides both visual and auditory stimulation.
5. *Printed material and programmed instructions.* All information should be discussed with the patient to clarify points and to elicit questions before assuming that the instructions are understood.

For example, you may start by telling the patient how to use crutches, followed by a demonstration, and finally, the patient may do a return demonstration. Patients also benefit from the use of teaching aids (drawings, charts, graphs, pamphlets) that they can take home and use as reference material. You can also use videos and audiocassettes to supplement the implementation process.

Miscommunication or misinterpretation can lead to serious complications or injury. For example, assume you are teaching a patient to use crutches. It is very important that you stress to the patient that the crutch must not press directly into the axilliary area. (There should be a two-finger distance between the crutch and the armpit.) If the patient does not comprehend the dangers of nerve damage to the axillary area from pressing the crutch into the armpit, a serious complication to the patient could occur. Miscommunication about medications can have fatal consequences.

The implementation stage may occur once or over a longer period. The disease process and the patient's ability to comprehend information will dictate the length of teaching. For example, teaching a patient about diabetes takes place over multiple sessions. The first session may focus on what diabetes is, while subsequent teachings may include topics such as diet, foot care, glucose monitoring, and insulin injection.

After implementation of a given skill or knowledge, you must determine whether your teaching was effective. This step is called evaluation.

Evaluation

Is the patient progressing? Did the teaching plan work? Does the plan need any changes? These are a few of the questions you may ask yourself when you begin to evaluate. **Evaluation is the process that indicates how well patients are adapting or applying new information to their lives.**

In the medical setting, where contact with patients is limited, part of the evaluation may have to be done by patients at home. For example, if office visits for direct observation are not scheduled, patients will be responsible for telephoning and reporting their status. In other words, can patients do the task they were taught, or are they having troubles? If they voice concern or appear unclear about their instructions, you should either redirect them on the phone or schedule them for an office appointment.

During the evaluation, you may discover noncompliance. **Noncompliance is the patient's inability or refusal to follow a prescribed order.** After determining that the given order is not being followed, your first step is to determine why the order is not being followed. It may be a misunderstanding. For example, a patient who is to take a certain medication twice a day may be taking it only twice a week because that is what he or she thought you said. If the noncompliance is because the patient refuses to follow these orders, however, you must notify the physician. Remember that the patient has the right to refuse medical treatment unless the patient is determined to be mentally incompetent. The physician will determine the next appropriate action in these cases. Evaluation is an ongoing process, so you should expect to update and modify your plan periodically.

Checkpoint Question

2. What is the purpose of evaluation during patient education?

Documentation

Documentation includes recording of all teachings that have occurred. It should consist of the following information:

- Date and time of teaching
- What information was taught, e.g., "Diabetes foot care was discussed. It consisted of the proper method for toenail cutting and regular examination by a podiatrist."
- How the information was taught, e.g., "ADA [American Diabetes Association] foot care video shown to the patient."
- Evaluation of teaching. For example, "Patient verbalized the need to make an appointment with a podiatrist."
- Any additional teaching planned, e.g., "Patient will return on Monday to the office with his wife for glucose monitoring instructions."

Box 4-2 has a charting example for patient education.

Your signature implies that you performed the teaching. If this is untrue or if another staff member assisted you in teaching, make sure that information is clearly noted. Also include the names of any interpreters who were used.

You must also document all telephone conversations, e.g., "I spoke with this patient via the telephone today and he said he is testing his blood sugar every morning without problem."

Box 4-2

CHARTING EXAMPLE

11/27/04

Patient arrived in the office for teaching on the glucose meter; brought meter from home. Following steps were demonstrated by me: calibration of meter strips, battery change, finger sticks, strip insertion into machine, use of the patient logbook. Normal BGM ranges were reviewed along with the treatment of low blood sugar. Pt returned demonstration without problem. Reviewed glucose meter instructions manual with pt. Pt. instructed to bring logbook to each MD appointment.—Bea Zame, CMA

Documentation is essential because from a legal viewpoint, procedures are only considered to have been done if they are recorded.

CONDITIONS NEEDED FOR PATIENT EDUCATION

Learning is the process of acquiring knowledge, wisdom, or skills through study or instruction. This process does not occur without certain conditions. Learning cannot occur without motivation or a perceived need to learn. For example, suppose you want to teach a patient about the need to adopt a low-sodium diet because of hypertension. Patients who feel that hypertension is not a problem, however, will not be motivated to learn the diet because they have not accepted the need for the teaching. For such patients to be taught, the following steps must occur:

1. The patient must accept that the hypertension has to be managed.
2. The patient must accept that there is a correlation between high sodium intake and hypertension.
3. The patient must accept and be willing to make this dietary change.

Only then can teaching begin.

In addition to patient motivation, basic human needs must be met first.

Maslow's Hierarchy of Needs

Abraham Maslow, an American psychiatrist, recognized that people are motivated by needs and that certain basic needs must be met before people can progress to higher needs, such as taking personal responsibility for their health (self-actualization). Maslow arranged human needs in the form of a pyramid, with basic needs at the bottom and the higher needs at the top. (Fig. 4-1). The patient progresses upward, fulfilling different levels of needs toward the highest level, which results in a state of health and well-being. In your responsibility as an educator, you need to be aware that patients must have the basic needs satisfied before they are willing or able to learn to take care of their own health. Not everyone will start at the bottom of the pyramid. Some patients will never reach the top, while others may be at the top and slide backward as a result of unfortunate circumstances.

Physiologic needs are air, water, food, rest, and comfort. If these basic needs are unmet, the patient cannot begin the process. Everyone has a different tolerance and expectation for these needs. For example, one person may expect that their food is served over three meals with full courses, while another person may accept that they will have one meal a day from a soup kitchen. If the patient perceives that these needs are met, we need to accept that and not judge the situation.

Safety and security needs include a safe environment and

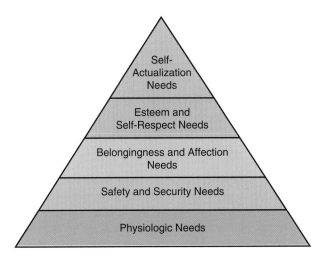

FIGURE 4–1. Maslow's hierarchy pyramid.

freedom from fear and anxiety. Patients are susceptible to fear and anxiety that accompany many medical conditions. For example, patients diagnosed with cancer may be so frightened that they are unable to think of anything but dying. Patients who have undergone some sort of trauma or disaster (hurricane, fire, motor vehicle accident) may place the need to feel safe above all other needs.

Affection needs, or the need for love and belonging, are essential for feeling connected and important to others. A sense of love or belonging can often be a powerful motivation for patients to try to regain good health.

Esteem needs involve our need to feel self-worth. Esteem can be self-generated, or it can come from those who admire us. If others value us or if we value ourselves, we are more likely to strive to maintain good health. Patients who lack self-esteem are less likely to want or accept education that targets improving their health. Thus, they will not see this as important information and will not be motivated to learn.

Self-actualization is the pinnacle of the pyramid, at which a person has satisfied all the other basic needs and feels personal responsibility and control over his or her own life. Self-actualized patients will strive to control their state of wellness by following all health directives and may even help others to achieve wellness. Not all patients will reach this level. Patients who have met this level will be ready to learn a multitude of health care skills and will strive to follow preventive health care maintenance guidelines.

After determining where on the pyramid the patient is, you can determine the appropriateness of education. For example, if the patient has not met the basic physiologic needs, you should help the patient meet these needs before beginning to teach. Patients who are in the middle levels may be able to focus and learn certain skills but may not be ready for complex teachings. If possible, you should involve family members or significant others in the teaching process.

Checkpoint Question

3. What are the basic physiologic needs outlined in Maslow's pyramid?

Environment

The environment where you teach must be conducive to learning. The room should be quiet and well lit and have limited distractions. It is not appropriate to teach patients a skill in a hallway, waiting room, or other high-traffic area. These areas produce distractions and prohibit confidentiality.

For patients to acquire knowledge, they must feel relaxed and comfortable. For example, it would be inappropriate to attempt to teach a patient who is sitting on an examination table with the stirrups in place. She will not feel comfortable. Reset the stirrups and direct the patient to have a seat in a chair. If the patient had a procedure done in the room and bloody dressings or suture equipment is still present, clean the area and then return for teaching.

Equipment

A common type of education is teaching patients to perform a **psychomotor** skill. A psychomotor skill requires the participant to physically perform a task. Some examples include crutch walking, glucose monitoring, eyedrop instillation, and dressing changes. The equipment for the skill must be present and functional. If possible, the equipment should be from the patient's home or be the exact replica of it.

The steps to teach a psychomotor skill are as follows:

1. Demonstrate the entire skill.
2. Demonstrate the skill step by step, explaining each step as you complete it.
3. Have the patient demonstrate the skill with your help.
4. Have the patient demonstrate the skill without your help.

Provide positive reinforcement throughout the steps. Always provide written step-by-step instructions along with the equipment. Always include instructions on maintenance of the equipment.

Knowledge

The person teaching the skill must have a solid knowledge of the material. Imagine how difficult it would be to learn to ski from an instructor who did not know how to put skis on. The same is true in medical assisting. If you are not comfortable or do not feel knowledgeable about the topic, ask for help before starting to teach a patient. Be reassured that you do not have to be an expert on the topic, but you do need to feel comfortable with the information. If you start teaching a given topic and the patient asks you a question that you are not able to answer, state that you are not sure about that specific piece but you will get the answer. Then either research

Box 4-3

TEACHING RESOURCES

Here are some teaching tools that you can use to help teach patients:

Audiocassettes   Models (heart, lungs)
Compact disks   Plastic food settings
Food labels   Pamphlets
Internet and websites   Videos
Manikins

the answer or ask for help from another health care professional. Never guess or imply that you know something that you do not know.

Resources

For patient education to be effective, it must consist of multiple techniques or approaches. The more techniques that are used, the more the patient will learn and retain. The three ways that we can learn are through hearing, seeing, and touch. If you can apply at least two of these senses in your teaching, your patient will be more stimulated to learn and will learn more information. For example, if you were teaching a patient about the dangers of smoking, which of the following would be more effective: (1) giving the patient a pamphlet that explains the dangers of smoking along with statistical data, or (2) showing a patient a diagram of how what a nonsmoker's lung looks like versus a smoker's and providing the patient with pamphlets about local smoking cessation programs? The teaching in the second approach would be more beneficial. The patient sees and hears the dangers of smoking and receives a brochure that contains practical hands-on information. Box 4-3 lists types of resources that you can use to help you teach patients.

In addition to the five conditions already discussed, these factors will be necessary for the patient to learn:

- Family or significant others should be present if the information is complex or if it will require their assistance. Family members are essential if the patient is confused or unreliable.
- Patients should be wearing any sensory devices that they need (glasses, hearing aids).
- Qualified interpreters should be present if needed.

FACTORS THAT CAN HINDER EDUCATION

Many factors or circumstances can hinder learning. It is important to recognize these factors and intervene as appropriate. In certain cases, teaching may have to be delayed, or your teaching plan may have to be revised.

Existing Illnesses

The type of illness that patients have will play a large role in their ability and willingness to learn. Generally, patients with acute short-term illnesses will be motivated to learn a skill that will accelerate healing. Examples of short-term illnesses are orthopedic injuries (uncomplicated fractures, sprains), colds, and viruses.

These are six examples of illnesses or conditions that will affect learning:

- *Any illness in which the patient has moderate to severe pain.* Examples of these illnesses include neuropathies, bone cancer, kidney stones, and recent surgical procedures. The patient's pain level must reach a tolerable stage before teaching can start and the patient can concentrate on learning.
- *Any illness or condition with a poor prognosis or limited rehabilitation potential.* Examples include progressive neurologic disorders, certain cancers, and large traumatic events. It is important that you assess such patients' readiness to learn and their level of acceptance of their illness before you proceed with your teaching.
- *Any illness or condition that results in weakness and general malaise as a primary symptom.* Examples include gastrointestinal disorders that cause vomiting and diarrhea, anemia, Lyme disease, and recent blood transfusion. For these patients, teaching should be limited to the essential information and expanded on as the patient regains strength.
- *Any illness or condition that impairs the patient's mental health or cognitive abilities.* Examples of these conditions include brain tumors, Alzheimer's disease, substance abuse, and psychiatric disorders. In these patients, education should be provided to patients at their ability level. Family members or significant others should be brought in to complement the learning process.
- *Any patient who has more than one chronic illness.* For example, patients with diabetes often have cardiac, renal, and integumentary complications. In patients with multiple system failures, it is important to prioritize the learning needs. Focus your education on the main problem and work from there.
- *Any illness or condition that results in respiratory distress or difficult breathing.* Examples of these conditions include chronic obstructive pulmonary disease, pneumonias, lung cancer, and asthma. The priority goal is first to establish optimal oxygenation for the patient. Once this is met, you can begin teaching. These patients tend to become exhausted easily during acute exacerbations of their illnesses. Keep the teaching time short and to the point and expand teachings as their activity tolerance allows.

4. List six types of conditions or illnesses that may hinder your ability to educate patients effectively.

Communication Barriers

Effective communication skills are essential for patient education. Any barriers to communication must be resolved before you can start teaching the patient. If an interpreter is needed for language translation or for hearing-impaired patients, schedule a time convenient to all parties. (See Chapter 3.)

Age

The age of the patient plays a very important part in the amount and type of education that you can do. Small children need to be educated at an age-appropriate level. For example, it would be inappropriate to teach a 2-year-old child how to assemble an asthma nebulizer. The parent or caregiver must be taught. It would be appropriate, however, to explain to the 2-year-old that the nebulizer is not a toy and that it contains medication. Safety education is a prime teaching focus for small children and their parents. Box 4-4 presents some tips for communicating with and teaching children.

As children mature at different speeds, you should assess what information this child can handle and what information should not be shared with the child. Communication with the parents is essential. They know the child's developmental stage. For example, a 7-year-old child who has just been diagnosed with diabetes needs to know the signs and symptoms of low blood sugar and how to treat it. The child may not be ready, however, to learn about the long-term complications (e.g., blindness, renal failure). It is important to teach the child

that the disease must be well controlled to prevent future problems, but not to the extent that the child develops fear.

The challenge in teaching adults is that they often have multiple responsibilities to their children, spouses, or aging parents. Obligations at work, school, church, and other activities may also limit their free time. These obligations and responsibilities can interfere with willingness to learn and attentiveness. Your teaching may have to occur in short sessions over long periods. This age group may benefit from electronic resources that they can access on their own time schedule.

Elderly patients can be a challenge to teach for a variety of reasons. These reasons include confusion, lack of interest, and overall poor health. Some older patients, however, can be the most attentive and curious learners. It is fairly common for this age group to address items that they have heard on the news. For example, a patient may hear an advertisement for a new medication for arthritis and request clarification from you regarding its effectiveness.

5. What is the primary teaching focus for small children and their parents?

Educational Background

Most initial health assessment forms ask patients what level of education they have obtained. This information may help you to determine the patient's ability to read. Caution is essential, because graduation alone does not guarantee that the patient can read. You will need to use your tact and diplomacy to evaluate the situation.

Patients who have completed some college courses, however, are likely to be interested in preventive health care. Patients with an educational background in health care will still need the same attention and teaching from you. Do not assume that since the patient is a nurse or a physician, you can skip teaching a skill. Their specialty may be in an unrelated area.

Physical Impairments

Numerous physical impairments may hinder learning. For example, patients with severe arthritis in their hands may have difficulty performing certain psychomotor skills, like giving themselves insulin. An occupational therapist is the best resource to assist you. Speak to the physician to obtain the proper referrals.

Other Factors

Other factors may hinder your ability to teach patients. The patient's culture may affect willingness to learn or the family's involvement in learning. Patients with financial troubles may not be ready to focus on learning new skills or knowledge. It is important that you assess the patient's readiness to learn and remove any obstacles that may be present.

Box 4-4

TIPS FOR TEACHING CHILDREN

Children require special communication skills and different teaching strategies. Here are a few tips to help you:

- Encourage the child to be part of the teaching process.
- Speak directly to the child.
- Avoid confusing medical terms.
- Avoid using baby language.
- Teach only age-appropriate information.
- Discuss with the parents the child's knowledge base about the illness and any feelings the parent may have regarding what they want the child to know. (This should not be done in front of the child.)
- Demonstrate skills on stuffed animals or dolls.

TEACHING SPECIFIC HEALTH CARE TOPICS

Your role in patient education will vary greatly. The topics that you will teach will depend on the patient, type of medical office, and physician's preferences. Next are some topics commonly taught by medical assistants.

Preventive Medicine

Preventing health problems is the key to living a long, healthy life. But the advantages to good preventive medicine extend much further. There are huge economical benefits to preventing illnesses. According to the American Hospital Association, approximately 34 million people are hospitalized each year. Caring for sick patients at home costs Medicare $200 billion annually. These statistics affect everyone. They lead to higher taxes, higher health care insurance premiums, and limited programs for low-income families.

These are some commonly recommended preventive health care tips that you should teach all of your patients:

- Regular physical examinations for all age groups
- Annual flu and regular pneumonia vaccinations
- Adult immunizations for tetanus and hepatitis B
- Childhood immunizations
- Regular dental examinations
- Monthly breast self-examinations for women and regular physician examinations
- Mammograms on a regular basis for certain groups of women
- Annual Papanicolaou tests
- Prostate-specific antigen blood tests for all men, along with need for regular digital rectal examinations

The frequency and age at which these procedures will be recommended to patients vary with the patient's medical history and genetics and the physician's preference. Some insurance will pay for these procedures, while others will not pay unless the procedure is deemed diagnostic. Many hospitals and clinics offer free preventive screenings to patients. Your office should have a list of which free screenings are available. Public health departments may also have this information available for your patients.

Your role as a medical assistant is to promote preventive screenings. The physician you work with will instruct you in his or her recommendations for these tests.

Another large part of preventive medicine is teaching safety tips. Preventable injury is the leading cause of death in persons aged 1 to 21. Approximately 25% of children will require at least one emergency room visit for treatment of a preventable accident during their childhood. Preventable injuries can arise from bicycle and car accidents, poisoning, fires, choking, falls, drownings, firearms, and lawn mowers. Toys can lead to injuries when they are broken or used by a child of an inappropriate age. The American Academy of Pe-

diatrics offers injury prevention tips for parents and health care providers. While working as a medical assistant, you will find valuable teaching tips to give to parents from their website. The AAP also provides numerous educational materials that can be mailed to physician offices and given to your patients.

One in three adults over age 65 will fall. These falls account for most of the 340,000 patients who are admitted to hospitals each year for hip fractures. Hip fractures require long hospitalizations and often rehabilitation in a nursing home. Most falls occur at home and are preventable. Fall prevention tips should be taught to all older patients or any patient who has a problem with maintaining balance or uses an ambulation device (cane, walker). Here are some tips that you can use to teach fall prevention:

- Encourage the patient to remove all scatter rugs in their home. Remind patients to keep hallways clutter free.
- Instruct the patient to ensure adequate lighting in all rooms and hallways.
- Encourage the patient to avoid steps. Encourage one-floor living.
- Ensure that the patient has well-soled shoes or sneakers. Advise the patient to avoid wearing heels.
- Instruct the patient to place nonskid surfaces in bathtubs or purchase a shower chair.
- Instruct the patient to install handrails or grab bars in hallways and stairwells.
- Encourage smoke detector installation and remind the patient to change the batteries twice a year.
- Advise patients taking medications that lower their blood pressure to stand up slowly and get their balance, then begin to walk.
- Advise patients to have regular eye examinations and have their glasses adjusted as needed.
- Encourage patients to have a plan for power outages and severe storms.

 Checkpoint Question

6. Which patients should you teach fall prevention tips?

Medications

With the increasing number of medications available, the possibilities for teaching patients in this area are virtually endless. Pharmaceutical companies offer in-depth medication information for health care providers and patients concerning the chemical makeup of the drug, physiologic reactions in the body, prescribed dosage and route, and possible side effects. This information comes from the pharmaceutical companies either by mail or from the sales support team. In addition, some of this information will come in package inserts. If this information is not available, the patient may not understand the importance of the medication therapy, and this could lead to noncompliance, drug interactions, or other serious side effects. You may be responsible for gathering the information needed and preparing teaching materials for your patients to help prevent such complications.

When preparing a medication therapy teaching tool, you must consider such factors as the patient's financial abilities, social or cultural demands, physical disabilities, and age. Be sure to include the following information in any teaching:

- Medication name (generic or brand)
- Dosage
- Route
- What the medication is for
- Why the medication must be taken as prescribed
- Possible changes in bodily functions (e.g., colored urine)
- Possible side effects
- Other medications (including over-the-counter ones) that might interfere with the action of this medication
- Foods or liquids to be avoided
- Activities to be avoided
- Telephone number to call for any questions or concerns

Figure 4-2 shows a medication therapy teaching tool that incorporates all of these elements.

Medication teaching should also include any over-the-counter medications the patient is taking. This information should consist of the same items listed above. Many patients have the misconception that over-the-counter medications (e.g., aspirin, ibuprofen, cough syrup) are 100% safe and no dangers are associated with them. Some of these medications may interact with their prescribed medications.

After assessing patients' understanding of all of their medications, you may find that scheduling is a prime concern. For example, the patient may be taking several types of medications at different times of the day or week. Before developing a medication schedule, evaluate the patient's daily routine to see how adhering to the schedule may affect the patient's lifestyle. For instance, you might ask the patient:

- How late do you sleep each morning?
- What time do you go to bed?
- When do you usually eat?

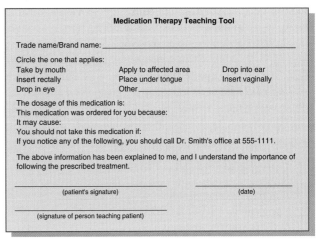

FIGURE 4-2. Medication therapy teaching tool.

Once you have collected this information, you can create a scheduling tool to serve as a reminder to the patient about what medications to take when. Pillboxes can also help to remind patients to take their medication. Pillboxes are plastic containers prelabeled with the days of the week and times. You may instruct the patient in how to fill them. Pillboxes are sold in most pharmacies.

Another patient education area that falls under the category of medication therapy includes how to administer medications—orally, vaginally, rectally, and so on. This information will be taught in the clinical part of your curriculum.

For more patient teaching information regarding safe and effective use of medications, you can contact the National Council on Patient Information and Education (NCPIE), a nonprofit organization, at 666 Eleventh Street, NW, Suite 810, Washington, DC 20001. NCPIE can provide you with literature and referrals to other sources.

Nutrition

Patients seen in the medical office have numerous reasons for being concerned about their **nutrition**. Nutrition is focused not only on what people consume but also on how the body uses the food it ingests to maintain and repair itself. Everyone needs to understand nutrition, not just people

Spanish Terminology

Tres veces al día.	Three times a day.
Antes/después de las comidas.	Before/after meals.
Al acostarse.	At bedtime.
Tómela con la comida.	Take this with food.
Dele la medicina cada cuatro horas.	Give him the medicine every 4 hours.

who are ill. People often turn to the medical profession to sort through the large amount of media hype pertaining to diets that bombards them each day. Whether the information pertains to the values of fast food or fad diets to lose weight, the media should not be the only source of guidelines for your patients. Materials are available to help you instruct patients about healthy eating.

Here are a few basic facts that you can teach all patients:

- There are no quick fixes to weight loss.
- Moderation is key. Total elimination of favorites (chips, ice cream, candy) is not necessary.
- A good dinner or meal will consist of a rainbow of colors.
- Limit salt and sodium intake.
- Eat three balanced meals a day.
- Avoid eating at least 2 hours before going to bed.
- Drink plenty of water. Avoid excessive soda and caffeine ingestion.

The Food Guide Pyramid

The U. S. Department of Agriculture (USDA) has developed a basic food group system and the Food Guide Pyramid (Fig. 4-3). The pyramid consists of five main food group categories and one "other" category:

1. Bread, cereal, grains, and pasta
2. Vegetables
3. Fruits
4. Milk, yogurt, and cheese (dairy)
5. Meat, poultry, fish, dry beans, eggs, and nuts (protein)
6. Fats, oils, sweets (other)

Next are listed some teaching tips for each of these categories.

Bread, Cereal, Grains, and Pasta

- Eat darker breads; avoid white. Avoid croissants, biscuits, sweet rolls, and pastries.
- The best cereals are oat, bran, and whole grain cereal. Avoid frosted or sweet types.
- Graham crackers, melba toast, and saltines are good cracker choices. Avoid cheese and butter crackers.
- Pasta and rice in limited portions are fine, but avoid the sauces.

Vegetables and Fruits

- Fresh or frozen is the best. Avoid dried fruits.
- Eat vegetables without butter or cream sauces.
- Limit boiling time for vegetables to prevent draining out the nutrients.

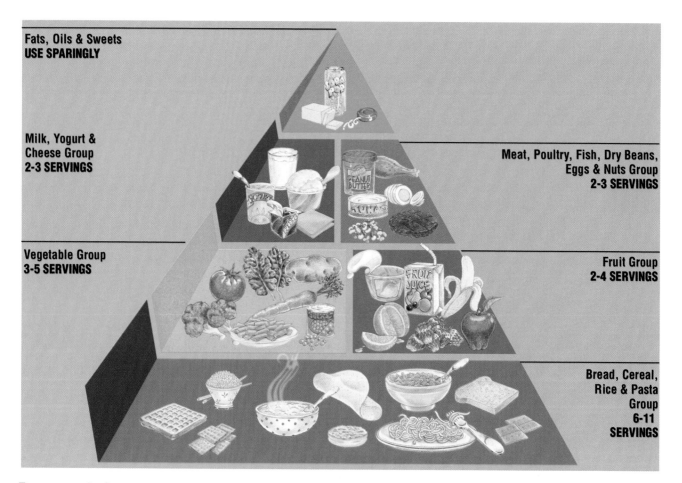

F I G U R E   4 - 3 .   General food pyramid.

Milk, Yogurt, and Cheese

- Milk: skim or 1%. Avoid creams and buttermilks.
- Yogurt: low fat or nonfat.
- Eat low-fat cheeses, 1% or 2% cottage cheese.

Meat, Poultry, and Fish

- Use USDA-select grade beef. Avoid beef with large amounts of marbling (indicates fat).
- Limit bacon to small serving sizes and limit its frequency.
- Fish should be fresh. Cook unbreaded and avoid sauces.

Fat, Oil, and Sweets

- Use oil sparingly.
- Avoid mayonnaise and salad dressings (unless low fat).
- Low-fat snacks: air-popped popcorn, pretzels, rice cakes are good choices.

In addition to the traditional food pyramid, the USDA has formed a variety of other pyramids to meet the needs of various groups. There is a special pyramid for children aged 2 to 6 (Fig. 4-4). This pyramid is visually appealing to children and provides parents with realistic serving size portions. The pyramid for people over age 70 focuses on the nutritional

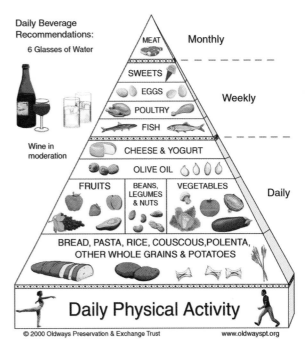

FIGURE 4-5. Food guide pyramid for a Mediterranean diet.

needs of older patients. A variety of ethnic pyramids have also been created to meet the needs of various cultures. For example, the Mediterranean diet pyramid (Fig. 4-5) varies in its recommended daily servings of the basic food groups. When you are teaching nutritional guidelines, provide the patient with a copy of the appropriate pyramid. Copies of pyramids can be obtained from the USDA website.

Checkpoint Question

7. What are the five main food groups listed in the USDA pyramids?

Dietary Guidelines

The USDA and U. S. Department of Health and Human Services also have guidelines to help improve our diets:

1. Eat a variety of foods from each of the five food groups.
2. Maintain a healthy weight by balancing the food you eat with physical activity.
3. Choose a diet low in fat, saturated fat, and cholesterol.

FIGURE 4-4. Food guide pyramid for children.

ñ Spanish Terminology

¿Qué comidas le gustan?	What foods do you like?
De dos a cuatro porciones de leche.	Two to four servings of milk.
De dos a tres porciones de carne, pescado o aves de corral.	Two to three servings of meat, fish, poultry.
De tres a cinco porciones de vegetales.	Three to five servings of vegetables.
Pan de trigo y cereales.	Wheat bread and cereals.

4. Choose a diet with plenty of vegetables, fruits, and grain products.
5. Use sugar and salt (sodium) in moderation.
6. Drink alcoholic beverages in moderation.

Encourage patients to read the labels on food containers; these labels provide important information on the nutritional value of the food, specific ingredients used, or any additives. All information on labels is based on the portion size. If you eat double the portion, you will need to double the nutritional facts. The serving size is at the top of the label. Below the serving size is the number of servings per container.

Total fat will be the first nutritional fact listed. This will give you the total grams of fat in a serving. The average diet consists of 2000 calories per day. On a 2000-calorie diet, the maximum grams of fat per day should be less than 65, with less than 20 g of saturated fat. Teach patients to add their total grams of fat per day. The label will list a percentage number as well. The percentage refers to what percent of the daily allowed fat is contained in one serving. Most patients find it easier to add up their total grams ingested. Explain that an item may be fat free or low fat but not healthy. Food manufacturers often add extra **carbohydrates** to low-fat foods to give them extra flavor and taste.

Total carbohydrates is the next fact listed on labels that patients should understand. This number tells the patient how many carbohydrates are in each serving. Carbohydrates are the prime energy source for our bodies. Carbohydrates are turned into sugar in the body. The unused portion of sugar is stored as fat. Based on a 2,000-calorie diet, the total carbohydrates per day should not exceed 300 g. Again, patients should add their total carbohydrate intake for 24 hours. It is essential that patients with diabetes learn to count carbohydrates.

Sodium, cholesterol, and protein facts are also listed on food labels. Large fast food chains, like McDonald's and Dunkin' Donuts, will have this information available at each of their stores. Patients should be encouraged to read this information.

In certain foods it is easy to determine the serving size. The label may say two cookies or one slice of bread. In other cases, however, it may be more difficult. Generally, serving sizes are listed in ounces. Here is a simple way to teach measuring: A thumb equals 1 ounce, the palm equals 3 ounces, a handful is 2 ounces, and a fist is approximately 1 cup.

After discussing healthy foods, give patients information about healthy food preparation. Here are a few guidelines on how to prepare healthy foods that you can teach your patients:

- Encourage patients to broil, boil, bake, roast, or grill.
- Trim the fat off of beef.
- Use a cooking rack so that fat drips away from the meat.
- Remove the skin from chicken. Use caution with raw chicken. Wash hands and cutting surfaces immediately.
- Homemade soups or gravies should be cooked, then chilled. Skim the fat off and then reheat.
- Use unsaturated oils (canola, corn, safflower). Use nonstick spray when possible. Avoid saturated oils (butter, lard).

Patients may ask you about vegetarian diets. There are three types of vegetarian diets. Lacto-ovovegetarian means that a diet of vegetables is supplemented with milk, eggs, and cheese. Lactovegetarian means the diet is supplemented only with milk and cheese; pure vegetarian is only vegetables and excludes all foods of animal origin. It is possible to eat healthy and obtain necessary nutrients with all three vegetarian diets. The USDA has created a vegetarian pyramid that will provide necessary education to your patients regarding serving sizes and meal planning.

Patients may ask you about vitamin and mineral supplements. If the patient maintains an appropriately balanced diet, adequate vitamins and minerals will be included in the foods consumed. A daily multipurpose vitamin can offer many benefits to patients. A common mineral supplement that patients are urged to take is calcium. Box 4-5 presents some important teaching tips on calcium supplements.

As with any patient teaching, you must consider many factors before sending the patient home with a preprinted diet form. The patient's age, culture, religion, geographic background, and social and financial circumstances may influence how well the patient complies with the diet modification. If necessary, the physician may refer the patient to a registered dietitian for in-depth nutritional education. Patients with di-

Box 4-5

CALCIUM TEACHING TIPS

Calcium is an essential mineral in everyone's diet. Here are a few teaching tips that you can your patients:

- Calcium keeps the bones and teeth strong. It is also necessary for muscle contraction and blood clotting.
- Calcium supplements are highly recommended for all women to prevent osteoporosis.
- Calcium is found in milk, yogurt, cheese, ice cream, dried beans, broccoli, and kale. Also, it can be added to cereals and some energy bars.
- Vegetables should be boiled in the least amount of water and for the shortest time to ensure nutrients are not lost.
- Daily recommended dosage is based on age: Children 1–3 should get 500 mg/day; children 4–8 should get 800 mg/day; children 9–18 should get 1200–1500 mg/day; Adults should get 1000 mg/day, and people over age 50 are recommended to get 1200 mg/day.
- Supplements can come in pills, chewable tables, or antacids.
- Calcium carbonate should be taken with meals. Vitamin D is needed to absorb calcium into the body.

- Benefits of the specific exercise
- How to get started
- How to choose a time to exercise
- How to choose a partner
- What clothing is best suited for the exercise
- How to warm up
- What a target heart rate zone is and how to achieve it
- Training program
- Calories used
- Checklist (a review of highlights from all of the above topics)

After physician clearance (if needed), you should review the information on the pamphlets with the patients. Answer any questions and document the teaching. Patients should be able to take the information in the AHA pamphlets and continue exercising on their own.

If patients are unable to perform exercises without assistance, it may be necessary to instruct them or their family members on **range-of-motion** (ROM) exercises. To perform ROM exercises, the patient moves the affected limb and joint through all of the movements that the joint is capable of making, until resistance is met. In most cases, ROM exercises are ordered by the physician to prevent further loss of motion or disfigurement after a musculoskeletal injury, surgery, or neurological damage.

When a stroke or other type of paralyzing injury is involved, ROM exercises are performed several times a day on each involved joint. If the patient is unable to perform the exercise on the affected area, passive ROM is performed. This requires someone else to perform the exer-

abetes, heart disease, and eating disorders are generally referred to dietitians. Remember to check your patient's progress during each return visit.

Exercise

Exercise is an activity using muscles, voluntary or otherwise, that helps maintain fitness. It is beneficial to the body for several reasons. If done in moderation, exercise can help relieve stress, maintain healthy body weight, and increase circulation and muscle tone. All patients should actively participate in some form of exercise on a regular basis. Box 4-6 discusses some common myths associated with exercising.

Patients who are under age 35 and in good health usually do not need a medical clearance before starting a routine exercise program. A physician consultation is recommended, however, for patients aged 35 or older who have not been active in several years. Patients with known medical disorders (e.g., hypertension, cardiovascular problems, or a family history of strokes) should check with the physician before exercising. Pregnant patients should consult their obstetrician prior to starting an exercise program.

The American Heart Association (AHA) offers information on exercise. The AHA has numerous frequently updated pamphlets available on various exercise activities and programs such as swimming, running, jogging, walking, and biking. Pamphlets cover the following information:

WHAT IF

A patient asks you about "crash" or "fad" diets. What should you say?

Patients often want to try fad diets, but they need to be taught about the potential dangers of these diets. Fad diets are advertised as "quick weight loss" fixes. These diets require precise meal plans and adherence to unhealthy portions and food selections. They are not balanced to meet all food group requirements. Most plans are targeted to a specific food, such as the grapefruit diet. Some of these diet plans can produce cardiac, renal, and digestive complications. Patients who want to lose weight should be instructed about eating regular small, balanced meals, counting calories, monitoring fat intake, and reading food package labels. Patients must also be taught that diet modification alone will not result in a significant long-term weight loss; regular exercise must also be included in any weight reduction plan.

MYTHS ABOUT EXERCISE

Here are some common myths about exercising that you can correct for your patients:

- "No pain, no gain." Patients should be instructed never to exercise to the point of exhaustion and pain. This can produce serious musculoskeletal injuries and cardiac complications.
- "I'm too old to exercise." Exercising at any age can help improve muscle tone, maintain joint flexibility, and prevent injuries.
- "Weight lifting is a man's sport." Weight lifting has been proved to help with weight reduction and limit the progression of osteoporosis.
- "The only good exercise is aerobic." Although aerobic exercise has many cardiovascular benefits, it can also lead to joint injuries. A combination of weight training, strength and resistance training, and a moderate aerobic workout is often most beneficial.

cises on the patient. Remember, ROM exercises are needed to promote circulation and maintain muscle tone. If they are not performed as ordered, the patient may not be able to regain use of the affected area. Patients with significant loss of motor skills will often be referred to physical therapy or occupational therapy for intense ROM teachings. In these cases, your role as a medical assistant will be to assess their compliance with attendance for physical therapy appointments and to provide positive reinforcement.

Checkpoint Question

8. Why is teaching range-of-motion (ROM) exercises important?

Alternative Medicine

Many ancient remedies that were once considered voodoo and dismissed by Western medicine have proven to be beneficial. Approximately $300 billion a year is spent on **alternative** medicine, and surveys have shown that about 50% of all Americans have used some form of unconventional medicine. In 1998, a federal agency was created to evaluate and monitor alternative medicine therapies. The name of the agency is National Center for Complementary and Alternative Medicine (NCCAM). The NCCAM also conducts clinical trials and training programs for practitioners of alternative medicine.

There are numerous types of alternative medicine therapies. Below is a discussion of four of the most common therapies.

Acupuncture

Acupuncture is one of the oldest forms of Chinese medicine. Acupuncture works on the principle that there are 2,000 acupuncture points in the human body. These 2,000 points are connected throughout the body by 12 pathways called meridians. The meridians conduct energy, or qi, in the body when they are triggered. The trigger comes in the form of a needle. When the meridian is stimulated, it prompts the brain to release certain chemicals and hormones.

Acupuncture is primarily used to treat addictions, fibromyalgia, osteoarthritis, asthma, and chronic back pain. It is sometimes used in treating children with attention-deficit/hyperactivity disorder.

In 1996, the Federal Drug Administration (FDA) required that all acupuncture needles be labeled single use. Only 40 states require that acupuncturists be licensed to practice. Training requirements vary among states.

Acupressure

Acupressure is a similar practice except that it does not use needles. The practitioner applies pressure to the meridians through direct touch. This method has shown great success in treating nausea and vomiting associated with chemotherapy. Some hospitals and clinics offer acupressure on an outpatient basis to cancer patients. Studies have shown that acupressure may help alleviate chronic pains and may even boost the immune system. Requirements for licensure and training vary among states.

Hypnosis

Hypnosis is portrayed on television as a magical method for reaching the inner workings of the brain. There is proof, however, that when conducted properly, it may provide some health care benefits. It is primarily used for weight reduction, for treatment of obsessive-compulsive disorders, and for smoking cessation. The training requirements vary greatly from state to state, and in most areas licensure is not required.

Yoga

Yoga has proved to be very beneficial for relieving stress and improving flexibility. Yoga consists of a comprehensive discipline of physical exercise, posture, breathing exercises, and meditation. There are a variety of types of yoga. Iyengar consists of motionless poses that emphasize posture and form. Once this method is learned, patients are able to practice this at home. This method may help patients who are recovering from injuries. Bikram consists of 26 poses that are conducted at 100°F. This method promotes muscle relaxation and stretching. Perspiration is thought to help cleanse the body of various toxins. Sivananda is a 5-step system that focuses on breathing exercises, relaxation, diet, and meditation.

Herbal Supplements

The use of herbal supplements is a multibillion-dollar business in the United States. The general public views herbal supplements as "natural," hence safe. This is a misconception. Herbal supplements, vitamins, and similar substances are not regulated by the FDA. The patient or consumer must understand that since there has been no formal government testing or approval of these substances, their dosages, side effects, interactions, and possible benefits are unclear. A classic example of an herbal supplement that has been shown to have dangerous side effects is ephedrine. This supplement was once thought to be the weight-loss miracle. It can, however, cause heart attacks and strokes. The FDA has issued many warnings about ephedrine and its dangers.

Furthermore, since these products are not regulated, there is no guarantee that what the label claims is in the bottle is actually there. The quality and the purity of the herbal supplements have shown to vary greatly from manufacturer to manufacturer. Patients should be advised to purchase only supplements that are stamped with a U. S. Pharmacopeia bar code. This bar code means that the manufacture site has met certain standards for distribution but does not mean that the supplement has been tested for health care benefits. Box 4-7 provides some general teaching tips for any patient using an herbal supplement.

Some of these substances have evolved through folklore, various cultures, or clinical research. In some cases, there is an element of **placebo** action involved. Placebo is the power of believing that something will make you better when there is no chemical reaction that warrants such improvement. Other supplements actually have scientific studies to document their effects. Table 4-1 lists some commonly used herbal supplements and their reported benefits.

Your role as a medical assistant is to assess whether patients are using any alternative therapies. Your assessment should include the length of time they have used these treatments and any side effects or benefits that the patient has noted, and you should report such information to the physician. Patients should be advised to verify the training and credentials of the practitioner they are using and to ascertain that the practitioner is appropriately licensed. Patients should be encouraged to look at the NCCAM website for safety updates and for more detailed information about alternative medicine. You should never recommend that a patient start taking herbal supplements or other alterative medicine therapies without a physician's approval.

Box 4-7

GENERAL TEACHING TIPS FOR HERBAL SUPPLEMENTS

Here are a few general teaching points on herbal supplements:

- Explain to patients the importance of always telling the physician or other health care provider about any herbal supplements that they are taking.
- Explain to patients that the fact that a product is "natural" does not mean it is safe. A good example is mushrooms. All mushrooms are natural, but some are very poisonous.
- Teach patients the importance of looking for the USP (United States Pharmacopeia) label. Teach patients to look for expiration dates on all supplements.
- Advise patients not to ask health store clerks for information on supplements but to speak to physicians or pharmacists.
- Advise patients to distrust advertisements that use words like magical or breakthrough or that claim to detoxify the whole body.
- Instruct patients to stop taking all herbal supplements at least 2 weeks prior to surgery and to tell their surgeon what supplement they have been using and how long. (Some supplements can increase bleeding time.)
- Warn diabetic patients that many supplements will interfere with blood sugar levels.
- Advise parents to avoid giving herbal supplements to their children unless approved by a physician.
- Advise pregnant or breast-feeding patients to consult with a pharmacist or physician before taking any supplements.

Checkpoint Question

9. What is a placebo?

Stress Management

Everyone is affected by an illness or injury at some time. Along with this often comes stress. **Stress** can come from forces such as fear, anger, anxiety, crisis, and joy. The stress may produce physiologic changes as well as psychologic effects. When faced with illness or injury, a patient usually must confront:

- Physical pain
- Inability to perform self-care
- Stress of treatments, procedures, and possible hospitalization
- Changes in role identity and self-image
- Loss of control and independence
- Changes in relationships with friends and family

Patients with chronic conditions may need more time to adjust than patients with acute illnesses. If patients are able to deal with stress factors, they are more likely to adapt and adjust to lifestyle changes.

Table 4-1   Herbal Supplements[a]

Supplement	Reported Benefits
Alfalfa	Relief from arthritis pain; strength
Anise	Relief of dry cough; treatment of flatulence
Black cohosh root	Relief of premenstrual symptoms; rheumatoid arthritis
Camomile	Treatment of migraines, gastric cramps
Cholestin	Lowers cholesterol and triglycerides
Echinacea	Treatment of colds; stimulates immune system; attacks viruses
Garlic	Treatment of colds; diuretic; prevention of cardiac diseases
Ginkgo	Increased blood flow to brain; treatment of Alzheimer's disease
Ginseng	Mood elevator, antihypertensive
Glucosamine	Treats arthritis symptoms; improves joint mobility
Kava	Treatment of anxiety, restlessness; tranquilizer
Licorice	Soothes coughs, treats chronic fatigue syndrome
St. John's wort	Treats depression, premenstrual symptoms; antiviral

[a] This box lists some commonly used herbal supplements and their reported benefits. Research is an ongoing process to document these findings. Some of these herbal supplements may have side effects or may interact with prescribed medications.

Many other causes besides illness or injury can place patients under stress. The best way to cope with stress is by living a healthy lifestyle. When the body is healthy, it can handle stress more easily. Unfortunately, most of the reasons that hinder learning are the same factors that hinder patients' ability to comply with patient education. Patients who are not capable of coping with stress on their own or with the help of instruction provided by the medical office staff may need professional counseling.

Positive and Negative Stress

Two types of stress affect all of us daily: positive stress and negative stress. Positive stress motivates individuals to work efficiently and perform to the best of their abilities. Examples of positive stress include working on a challenging new job or assignment, getting married, and giving a speech or performance. In fact, many people work best under positive stress. Under positive stress the brain releases chemicals that increase the heart rate and breathing capacity. The body also releases stored glucose that gives an energy boost. Once the job (or wedding) is over, though, time must be taken to relax and prepare for the next project. If relaxation techniques are not incorporated into the daily routine, positive stress can become negative stress.

Negative stress is the inability to relax after a stressful encounter. Left unchecked, it can lead to such physiologic responses as

- Headache
- Nausea, diarrhea
- Sweating palms
- Insomnia

- Malaise
- Rapid heart rate

Long-term physical effects of unrelieved stress include increases in blood pressure, glucose levels, metabolism, intraocular pressure, and finally exhaustion. There is also an increased risk of heart attack, stroke, diabetes, certain cancers, and immune system failure. If the stress is not relieved, patients will progress to higher anxiety levels and will require all of their energy and attention to focus solely on the problem at hand. Most mental and physical activity will be directed at relief of the stress to avoid the ultimate anxiety level known as panic—a sudden, overwhelming state of anxiety or terror.

Most people have developed methods of alleviating intense stressors called **coping mechanisms**, which are usually beyond our conscious ability to direct. Coping mechanisms are a psychologic defense against unpleasant situations. Some common coping mechanisms are repression, denial, and rationalization.

It may be difficult to escape completely from stress-causing factors, but management of them is possible. For a patient suffering from the physiologic effects of negative stress, you can offer the following coping strategies:

- Encourage patients to attempt to reduce stressors, but emphasize that it is not possible to remove all stressors. Warn them to avoid attempting to make everything perfect; perfectionism adds its own stress.
- Encourage patients to organize and limit activities as needed.
- Try to lessen patients' fear of failure so they just do the best they can.

- When they are feeling anxious, encourage them to talk to someone about their problems and let off steam.

Any one of these tips may help patients to regain control over stressors. In addition, a number of relaxation techniques described in the following sections may help.

Relaxation Techniques

Patients can use any of several types of relaxation techniques. To determine what works best for them, they must first consider how much time they have and what type of relaxation they need. Next are three examples of relaxation techniques.

Breathing Techniques. Breathing exercises can be done anywhere. Most people are shallow breathers and need to be instructed on deep-breathing techniques. To perform these breathing exercises, the patient should sit up straight with hands placed on the stomach and take a deep breath in through the nose, feeling the hands being pushed away by the stomach. (This may feel awkward because most people do just the opposite.) The patient holds the breath for a few seconds, then exhales through pursed lips as the hands are felt being pulled in. This exercise allows for good control of the rate of exhalation. Sometimes, getting the oxygen flowing through the body at a faster rate is all that is needed to relieve boredom, tension, and stress.

Visualization. Visualization is a relaxation technique that involves allowing the mind to wander and the imagination to run free and focus on positive and relaxing situations. It is similar to daydreaming. It can "remove" the patient from a stressful situation and put him or her in a place where, if nothing else, the mind can relax. Instruct the patient to find a quiet place, close the eyes, and then visualize a soothing scene. Sometimes, background music helps. Remind the patient that it is important to choose appropriate times for this daydreaming technique. For example, it would be dangerous to use this technique when driving a car or operating heavy equipment.

Physical Exercise. There is no better tranquilizer than physical exercise. Most people who exercise regularly say that it helps them reduce tension, relax, and rest better at night.

Smoking Cessation

The health risks associated with smoking have been well documented for many years. Nicotine is highly addictive whether ingested by inhaling or chewing. This drug reaches the brain in 6 seconds, damages the blood vessels, decreases heart strength, and is associated with many cancers. The withdrawal symptoms include anxiety, progressive restlessness, irritability, and sleep disturbances. There are numerous methods to try to stop smoking. The methods vary greatly. Some programs have the patient gradually stop, while other programs seek a total, abrupt stoppage. There is research data to support both methods.

Here are some suggestions to help patients stop smoking:

- Find local smoking cessation support groups. Provide phone numbers and contact names of these groups to your patients.
- If you do not have a local connection, the American Heart Association, American Lung Association, or American Cancer Society may help. Websites are provided at the end of this chapter.
- Discuss with the physician the options of prescribing various patches, gums, or other interventions for the patient. Some products have side effects, and the physician may opt not to order them based on the patient's age or other medical illnesses.

Substance Abuse

Substance abuse is excessive use of and dependency on drugs. Some abused substances are legal (e.g., alcohol, nicotine), whereas others are illegal (e.g., marijuana, cocaine). Patients affected by commonly abused substances usually work with trained specialists or counselors. Substance abuse can be highly detrimental to your patients' health, so it is important that you give them information about substance abuse if they should ask. This information may come from various national organizations. You should have information available for patients on any local chapters or organizations that may help these patients. Following is a brief outline of abused drugs and some of the consequences of using them.

Alcohol is the most commonly abused drug in our society. Alcohol is chemically classified as a mind-altering substance because it contains ethanol, which has the chemical power to depress the action of the central nervous system. This depression affects motor coordination, speech, and vision. In large amounts, alcohol can affect respiration and heart rate. The long-term effects of excessive alcohol use are liver failure, certain cancers, strokes, and nutritional deficiencies.

Alcoholics Anonymous (AA) was founded in 1935 and has approximately 2 million members. It is the leading organization in treating alcoholism. The success of the AA program is based on the patient's completion of a 12-step program. Recovering alcoholics provide many of the support services. The AA has numerous chapters and support services throughout the country for both the patient and the family. There are also special services for teenage alcoholics.

Marijuana and hashish impair short-term memory and comprehension. They alter the user's sense of time and reduce the ability to perform tasks requiring concentration and coordination. They also increase the heart rate and appetite. Long-term users may develop psychologic dependence. Because these drugs are inhaled as unfiltered smoke, users take in more cancer-causing agents and do more damage to the respiratory system than with regular filtered tobacco smoke.

Cocaine and crack cocaine stimulate the central nervous system and are extremely addictive. Crack cocaine is particularly dangerous because this pure form of cocaine is usually smoked and absorbed rapidly in the bloodstream. It can cause sudden death. Use of cocaine can cause psychologic and physical dependency. Side effects include dilated pupils, increased pulse rate, elevated blood pressure, insomnia, loss of appetite, paranoia, and seizures. It can also cause death by disrupting the brain's control of the heart and respiration.

Stimulants and amphetamines can have the same effect as cocaine, causing increased heart rate and blood pressure. Symptoms of stimulant use include dizziness, sleeplessness, and anxiety; these substances can cause psychosis, hallucinations, paranoia, and even physical collapse. The long-term effects of these substances include hypertension, heart disease, stroke, and renal and liver failure.

Depressants and barbiturates can cause physical and psychologic dependence. Abuse of these drugs can lead to respiratory depression, coma, and death, especially when they are taken with alcohol. Withdrawal can lead to restlessness, insomnia, convulsions, and death.

Hallucinogens such as lysergic acid diethylamide (LSD), phencyclidine ("angel dust" or PCP), mescaline, and peyote all interrupt brain messages that control the intellect and keep instincts in check. Large doses can produce seizures, coma, and heart and lung failure. Chronic users complain of persistent memory problems and speech difficulties for up to a year after discontinuing use. Because hallucinogens stop the brain's pain sensors, drug experiences may result in severe self-inflicted injuries.

Narcotics such as heroin, codeine, morphine, and opium are addictive drugs. These drugs can produce euphoria, drowsiness, and blood pressure and pulse fluctuations. An overdose can lead to seizures, coma, cardiac arrest, and death.

Any of these substances can impair a fetus's health. Two such common illnesses are fetal alcohol syndrome and crack baby (cocaine dependency). You will learn more about these conditions in the clinical portion of your program. It is important to teach all pregnant women the damage substance abuse may do to their unborn child and to refer pregnant patients to support services.

Patients with a substance abuse problem may require **detoxification** before counseling. Detoxification is the process of clearing drugs out of the patient's body and treating the withdrawal symptoms. This process varies with the type of substance, length of abusing the substance, and the patient's overall health. In certain cases, hospitalization will be needed.

The most important role of the medical assistant in educating patients about any type of substance abuse is to be supportive. Provide positive reinforcements as appropriate. Offer services to patients for cessation programs. Never condemn a patient for not seeking help. Always be nonjudgmental.

Checkpoint Question

10. What is the most commonly abused drug in our society? What does the term detoxification mean?

PATIENT TEACHING PLANS

Developing a Plan

Because medical assistants are usually allotted only minimal time for patient teaching, you may often find yourself teaching without a written plan. To ensure that teaching is done logically, always use the education process to help you formulate a plan in your mind. Also remember to document in the patient's record whatever teaching you perform and the patient's response.

Many facilities use preprinted teaching plans for common problem areas, such as "Controlling Diabetes," "Living With Multiple Sclerosis," and "Coping With Hearing Loss." Although these save time, they are not individualized to the patient. If you use preprinted teaching plans, be sure to adapt them to your particular patient's learning needs and abilities.

If preprinted plans are not an option, consult teaching plan resource books, which contain the necessary information in outline form. You can take the plans from these sources and transfer them as needed to your facility-approved teaching plan format, adding your own comments to fit the patient's needs.

All teaching plans, no matter what the design, should contain the following elements:

- *Learning goal.* A description of what the patient should learn from implementation of the teaching plan.
- *Material to be covered.* All major topics to be discussed.
- *Learning objectives.* Steps or procedures the patient must understand or demonstrate to accomplish the learning goal.
- *Evaluation.* Appraisal of the patient's progress.
- *Comments.* Remarks concerning circumstances that may be preventing successful completion of the objectives.

Teaching plans must also include an area for documenting when the information was presented to the patient and when the patient successfully completed each objective. Figure 4-6 is an example of a teaching plan.

Selecting and Adapting Teaching Material

An enormous amount of teaching material is available. Although the physician or institution may select much of the material you will use, you may be responsible for selecting some teaching aids. Assess your patients' general level of understanding to choose materials appropriately. When using preprinted material, consider the format, headings, illus-

Teaching Plan: 32-year-old female with Iron Deficiency Anemia
Patient Learning Goal: Increase patient's knowledge of Iron Deficiency Anemia, its complications and treatments
Material to be Covered: Description of disorder, complications, diet, medications, procedures

Learning Objectives Comments	Teaching Methods/Tools	Procedure Explained/Demonstrated Date/Initial	PT Demonstrated/ Objectives Met Date/Initial
1. Patient describes what happens when body's demand for oxygen is not met. a. oxygen and hgb concentration decrease b. signs/symptoms of anemia c. anemia occurs only after body stores of iron are depleted	Instruction		
2. Patient describes complications caused by decrease of oxygen concentration a. chronic fatigue b. dyspnea c. inability to concentrate, think d. decrease in tissue repair e. increase of infection f. increase in heart rate	Instruction		
3. Patient discusses importance of diet in prevention of iron deficiency anemia a. including iron-rich foods in diet (beef, poultry, green vegetables) b. including foods that contain ascorbic acid to assist in absorbing iron in body (fruits) c. importance of limiting large meals if fatigued; stress importance of several small meals	Instruction/Video: "Your Diet: Why It Is Important"		
4. Patient describes prescribed medication, its purpose, dosage, route, and side effects	Instruction/Pamphlet: *Taking Your Iron Supplements*		
5. Patient aware of importance of follow-up appointments for evaluation of prescribed plan of treatment	Instruction/Appointment slip with next scheduled appointment		

FIGURE 4–6. Teaching plan.

trations, vocabulary, and writing style for overall clarity and readability. Also, ensure that the information provided on commercial materials is truthful and in agreement with the policies and procedures of your facility. A good rule of thumb is to use commercial material only from nationally recognized organizations or government agencies.

Many patient education textbooks are available from your clinic library. If you do not have access to a library, you can order most texts from local bookstores or through the Internet. Many of these sources list addresses for other patient education materials available from companies or associations. These materials commonly include printed items as well as videos, audiocassettes, and compact discs. Use commercially prepared materials to start a patient teaching library in the physician's office so you will have information at your fingertips when needed.

Developing Your Own Material

Sometimes, you may need to create your own teaching materials. Review available resources and teaching aids and adapt the information to benefit your patients. When developing teaching material, remember to do the following:

- Indicate the objective of the information.
- Personalize the information so the patient wants to learn.
- Make sure information is clear and well organized.
- Use lists and outlines, which are easier to read and remember than paragraphs.
- Avoid medical jargon as much as possible.
- Focus on the key points.
- Select appropriate printing type.
- Use diagrams that are simple, clear, and well labeled.
- Include the names and telephone numbers of people or organizations that patients can call with further questions or concerns.

After patients have been using the material for a while, periodically evaluate its effectiveness and modify your teaching plan as needed.

Not all of the patient teaching materials you create will have to be in print form. Patients must be motivated to read, but many will be more receptive to audiovisual instruction. Take advantage of any opportunity to develop teaching materials in other media.

CHAPTER SUMMARY

Your role in teaching depends on the clinical setting in which you work. Some facilities hire professional staff to teach patients. If that is the case in your facility, your teaching role may be limited. Even so, never pass up an opportunity to teach. Encourage patients to ask questions. Always provide a telephone number that patients can call if they have additional information. Periodically check to ensure that your teaching has been effective.

Remember, do not overstep your role as a medical assistant. The teaching you provide should clarify and complement information provided by the physician. A well-planned patient education program helps ensure that patients receive the high-quality health care they deserve.

Critical Thinking Challenges

1. Look at the Maslow's hierarchy pyramid. What level are you on? What steps can you take to reach the self-actualization level? If you are at that level, what steps can you take to ensure that you remain there?
2. Keep track of all of the food that you consume over a 24-hour period. Calculate your total fat and total carbohydrate intake. Do your meals follow the general food pyramid? If not, what do you need to do to improve your nutritional status? Using pictures from magazines, create well-balanced breakfast, lunch, and dinner plates. Hint: your plate should have many colors in the rainbow.
3. Review the list of information that you should teach patients about their medications. Choose two medications, herbal supplements, or vitamins that you have taken. (The medication can be over-the-counter or prescribed.) Using all available resources, write the information for these two medications or supplements.
4. Review the material on fall prevention and preventing childhood injuries. Make a checklist of at least 10 safety tips for both groups. Take your list and visit your neighbor's home. Review these tips with your neighbor. What safety improvements or recommendations were you able to provide?
5. Make a list of preprinted educational materials that every office should have. What professional organizations (e.g., American Heart Association, American Cancer Society) could help provide these materials?

Answers to Checkpoint Questions

1. The purpose of the assessment step in teaching patients is to allow you to gather information about the patient's health care needs and abilities.
2. The purpose of the evaluation step in teaching patients is to allow you to determine how well pa-

tients are adapting or applying the new information to their lives.
3. The basic physiologic needs are for air, food, water, rest, and comfort.
4. Six types of conditions or illnesses that may hinder patients' ability to learn effectively are illnesses with moderate to severe pain; illnesses with a poor prognosis or limited rehabilitation; illnesses resulting in weakness or general malaise as a primary symptom; illnesses that impair the patient's mental health or cognitive ability; more than one chronic illness; illnesses that result in respiratory distress or difficulty in breathing.
5. The primary teaching focus for small children and their parents is safety and injury prevention.
6. Any patient who has trouble maintaining balance or uses an ambulation device should be taught fall prevention tips.
7. The five major food groups are bread, cereals, grains, pasta; vegetables; fruits; meat, poultry, fish; and milk, yogurt, cheese.
8. It is important to teach ROM exercises to patients to prevent further loss of motion or disfigurement to their joints.
9. A placebo is the power in believing that a substance or action will help you when there is no chemical reaction that warrants such improvement.
10. The most commonly abused drug is alcohol. Detoxification is the process of clearing drugs out of the patient's body system and treating the withdrawal symptoms.

 Websites

Here are some websites that you can search for additional information:

Alcoholics Anonymous
    www.alcoholics-anonymous.org
American Academy of Pediatrics
    www.aap.org
American Cancer Society
    www.cancer.org
American Heart Association
    www.americanheart.org
American Lung Association
    www.lungusa.org
Food and Drug Administration
    www.fda.gov
Food and Nutrition Information Center
    www.nal.usda.gov/fnic
National Center for Complementary and Alternative Medicine
    www.nccam.nih.gov
National Institute of Drug Abuse
    www.nida.nih.gov

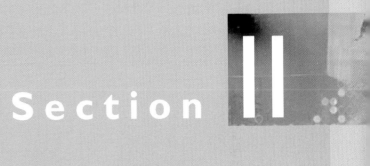

The Administrative Assistant

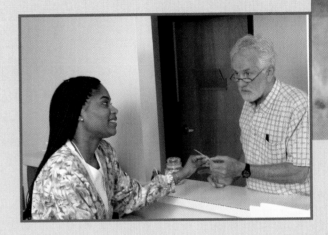

Performing Administrative Duties

A well-run medical office requires that everyone works together as a team. Unit three consists of eight chapters that address administrative duties performed in the medical office. These duties include telephone and reception, appointment management, written communications, medical record management, transcription, computer use, quality improvement, and medical office management. Some of these duties are shared with clinical personnel. This unit will help you to perform these duties whether you work in the front desk area or in the clinical area.

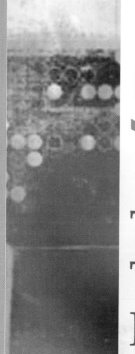

5

The First Contact: Telephone and Reception

CHAPTER OUTLINE

PROFESSIONAL IMAGE
Importance of a Good Attitude
The Medical Assistant as a Role Model
Courtesy and Diplomacy in the Medical Office
First Impressions

RECEPTION
Definition of a Receptionist
Duties and Responsibilities of the Receptionist
Ergonomic Concerns for the Receptionist
The Waiting Room Environment
The End of the Patient Visit

TELEPHONE
Importance of the Telephone in the Medical Office
Basic Guidelines for Telephone Use
Routine Incoming Calls
Challenging Incoming Calls
Triaging Incoming Calls
Taking Messages
Outgoing Calls
Services and Special Features

ROLE DELINEATION COMPONENTS

GENERAL: Professionalism
- Display a professional manner and image
- Prioritize and perform multiple tasks
- Treat all patients with compassion and empathy

GENERAL: Communication Skills
- Adapt communication to individual's ability to understand
- Use professional telephone technique

ADMINISTRATIVE: Administrative Procedures
- Perform basic administrative medical assisting functions

CHAPTER COMPETENCIES

LEARNING OBJECTIVES

Upon successfully completing this chapter, you will be able to:

1. Spell and define the key terms
2. Explain the importance of displaying a professional image to all patients
3. List six duties of the medical office receptionist
4. List four sources from which messages can be retrieved
5. Discuss various steps that can be taken to promote good ergonomics
6. Describe the basic guidelines for waiting room environments
7. Describe the proper method for maintaining infection control standards in the waiting room
8. Discuss the five basic guidelines for telephone use
9. Describe the types of incoming telephone calls received by the medical office
10. Describe how to triage incoming calls
11. Discuss how to identify and handle callers with medical emergencies
12. List the information that should be given to an emergency medical service dispatcher
13. Describe the types of telephone services and special features

KEY TERMS

attitude	diplomacy	ergonomic	teletypewriter (TTY)
closed captioning	emergency medical service	receptionist	triage
diction	(EMS)		

As a MEDICAL ASSISTANT, YOU are the patient's primary contact with the physician. In certain situations, the patient may spend more time with you than with the physician. Your interaction with the patient sets the tone for the visit and directly influences the patient's perception of the office and the quality of care the patient will receive. Therefore, it is vital that you project a caring and competent professional image at all times. You will have various responsibilities and duties when working as a receptionist. These duties will vary among physician offices. Proper telephone etiquette and use is an essential skill for all medical assistants. You must be able to handle incoming and outgoing calls correctly and efficiently.

PROFESSIONAL IMAGE

Importance of a Good Attitude

An **attitude** is a state of mind or feeling regarding some matter. It can be either positive or negative. Attitudes can be formed by past or present experiences; they can be transmitted from one person to another. How you feel influences how you act; thus, your attitude shapes your behavior. You transmit your attitude to others through your behavior, thereby influencing their attitudes and behaviors.

The medical assistant must be able to transmit a positive attitude to the patient. This requires acceptance of the patient as a unique individual who has the right to be treated with dignity and compassion in a nonjudgmental manner. Ask yourself how you would feel in a similar situation, how you would want to be treated. By demonstrating empathy, interest, and concern, you tell the patient that he or she is important to you and that you care. This exerts a positive influence on the patient's own attitude, behavior, and response.

For example, let's assume that you are working as a receptionist in a busy family practice office. It is the peak of the flu and cold season. Which of the following interactions between the medical assistant and the patient transmits a positive attitude to the patient:

- "I know you feel terrible, Mr. Smith, but so does everyone else in the waiting room. It's the flu season. Just have a seat, and the doctor will see you shortly."
- "I'm sorry you don't feel well. Do you feel well enough to sit in the waiting room for about 10 minutes? The doctor will be ready to see you then."

The second interaction shows the patient that you care about how he feels and reassures him that he will be seen by the physician shortly. In the first interaction, the attitude that was transmitted made Mr. Smith feel like just another sick patient. Your positive attitude will influence the patient's attitude, behavior, and response.

The Medical Assistant as a Role Model

Another way in which you as a medical assistant influence the patient's perception of the medical office is your personal appearance. Good health and good grooming present a positive image to the patient. Taking care of yourself by eating well, exercising regularly, and getting enough rest is important not only for your appearance but also for your job performance. If you are tired or sluggish, you cannot give good patient care.

Pay particular attention to your personal hygiene to avoid offending your patients. A person who is ill is often acutely sensitive to odors, even those normally considered pleasant. A daily bath or shower is essential, followed by an unscented deodorant. Keep your hair clean and styled. Good oral hygiene is important, and during the day you should avoid foods that may give an offensive odor. Keep your fingernails clean and trimmed, with clear or neutral polish. Long nails polished with vivid colors are not appropriate for the medical office. Natural nail tips must be less than a quarter inch long, according to the Centers for Disease Control (CDC). Artificial nails may increase the potential for infection transmission to you and your patients. The CDC recommendation is for health care providers not to wear artificial nails if high-risk patient care is required. If you wear makeup, keep it natural and apply it lightly. Do not wear perfume, cologne, scented lotion, hair spray, or the like.

Most offices have a dress code. Whether you wear a uniform or street clothes, they should be clean, neat, pressed, and in good repair (Fig. 5-1). Wrinkles, missing buttons, split seams, torn hems, and stains project a negative image. Always wear clean, polished shoes. Stockings should be full length, of a neutral shade, and free from runs and holes. Jewelry such as dangling earrings, large rings, long chains, and ornate or multiple bracelets are not appropriate in the health care environment.

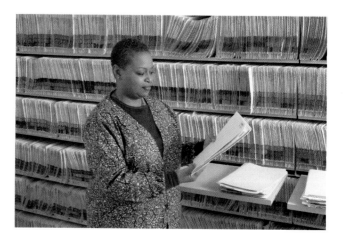

FIGURE 5–1.   The properly dressed medical assistant presents a professional and positive image to patients.

Courtesy and Diplomacy in the Medical Office

Being a medical assistant requires excellent human relations skills. In the course of a day you will interact with a variety of personalities in a variety of situations, and you must be able to maintain a positive professional attitude regardless of how difficult the encounter may be. For example, you may have to interact with a person who has done domestic violence to a patient. It is important that you treat him or her with the same courtesy and respect that you offer all patients. Courtesy and diplomacy are fundamental to successful human relations.

Courtesy is based on sensitivity to the needs and feelings of others and demands that everyone be treated with respect and dignity. It is disrespectful to refer to physicians by first name or title only. Always use the title and last name. It is permissible to call a physician by his or her first name outside of clinical areas if the physician so requests. Be courteous to your coworkers as well as your employer and your patients. Do not borrow supplies or use someone else's desk without asking permission. Always knock before entering an office, even if the door is open.

Diplomacy is the art of handling people with tact and genuine concern. Use diplomacy in difficult situations. Patients may be curious about other patients; family members may want to know what the doctor said to the patient—such questions must be met with a polite refusal to disclose confidential information. Pain, worry, and waiting can make a patient unreasonable or irritable. You must exercise self-control and understanding and maintain your professional attitude. Never argue with a patient. Try to calm the patient and communicate your desire to help. Table 5-1 lists three common problems with patients and the diplomatic way to control each situation.

First Impressions

First impressions are lasting. Remember, you have only one chance to make a first impression on patients and other health care professionals. The patient's perception of the medical office is based in part on the impression you make. A negative perception can adversely affect the patient's health. A positive perception contributes to a successful doctor–patient relationship. Patients who feel positive about their relationship with health care providers are likely to follow treatment regimens.

Physician offices must operate as a business to remain financially sound. Patients who are not satisfied with their care may opt to leave the practice. Loss of patients will result in loss of revenue for the practice. As a medical assistant, you play a key role in promoting a positive image for the physician's practice.

Checkpoint Question

1. What are four ways that you can demonstrate a professional image to patients?

RECEPTION

Definition of a Receptionist

The definition of a receptionist will vary greatly among offices. According to the 10th edition of Merriam-Webster's Collegiate Dictionary, a **receptionist** is a person employed to

Table 5-1 DIPLOMACY TABLE		
Common Problem	**Example of What to Say**	**Example of What Not to Say**
Prolonged Waiting Time "My appointment was for 9:30, and it is now 10. When am I going to be seen?"	"The doctor will see you in about 30 minutes. Would you like to wait or reschedule your visit?"	"We have had some emergencies." "It's flu season. Everyone is sick. Please sit down."
Patient Confidentiality "I am worried about my neighbor. He was seen here yesterday and sent to the hospital by ambulance. What happened?"	"We appreciate your concern, but it is against our office policy to give out patient information."	"He was having some chest pain, but he is fine now." "Yes, we sent him by ambulance because he was very sick."
Patient Discomfort "I am in a lot of pain. I want to see the doctor now!" "I have been vomiting all day. I won't sit in the waiting room. I want to be seen now!"	"I can see that you are in pain. Please have a seat for 1 minute. I will find a room for you to lie down."	"You are going to have to wait your turn. There are three patients ahead of you." "If you need to vomit, the rest room is to your left. You will have about a 20-minute wait."

greet telephone callers, visitors, patients, or clients. In certain physician offices the receptionist may be a non–medically trained professional whose primary task is to greet patients, alert staff members when patients are present, and serve as a telephone operator. This situation is generally found in large, multiphysician practices. If you are working in this type of setting, your role as a medical assistant will be to provide coverage while the receptionist is on break or at lunch.

In other office settings, however, you may work as the receptionist. These offices may also have multiple physicians but choose to have a medically trained person as the receptionist. No matter which type of office you work in, you will need to know and be able to assume the duties and responsibilities of a receptionist.

Duties and Responsibilities of the Receptionist

The duties of the receptionist begin long before the first appointment of the day. Most offices have the receptionist arrive at least 30 minutes prior to the first appointment. Your first task will be to prepare the office for patient arrivals.

Prepare the Office

As receptionist, you are responsible for preparing the office for patients and for other employee arrivals. These tasks should be done first:

- Unlock doors as appropriate.
- Disengage the alarm system.
- Turn on appropriate lights.
- Turn on computers, printers, copiers, and other electronic devices.
- If the office uses a drop box to leave specimens for evening pickups, check the box to ensure that the specimens were taken.

After those five tasks are done, do a systematic check of the office. The reception area should be clean and tidy. The reception desk should be free from clutter with confidential material safely out of sight (Fig. 5-2). Restock your desk with necessary forms and office supplies before patients arrive. In smaller offices you may be responsible for checking the examination rooms.

This process should not take long. The office should never be left messy or in disarray at the end of the day. Stocking of supplies and cleaning and disinfecting examination rooms should be done before the staff leaves at night. The office should be left in a professional manner.

Retrieve Messages

Another responsibility you may have as a receptionist is to retrieve messages that were left while the office was closed. All physician offices have a method for communicating with their patients after hours. Most offices leave a voice message

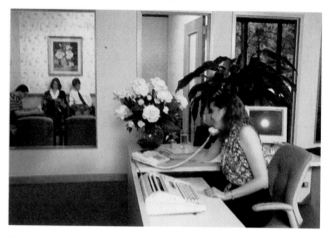

F I G U R E   5 – 2.   The receptionist desk and waiting room area must be easily accessible at all times.

on their main incoming line that directs patients to call a given number (answering service) for acute medical problems. Usually, this message also instructs patients to leave nonemergency messages on the voice mail.

Messages may be obtained from four sources:

- Answering service
- Voice mail system
- Electronic mail
- Facsimile machine

No matter how a message has been sent, however, all information must be treated confidentially.

Messages should be checked as soon as the office opens, at midday, after breaks, and periodically throughout the day. After retrieving the messages, forward them to the appropriate staff for resolution.

Answering Service.   Answering services receive calls from patients, hospital staff, and other physicians and communicate the emergency messages to the physician, generally by beeper. Other messages are left for the office staff to obtain the following morning. Examples of messages that could be left here:

- Patients calling the office for a sick appointment (not an emergency) (such as an earache, flulike symptoms)
- Calls from hospitals or skilled nursing facilities about changes in patient status (new wounds or bed sores, patient falls without injury)

Voice Mail Systems.   A voice mailbox is a type of answering machine in which the caller can leave a detailed message. You will need to know the security access code to obtain messages. After you obtain the messages, delete them from the recorder unless otherwise directed by office policy. Examples of messages that could be left here are

- Patients wishing to change or cancel their appointment
- Patients requesting prescription refills

- Family members or patients calling to ask for additional information or clarification about their medical care or test results

Electronic Mail. The computer is a vital link for physicians to communicate with all health care professionals. E-mail messages are sent from other physicians, professional organizations, and hospital personnel. Some physician offices provide patients with their E-mail address. Examples of messages left here are

- Memos from professional organizations
- Pharmaceutical representatives' updates or announcements
- Medical staff meeting minutes, announcements from hospital administration
- Upcoming continuing education courses for physicians
- Insurance representatives regarding billing issues

Facsimile Machines. All physician offices have a fax machine. The most common messages left here are

- Patient referrals
- Consultation reports
- Laboratory and radiology reports

 Checkpoint Question

2. What four locations should you retrieve messages from?

Prepare the Charts

Your next duty will be to gather charts. Gather the charts of all of the patients scheduled to be seen for the day and put them in order by appointment. Review each chart to ensure that it is complete and up to date. Check that adequate clinical data sheets are available for the doctor to record any notes. Test results received since the patient's last appointment and any other new information are placed in the front of the chart for the doctor's review. Make up a chart for each new patient and have the appropriate registration forms ready for the patient to complete. Once the charts are prepared, they are usually kept at the reception desk and given to the doctor or clinical assistant as the patient arrives, although some doctors prefer to have all charts on their desk at the start of the day. (See Chapter 8.)

Welcome Patients and Visitors

Make every attempt to greet patients personally and by name, e.g., "Good morning, Ms. Misko." A smile and cheerful greeting promote a positive image and make the patient feel welcome. Try to remember something personal about each patient, such as hobbies, pets, or special interests about which you can ask. Sometimes, you will not be at your desk when a patient arrives. Check the waiting room for new arrivals upon your return. Many offices install a bell or chime on the door and post a sign requesting patients to check in with the receptionist.

Register and Orient Patients

Patients who are new to the office will have to complete a registration form, also called a patient information sheet. On this form the patient provides name, address, and telephone number; the name, address, and telephone number of the insurance company or other party responsible for payment; employer names and addresses; marital status; spouse's name; social security number; and name of the person who referred the patient. Some information sheets include ques-

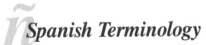 ## Spanish Terminology

¡Hola!	*Hello!*
¿Cómo se llama usted?	*What is your name?*
¿En qué puedo servirle?	*May I help you?*
¿Cuál es su dirección?	*What is your address?*
¿Cuál es el código postal?	*What is the zip code?*
¿Cuál es su número de teléfono?	*What is your phone number?*
¿Fecha de nacimiento?	*What is your birth date?*
¿Cuántos años tiene?	*How old are you?*
Por favor, siéntese en la sala de espera.	*Please have a seat in the waiting room.*
Necesito hacerle unas preguntas.	*I need to ask you some questions.*
Por favor, llene estos papeles.	*Please fill out these papers.*

tions about medical history. In some cases, you may complete the form while interviewing the patient. Most offices have the patients fill in these forms and ask for your help if questions arise.

After registration, orient the patient to the office. Brochures that give the names of the doctor and staff, office hours, and telephone numbers are helpful. Explain any pertinent office policies or procedures, such as billing procedures, how to make or cancel appointments, and parking. Ask if the patient has any questions. Tell the patient where the water fountain and restrooms are, but caution the patient against using the restroom without checking with you to determine whether a urine specimen is needed. Urine specimens are generally needed for pregnant patients, patients with lower back or abdominal pain or back injuries, and patients being seen for drug or preemployment health examinations. At the appropriate time, you may be responsible for taking patients to the examination room unless another health care worker escorts the patients.

Manage Waiting Time

Patients expect to be seen at the appointed time. They have allotted time in their schedule to see the doctor and do not want to be kept waiting. One of the major complaints of patients is the length of time they must wait to see the physician. Be sure to tell the patients if the doctor is behind schedule. If you expect the wait to be 30 minutes or more past the scheduled time, offer waiting patients some choices. Some choose to leave and come back in an hour, and some choose to reschedule the appointment for another time.

Ergonomic Concerns for the Receptionist

For most of the day you will be sitting at your desk performing these tasks. Occasional lifting of delivery boxes, paper supplies, and so on is required. The duties of the receptionist require you to twist from your primary desk to other areas to reach for files or to answer the telephone. These actions can lead to back injuries and other musculoskeletal disorders. Medical professionals are at high risk for such injuries. Having a good **ergonomic** workstation and good body mechanics, however, can prevent most injuries.

An ergonomic workstation is designed specifically to prevent injuries and often results in increased employee satisfaction and work efficiency. The Occupational Safety and Health Administration (OSHA) has many recommendations for preventing such injuries. Box 5-1 offers workstation recommendations. Here are some other suggestions to prevent injuries:

- Keep items that you must lift at waist level when possible. Keep the load close to the body. Bend at your hips.
- Instruct delivery people to place packages in locations that will not require movement.
- Carry only small loads of paper. Make additional trips as needed.

Box 5-1

ERGONOMIC WORKSTATION RECOMMENDATIONS

The following is a list of recommendations to prevent injuries:

- Your head and neck should be upright, not bent down. All desks should lead you to face forward, not twist. Objects should be within reach to allow your arms to stay close to your body, not extended. Forearms, wrists, and hands should be parallel to the ground. Your thighs should be parallel and your legs perpendicular to the floor.
- Chairs should be appropriate size. The backrest should touch the lumbar area and be strong enough to provide lumbar support. Seats should be cushioned and rounded. The seat should press against the back of your legs or knees. Armrests should support both forearms and not interfere with movement. Your feet should rest flat on the floor or on a stable footrest.
- Desks should be large enough to accommodate all needed equipment. There should be clearance between your thighs and the desk. Nothing should be stored under the desk if it limits your mobility.
- Carpets should be flat and not have a thick pile.
- Upper drawers of file cabinets should not be used if they are above your head and require reaching. Lower drawers should not hold files that require constant access, as this causes excessive bending.

- Place items that you frequently use within easy reach. Moves from side to side are safer than twisting to a desk behind you. Avoiding storing charts above chest level to limit reaching over your head. Use a step stool to reach high shelves instead of stretching.
- Telephones with headsets will keep your head upright and allow your shoulders to relax. If you use a stationary phone, a long handset cord can reduce muscle strain. Do not rest the telephone on your shoulder while talking, since this causes neck and back injuries.

 Checkpoint Question

3. What is the purpose of having an ergonomic workstation?

The Waiting Room Environment

General Guidelines for Waiting Rooms

The reception area should be designed for the comfort, safety, and enjoyment of all patients. It should be kept clean and uncluttered, with the furniture arranged to allow ample room for walking. A coat rack and umbrella stand should be present. Restrooms and a water fountain should be easily accessible.

Furniture should be aesthetically pleasing, comfortable, and durable. Chairs are preferable to sofas because most people find sharing a sofa with strangers uncomfortable. Chairs allow patients to maintain a degree of privacy and personal space. There should be a variety of soft chairs and firm chairs and chairs with and without arms. Some patients find it hard to stand up from a soft chair; others prefer the comfort. Some need chair arms to push themselves up, and others are more comfortable without chair arms.

A low-key color scheme is advisable. Muted pastels are preferable to bright primary colors, although the latter work well in pediatric offices. Lighting should be bright but not harsh. The room should be well ventilated and kept at a comfortable temperature. Many offices provide soothing background music.

Landscapes, waterscapes, and floral and animal pictures make better wall décor than abstract art. Lamps and plants can add interest to corners. Keep plants in good condition and remove any dead leaves. An office with dead or dying plants does not project a comforting image.

A good selection of reading material should be available. Have a variety of current magazines that are appropriate for your patients. The doctor's professional journals should not be included. The reception area is a good place to set out patient education materials.

Some offices provide television for patients who prefer not to read. Most patients find television relaxing and entertaining, but other patients find it annoying. Television can serve as an education tool. Here are a few tips that you should follow regarding television:

- The volume should be set to allow a group of people to hear the television but not at a distracting volume for the whole waiting room.
- A simple sign placed on the television, "Please do not touch the controls; see the receptionist for channel changes" will prevent patients from selecting inappropriate programs.
- Only family-oriented programs should be shown. It is acceptable to select a news channel. No shows with violence, strong language, or sexual content should be on. Soap operas are not suitable for medical office waiting rooms.
- Some offices leave the television off unless a patient asks to have it on.
- Patients with hearing impairments must be offered the option of **closed captioning** if they choose to watch television. (Closed captioning is the translation of the spoken word into a written format. Most televisions have this capability under their options menu.)

You should check the waiting room several times during the day to make sure it is clean and tidy. Also check the entrance, hallways, and stairs. These areas too must be well

PATIENT EDUCATION

Television as a Teaching Tool

A television in the reception area can entertain patients while they wait for an appointment, but it can also be a patient education tool. By using a television in conjunction with a VCR, you can play a variety of educational videos. Here are some points to keep in mind:

- Be sure all videos have been previewed by the physician.
- Select videos that are geared toward the specialty of the practice (e.g., a video about heart attacks is appropriate for a cardiologist's office but not for a dermatologist's office).
- Carefully assess the graphic nature of certain videos. (A picture of the birth of a child may interest you but be too much for certain patients.)
- Keep in mind the age of the patients and family members who will be in the waiting room. Caution must be used if small children are often in the area. For example, a video about preventing sexually transmitted diseases may provide information appropriate for a family practice office, but it would not be appropriate to show the video in the reception area.

lighted and maintained. Liability is a concern if patients slip on ice or snow coming into the office.

Checkpoint Question

4. What option should you offer hearing impaired patients if they wish to watch television?

Guidelines for Pediatric Waiting Rooms

Pediatric offices tend to be very busy practices with a multitude of reasons for patient visits. Generally, visits to the pediatrician can be divided into three types: well child checks, sick child visits, and follow-up visits. Because of the large volume of sick child visits, most pediatric waiting room areas are broken into two sections, one for well children and the other for sick children. Parents may have to be instructed by you as to which side of the waiting room they should sit in. According to the American Academy of Pediatrics (AAP), no studies document the effectiveness of segregated waiting room areas. The recommendation of the AAP is to move children with a communicable disease into an examination room as quickly as possible. Your employer will provide you with instructions and guidelines for dealing with sick children.

A children's play area must be closely watched and monitored. Toys should be kept away from the general seating area. Here are some guidelines for toys:

- Toys should be simple and easy to clean, without sharp edges.
- A policy must be in place for routine cleaning of these toys.
- Toys should be checked daily to ensure that they are not broken. Toys that are broken must be thrown away. Toys should never be glued or taped together.
- Battery-powered toys that make loud noises are not permissible.
- Toys can be a choking hazard. According to the American Heart Association, small children should never to be given toys that can fit inside a standard toilet paper roll. Although older children would like to play with toys like Legos, these toys should not be present. Older children should be expected to sit quietly while waiting for their appointment.

A good selection of books should be present for parents to read to their children. Books must be checked periodically to ensure that they are clean and no pages have been torn out. A small table and chairs will give children a place to read or color.

Americans with Disabilities Act Requirements

The U. S. Department of Justice is responsible for ensuring that all people are treated without discrimination of any kind. Under this department is the Americans with Disabilities Act (ADA). This act prohibits discrimination on the basis of a person's disability. The ADA Title III act requires that all public accommodations be accessible to everyone. This includes access into medical facilities. It is important that you be aware of the basic concept of the ADA rules. Table 5-2 lists some of the basic facility requirements. Additional information is available on the ADA website.

The existing structural dimensions are not something that you have control of, but you need to ensure that there is a clear path to the physician's office at all times. Here are some steps that you can take to ensure this:

- Check that deliveries are left in a safe place. They must not be left in the waiting area or block the door.
- Keep toys clear of entrance pathways.
- Check that chairs are not moved, creating obstacles that might limit wheelchair accessibility.
- Ensure that doors are not blocked or propped opened with objects.

Table 5-2   SUMMARY OF ADA REQUIREMENTS FOR PUBLIC BUILDINGS

Area	Specifics
Access	Route must be stable, firm, and slip resistant.
	Route must be 36 inches wide.
Ramps	Ramps longer than 6 feet must have two railings.
	Railings must be 34–38 inches high.
	Ramp must be 36 inches wide.
	Ramps and elevators must be available to all public levels.
Entrance and door	Door must be 32 inches wide.
	Door handle must be no higher than 48 inches and must be operable with a closed fist.
	Interior doors must open without excessive force.
Miscellaneous	Carpeting must be no more than 0.5 inch high.
	Emergency egress system must have flashing lights and audible signals.
	Space for wheelchair seating must be available.
	Tables or counters must be 28–34 inches high.
Restrooms	Tactile signs must identify restrooms.
	Doorway must be at least 32 inches wide.
	All doors (including stall doors), soap dispensers, hand dryers, and faucets must be operable with a closed fist.
	Wheelchair stall is required and must be at least 5 feet by 5 feet.

WHAT IF

A patient brings in his seeing eye dog and asks, "Can I keep the dog with me in the office?" What would you say?

The Americans with Disabilities Act (ADA) prohibits businesses from banning service animals. A service animal is defined as any guide dog or other animal that is trained to provide assistance to a person with a disability. The animal does not have to be licensed or certified by the state as a service animal. Examples of duties that service animals perform include alerting to sounds patients with hearing impairments, pulling wheelchairs for spinal cord injury patients, picking up items for patients with mobility impairments, sensing smells or auras for seizure patients, and assisting patients with visual impairments. The service animal should not be separated from its owner and must be allowed to enter the examination room with the patient. The ADA law supersedes local health department regulations that ban animals in health care centers. The care of the service animal is the sole responsibility of its owner.

- Limit the amount of stacked papers on counters that may limit the patient's access to you.
- Check the restroom regularly to make sure the entrance is open and not obstructed.

Checkpoint Question

5. What act prohibits discrimination of patients with disabilities?

Infection Control Issues

To prevent the spread of disease, aseptic technique must be used in every aspect of work in the medical office. During the clinical portion of your training, you will learn detailed information about infection control. As a receptionist, however, you need to be aware of a few key points:

- Always follow standard precautions. This means that you must treat all body fluids with precautionary measures.
- Handwashing is the most important practice for preventing the transmission of diseases. You must wash your hands following all direct patient contact (touching the patient) (Fig. 5-3). Since it is not always possible to leave the desk to wash your hands, the CDC has

approved the use of alcohol-based antiseptic hand-washing solutions for health care providers.

- Patients are often told to bring specimens to the office. Never touch a specimen container without proper gloves and personal protective equipment.
- Patients who arrive coughing and sneezing should be given tissues and instructed to cover their mouth and nose when coughing. Communicate with the clinical staff to have these patients taken directly into examination rooms. Patients who are vomiting, bleeding, or discharging other body fluids must not be left in the waiting room.

Biohazard Waste. All body fluids must be considered infectious and be managed appropriately. All body fluid spills and blood-stained papers must be disposed of in a biohazard container. The spills must be cleaned with an approved germicidal solution. If you have not been trained in handling such waste, do not touch it. Allow the clinical staff to handle the waste. If possible, contain the spill and prevent other pa-

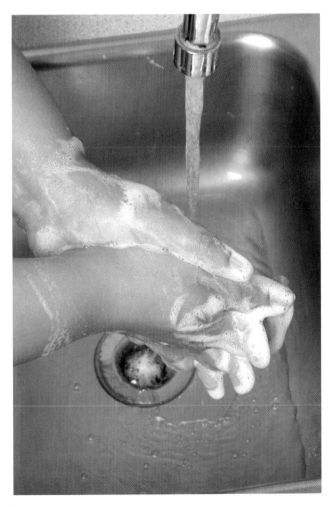

FIGURE 5-3. Good handwashing skills are essential to prevent disease transmission.

tients from touching the area. Here are some examples of biohazard waste that you may encounter:

- Dressing supplies with bloodstains from cuts or wounds
- Tissues from patients with acute nosebleeds
- Urine-saturated diapers left in the restroom
- Vomit
- Saturated tissues with sputum

Communicable Diseases. Depending on the type of office you work in, the amount of exposure to communicable diseases will vary. Family practice physicians and pediatricians, for example, treat acute communicable diseases regularly. If you work as a receptionist for a pediatrician, you will need to learn how to look at rashes and determine whether they are contagious.

Good communication between you and the clinical staff is essential to manage patients with communicable diseases. The clinical staff is often aware of patients with such diseases and will communicate it to you. Most infectious diseases can't be transmitted with routine physical contact (handshaking, talking, touching, sharing pencils, using the telephone). Examples of infectious diseases that can't be transmitted by routine physical contact include HIV, hepatitis, and the common cold. Some diseases can be easily transmitted, however, and patients with these diseases should not be left in the waiting room. Box 5-2 lists patients who should not be left in the waiting room.

Patients who have an impaired immune system or are taking medications that hinder their immune system (chemotherapy agents) may require immediate placement in an exami-

nation room to prevent exposure to otherwise benign organisms. The clinical staff will alert you to these patients.

Checkpoint Question

6. What is the most antiseptic technique for preventing the transmission of diseases?

The End of the Patient Visit

After physicians have completed the examination or other procedures, they generally direct patients to get dressed and wait for their discharge information. In some offices, physicians provide all discharge instructions, while in other office settings nurses or medical assistants may be assigned to discharge patients. Chapter 4 discusses the information you need to teach your patients. After the medical portion is completed, the patient is escorted to the front desk. It is generally at this time that any fees or copayments are collected by the receptionist. If the doctor has requested a follow-up visit, the appointment should be scheduled. An appointment reminder card is helpful for the patient. You or other administrative personnel may do these tasks. You should bid the patient goodbye in a warm and friendly manner. As patients leave the office, they should feel they have been well cared for by a competent and courteous staff.

TELEPHONE

Importance of the Telephone in the Medical Office

The medical office is filled with expensive scientific equipment used in the diagnosis and treatment of disease, but one of the most important instruments is the telephone. It allows the patient rapid and easy access to medical care. A patient can schedule an appointment, seek medical advice, request prescription refills, obtain test results, question a bill, or report an emergency simply by picking up the telephone. The telephone also links the physician's office to the rest of the medical community, including hospitals, pharmacies, and other doctors.

You must be able to communicate a positive image of the physician and staff over the telephone without the aid of nonverbal cues such as appearance, facial expressions, body language, and gestures. You must be able to use the tone and quality of your voice and speech to project a competent and caring attitude over the telephone.

Basic Guidelines for Telephone Use

Telephone communication is not effective if either party does not fully understand what is being said. Misunderstandings can be embarrassing, frustrating, or even life-threatening. To have effective telephone communication, you must be able to overcome various obstacles, such as a

---

Box 5-2

PATIENTS WHO SHOULD NOT BE LEFT IN THE WAITING ROOM

Patients with any of the following diseases or conditions should not be left in the waiting room. These patients should be taken to an examination room as soon as possible:
- Chickenpox
- Conjunctivitis
- Influenza
- Measles and rubella
- Meningitis (or suspected cases)
- Mumps
- Pertussis
- Pneumonia (if patient is coughing)
- Smallpox
- Tuberculosis
- Wounds (if open and draining)

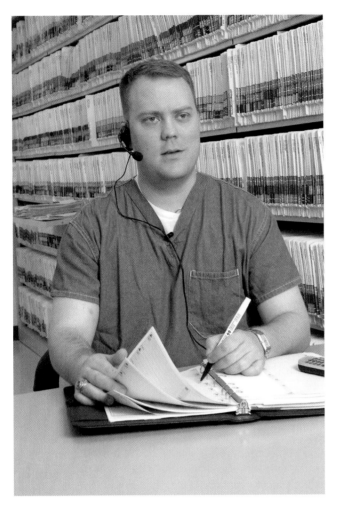

FIGURE 5-4. While speaking on the telephone, be courteous and professional.

noisy environment, a poor telephone connection, a patient's emotional distress, or a patient's hearing or speech impairments (Fig. 5-4).

Diction

Diction refers to how words are spoken and enunciated. You should speak clearly and distinctly. Talk clearly into the mouthpiece; do not prop the handset between your chin and shoulder. Never chew gum or eat while you speak on the telephone. Speak at a moderate pace to avoid slurring your words.

Pronunciation

Make sure you pronounce words correctly to avoid misunderstandings. Avoid using unfamiliar words, slang, and idiomatic expressions. Most patients do not understand medical terminology, so it is best to use lay terms whenever possible. For example, do not ask the patient, "Are you dyspneic?" Instead ask, "Are you having trouble breathing?"

Expression

Put a smile in your voice by sitting up straight and putting a smile on your lips. Speak with a modulated pitch and volume. Use proper inflection to avoid a droning, monotonous speaking style.

Listening

Be an attentive listener. Focus on the conversation and ignore outside distractions. Do not interrupt the speaker. You may have to ask the caller to repeat what was said. Verify your understanding by repeating the message.

Courtesy

Always speak politely and courteously. Address the caller by title and last name. Although many telephone calls interrupt your work, do not allow your voice to betray impatience or irritation. Remember that you are there to help the patient.

Never answer the telephone and immediately put the caller on hold. If you need to answer another line or finish a task before you can engage in conversation, ask if the caller would mind holding. Courtesy demands that you wait for an answer before you place the call on hold. Also of great importance, you must determine whether the call is an emergency. If you are unable to take the call after 90 seconds, check back with the caller and ask whether he or she would like to continue holding. Again, wait for an answer before you place the call on hold. If the hold exceeds 3 minutes, you should apologize to the caller for the delay and offer to return the call as soon as you are available.

If you are already engaged in a telephone conversation and have to answer another line, ask the party with whom you are speaking if he or she would mind holding. Again, wait for a reply before answering the second call. Explain to the second caller that you are on the other line and need to complete that call. Do not handle the second call while the first party waits unless the second call is an emergency, a long distance call that cannot be referred to another worker, or a physician calling to speak with your physician.

Quite often you will find that you are juggling the telephones and patients who are in the office. Exercise your best judgment in balancing the two tasks. If the call is going to take a long time, ask the caller to wait a moment, address the needs of the patient in the office, and then return to the call. Use caution when talking on the telephone in front of patients. Remember, all information about and conversations with patients are confidential.

Checkpoint Question

7. What are the five basic guidelines for telephone use?

Routine Incoming Calls

An incoming call should be given the same courtesy and attention as an arriving visitor. Just as you would not keep a patient waiting without acknowledging his or her presence, so you must acknowledge an incoming call promptly. Answer the telephone by the second ring if at all possible. Identify both the office and yourself to assure the caller that the correct number has been reached, and offer your assistance. The following are examples of common calls that come into a medical office.

Appointments

New patients call to make appointments and established patients call to schedule return visits. (See Chapter 6.)

Billing Inquiries

In some offices you may be responsible for handling routine inquiries concerning billing, fees, services, and insurance. You may be asked for specific information concerning the cost of services; do not quote exact prices but tell the patient that costs depend on the type of examination and diagnostic tests performed. Sometimes, third-party callers request information about the patient; remember that no patient information can be given to anyone without a specific release from the patient.

Diagnostic Test Results

Many laboratory and radiology reports are called in to the physician's office before the written copy is sent. Record the information and post it on the front of the chart for the physician to review. If the results are needed at once, bring the information to the physician's attention immediately upon receiving the report. Having at hand a blank laboratory slip or specially designed forms listing the most frequently ordered reports for your office will save time and make it easier to accurately record the results as they are relayed from the laboratory or radiology department. Administrative personnel will place a written copy of test results in the patient's chart.

Routine and Satisfactory Progress Reports

At the end of an office visit a patient may be told to call in a progress report within a few days. If the patient says he or she is feeling better or getting stronger or the symptoms have resolved, take down the information, record it in the patient's chart, and place it on the physician's desk for review. You may also handle routine progress reports from hospitals, home health agencies, and other allied health professionals. For example, a home care nurse may call and report that a patient's blood pressure is now within normal limits, or a phys-ical therapist may call the office and to say that a patient's range of motion is improving. Again, record the information and place it on the physician's desk for review.

Test Results

Patients often call for their test results, and many doctors allow the medical assistant to report favorable test results to patients. Your office will have a specific policy for handling these calls. It is illegal to give information to anyone other than the patient without the patient's specific consent.

Unsatisfactory Progress Reports and Test Results

The doctor must speak with patients whose progress or test results are unsatisfactory. The urgency of the patient's condition determines whether the call requires the physician's immediate attention. The physician will discuss serious unsatisfactory test results with the patient. In less serious cases, the physician may ask you to speak with the patient. Never discuss unsatisfactory test results with a patient unless the doctor directs you to do so.

Prescription Refills

As a medical assistant, you can handle requests for prescription refills if they are indicated on the chart. If there is any doubt, tell the pharmacy or the patient that you will check with the doctor and call back.

Other Calls

Other calls you ordinarily handle include requests for referrals to other physicians, clarifying instructions for patients, and calls concerning routine administrative matters.

Ask the physician which calls he or she prefers to have transferred immediately and which calls can be returned later. Calls from other physicians should be directed to the physician immediately or according to office policy. Physicians also receive personal calls. Your employer will tell you which calls should be put through immediately. Otherwise, take a message and tell the caller that the doctor will return the call.

Challenging Incoming Calls

Unidentified Callers

Sometimes, callers who ask to speak with the physician refuse to state their name or the nature of their business. In such instances you should politely but firmly tell the caller that you can't interrupt the physician and politely explain that you would be happy to take a message. If the caller persists, ask the caller to call back at a specific time when the physician will be available. Alert the physician that there

Procedure 5-1

Handling Incoming Calls

Equipment/Supplies

- Telephone
- Telephone message pad
- Writing utensil (pen or pencil)
- Headset (if applicable)

Steps	Purpose
1. Gather the needed equipment.	Ensures that all materials are available and ready for use.
2. Answer the phone within two rings.	Demonstrates professionalism and courtesy to the caller.
3. Greet caller with proper identification (your name and the name of the office).	Demonstrates professionalism and courtesy to the caller.
4. Identify the nature or reason for the call in a timely manner.	Allows the call to be appropriately managed.
5. Triage the call appropriately.	Prompt identification of emergency calls is important for good patient care.
6. Communicate in a professional manner and with unhurried speech.	Demonstrates compassion and caring for the patient. An unhurried speech pattern is reassuring to the patient.
7. Clarify information as needed.	Prevents errors in communication.
8. Record the message on a message pad. Include name of caller, date, time, telephone number where the caller can be reached, description of the caller's concerns, and person to whom the message is routed.	Promotes good communication between you and the recipient of the message.
9. Give the caller an approximate time for a return call.	Provides reassurance to the patient that the call will be handled promptly and timely.
10. Ask the caller whether he or she has any additional questions or needs any other help.	Confirms that the patient's needs have been met.
11. Allow the caller to disconnect first.	Ensures that the caller has completed the communication.
12. Put the message in an appropriate place.	Ensures that the call will be handled correctly and the intended recipient gets the information.
13. Complete the task within 10 minutes.	Ensures that the call is handled promptly and efficiently.

will be a call for him or her at the specified time. Unidentified callers may be sales representatives.

Irate Patients

When a caller is angry, you must be careful to keep your own temper in check. Try to calm the patient and offer assurance that you want to help. Listen carefully and take notes. If you cannot resolve the situation, let the patient know you must consult with the physician and offer to call back. The physician will probably want to speak with the patient personally. Always tell the physician about complaints regarding fees or care.

Medical Emergencies

As a medical assistant, you must be able to differentiate between routine calls and emergencies. To do this, first try to calm the caller and ask specific questions concerning the patient's condition. Severe pain, profuse bleeding, respiratory distress, chest pain, loss of consciousness, severe vomiting or diarrhea, and a temperature above 102.0°F are all emergencies, and you should immediately put the call through to the physician or an appropriate health care professional. In some offices, nurses will be assigned to handle these calls.

Determine the patient's name, location, and telephone number as quickly as possible in case you are disconnected or the patient is unable to continue the conversation. This will allow you to direct emergency personnel to the patient's aid. The office should have a policy for handling emergency calls when the doctor is not in the office. Most policies advise you to direct patients to go to the nearest emergency room or walk-in center.

Ask the physician to list instances that might constitute an emergency in his or her specialty and to describe how they should be handled. For example, if you work for a cardiologist, most of your emergency calls will be patients with chest pain and trouble breathing. The cardiologist may instruct you to ask the patient standard questions, have you instruct patients to take certain medications, and then instruct the patient to dial for an ambulance. If you are working for an obstetrician, your emergency calls will be related to patients who have labor concerns or sudden onset of bleeding. Most obstetricians have precise recommendations for when patients in labor should go to the hospital (e.g., contractions lasting more than 1 minute with a frequency of every 5 minutes). Once you have the list of the most common calls and what your response should be, put the list in a prominent place near the telephone.

Triaging Incoming Calls

Usually the office telephone has multiple lines, and frequently several patients call at the same time. You must be able to **triage** (sort) them into a priority order. How would you sort these four calls?

- Line 1: Caller wants to make an appointment for her son, who has a 101.3°F fever.
- Line 2: Caller wants to see the doctor this afternoon because he is having chest pain.
- Line 3: Caller is upset because she has been disconnected 3 times and has a question about her bill.
- Line 4: Caller needs a prescription refill.

Who would you take first? Why? Last? Why?

Any patient with a potentially life-threatening problem needs to be taken first. Therefore, talk first to caller 2. Follow your office policy for emergencies. Sometimes, a nurse will further assess the emergency or the patient may be directed to call 911. The caller on line 3 needs attention next. The longer she waits, the more upset and difficult to please she will be. Explain to the patient that you have to get the bill and chart, and ask for a phone number where you can call her back. Make the appointment for the caller on line 1. Again, follow your office policies regarding patient care issues. Caller 4 is last. Remember, you need to get back to caller 3 promptly. Do not leave messages unresolved.

Taking Messages

Taking messages for the physician or other health care professionals will be a large part of your daily responsibilities. Taking messages is easier using notepads designed for this

task. Office supply companies have an assortment of pads, or your physician may choose to design his or her own. Carbonless copies give you a record of the messages taken during the day and the action taken.

The minimum information needed for a telephone message includes the name of the caller, date and time of the call, telephone number where the caller can be reached, a short description of the caller's concern, and the person to whom the message is routed.

Before you end the call, tell the patient when to expect a return call. Callback times vary from office to office. Some physicians return calls only at the end of the day, while others return calls randomly. Learn the policy of the office in which you are working.

The patient's chart must document all calls. If you return the call to the patient, document your conversation in the medical record. Some message pads are designed to be added to the progress note on the patient's chart when the call is complete.

Checkpoint Question

8. What is the minimum information needed for taking messages?

Outgoing Calls

General Guidelines for Outgoing Calls

You will make outgoing calls as well as receive incoming calls. You should prepare for your calls carefully; have all information gathered and know what you want to say before you dial the number. If you are calling a patient to reschedule an appointment, be able to explain why the change is necessary and be prepared to offer a new appointment time.

At times you may have to make long distance calls. Keep in mind the difference in time zones; if you do not know the time zone of the city you are calling, check the front of the telephone directory. Long distance calls should be dialed directly, without operator assistance. If you dial a wrong number or become disconnected during the call, notify the long distance operator immediately to avoid charges.

Your employer may ask you to place a conference call, which connects three or more people. Notify all parties of the date and time the call will be made to ensure that everyone will be available to participate. Participants should be given the access phone number and the access code in advance of the scheduled call.

Calling Emergency Medical Services

Some patients will need immediate transport to a hospital. When emergencies occur in the physician's office, the clinical staff will be busy providing lifesaving procedures to the patient. As a receptionist, you will be directed to call the local **emergency medical service (EMS)** for transport. In most areas of the United States, the emergency number is 911. Prior to placing the call, obtain the following information:

- Patient's name, age, and sex. (Age is important, especially if the patient is a newborn or child. This will allow the dispatcher to send the most appropriate responders.)
- Nature of the medical problem (chest pain, abdominal pain, bleeding).
- Type of service the physician is requesting. Generally, there are two levels of care: basic and advanced life support. Types of services will vary from community to community.
- Any specific instructions or requests the physician may have. Generally, patients are taken to the nearest hospital; the physician may have made arrangements for the patient to be admitted at a specific hospital, however, because of a condition or diagnosis. For example, an patient with a high-risk pregnancy may be sent to a hospital with an appropriate newborn nursery instead of the community hospital. It is important that this information be told to the dispatcher so the appropriate team can be sent.
- The location of the office and any specific instructions for access, e.g., 92 Main Street, Medical Office Group, third floor, last door on the left.

After gathering the information, dial the emergency medical service number. Speak in a slow, calm voice to the dispatcher. Give the information. If the dispatcher has additional questions, answer them. Ask the dispatcher the approximate arrival time for the ambulance. Do not end the call until instructed to do so by the dispatcher.

After placing the call, alert the staff to the approximate arrival time and any other pertinent information. Ensure that the path for the ambulance personnel is unobstructed and accessible. Reassure other patients in the waiting room. If the patient has any family members present, offer them assistance and reassurance.

Checkpoint Question

9. What patient information should you know before calling emergency medical services?

Services and Special Features

The telephone system that is used for physician offices should be large enough to serve the needs of the office. For example, if you are working for a single dermatologist, two

---

Procedure 5-2

Calling Emergency Medical Services

Equipment/Supplies

- Telephone
- Patient information
- Writing utensil (pen, pencil)

Steps	Purpose
1. Obtain the following the information before dialing: patient's name, age, sex, nature of medical condition, type of service the physician is requesting, any special instructions or requests the physician may have, your location and any special information for access.	Information is necessary for quick and correct dispatch of EMS personnel. Certain types of patients require special teams for transport.
2. Dial 911 or other EMS number.	Call can't be placed if number is not dialed correctly.
3. Calmly provide the dispatcher with the above information.	Allows information to be communicated quickly and professionally.
4. Answer the dispatcher's questions calmly and professionally.	Allows dispatcher to obtain any additional information and verify the message.
5. Follow the dispatcher's instructions, if applicable.	Following instructions provides good patient care.
6. End the call as per dispatcher instructions.	Ensures that all communication needs have been met.
7. Complete the task within 10 minutes.	Prompt access to EMS promotes good patient care and is essential for good outcomes.

incoming phone lines may be enough. If you are a receptionist for a large family practice with multiple physicians and other practitioners, however, the number of incoming lines will be greater. Most offices also have unpublished incoming numbers or lines. Staff members, families, and other physicians primarily use these private lines. In addition, most offices have a direct line to the local hospital. A wide variety of communication equipment is available today, and communications consultants can help determine the appropriate services and equipment for your office. At minimum, the phone system should have recall, volume control, intercom, call forwarding, and caller identification. Cordless headsets prevent neck injuries and allow for mobility.

Most physicians have a cellular telephone. This number should never be given to anyone, although it should be readily accessible for staff members. Physicians and other health care professionals also have pager systems. Most pager systems allow you to send typed messages to the recipient via the computer. These messages are displayed on the pager, e.g., "Kate Larke's blood sugar was 420," or "Please call Dr. Harrison about Patrick Burke." Typing messages directly into a pager system is good time management.

Telecommunication Relay Systems

Patients with hearing or speech impairments often have difficulty communicating with a standard telephone. The ADA requires that telephone companies have telecommunication relay systems (TRS) available 24 hours a day (Fig. 5-5). A relay system allows the caller to type messages into a special telephone that transmits the message across the lines to the other party. The other party reads the message and types a response. The communication continues through written messages. A telephone with an attachment for typing messages is called a **teletypewriter** (TTY). If the other party does not have the capabilities to read the message, an operator can be used to translate the message. Most physician offices have a TTY phone or access to one. The Federal Communication Commission has set minimum standards for TRS and TTY

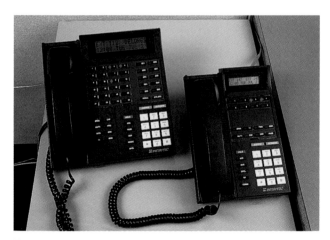

FIGURE 5-5. Various telephone systems.

systems for public buildings. These standards can be found on their website.

CHAPTER SUMMARY

As the receptionist, you are the most visible and accessible representative of the medical practice. Duties and responsibilities of a receptionist vary among office settings. The key to being a good receptionist is to demonstrate tact and diplomacy in all interactions with patients. Providing a positive attitude will ease the patient's anxiety and ensure the best and most confident image of the practice is projected. Proper telephone etiquette and manners are essential for good patient care and to achieve effective communication among various health care providers. Triaging incoming calls is a skill that you must master if you are to be an effective receptionist.

Critical Thinking Challenges

1. How would you calm an irate patient on the telephone? Identify some phrases that you might use to calm the caller. What phrases may make the situation worse?
2. Assume you are working in an obstetrician's office. What kinds of educational videos might be appropriate for the waiting room? What if you were working in an orthopedic office or for a surgeon?
3. Here is a triage scenario. Line 1 is a home care nurse calling the office with a patient status update. Line 2 is a pharmacist questioning a prescription. Line 3 is a mother of a 3-year-old child who has been vomiting for 24 hours. Line 4 is a patient who is having trouble breathing. Sort these calls. Who would you take first and last? Why? Explain your choices.
4. Describe how you would handle a patient who is vomiting in the waiting room. What would you do if a patient had a loud, congested cough?
5. Assume you are working for a pediatrician. A mother arrives carrying an 18-month-old child with symptoms of a respiratory illness. As per office policy, you direct her to sit in the sick child area. The mother refuses. What do you do?

Answers to Checkpoint Questions

1. You can demonstrate a professional image by transmitting a positive attitude, acting as a role model, using courtesy and diplomacy, and making a positive first impression.
2. Messages can be retrieved from answering services, voice mail, electronic mail, and facsimile machines.

3. The purpose of an ergonomic workstation is to prevent injuries to employees and to increase employee satisfaction and work efficiency.
4. Patients who are hearing impaired should be offered closed captioning if they are requesting to watch television.
5. The Americans with Disabilities Act prohibits discrimination against people with disabilities.
6. The most antiseptic technique for preventing the transmission of diseases is handwashing.
7. The five basic guidelines for proper telephone use are good diction, pronunciation, expression, listening, and courtesy.
8. The minimum information needed for a telephone message includes name of the caller, date and time of the call, telephone number where the caller can be reached, a short description of the caller's concern, and the person to whom the message is routed.
9. Before calling emergency medical services, you should know the name, age, and sex of the patient, nature of the medical problem, type of service the physician is requesting, and any special instructions the physician may have.

 Websites

These websites can provide you with some additional information:

American Academy of Pediatrics
www.aap.org

American Heart Association
www.americanheart.org

CDC
www.cdc.gov

Federal Communications Commission
www.fcc.gov/cib/dro

Institute for Disabilities Research and Training
www.idrt.com

Online Yellow Pages
www.smartpages.com

OSHA
www.osha.gov

Telecommunications for the Deaf
www.amrad.org

U. S. Department of Justice/Americans with Disabilities Act
www.usdoj.gov/crt/ada

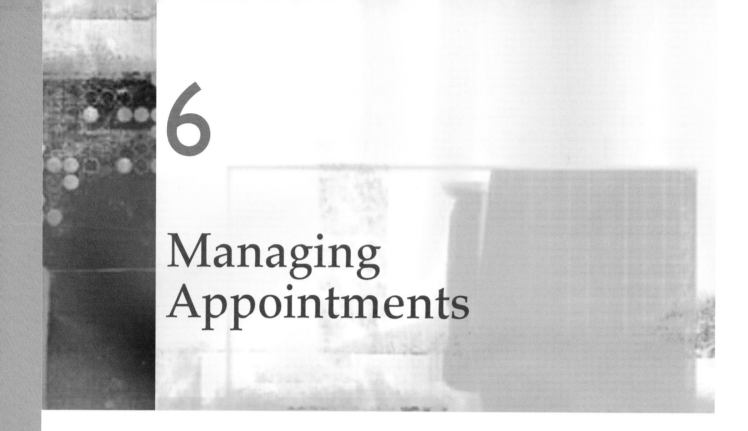

6

Managing Appointments

CHAPTER OUTLINE

ROLE DELINEATION COMPONENTS

GENERAL: Professionalism
- Display a professional manner and image
- Prioritize and perform multiple tasks
- Treat all patients with compassion and empathy

GENERAL: Communication Skills
- Use professional telephone technique
- Utilize electronic technology to receive, organize, prioritize, and transmit information
- Serve as a liaison

GENERAL: Instruction
- Explain office policies and procedures

ADMINISTRATIVE: Administrative Procedures
- Perform basic administrative medical assisting functions
- Schedule, coordinate, and monitor appointments
- Schedule inpatient/outpatient admissions and procedures
- Understand and apply third-party guidance
- Understand and adhere to managed care policies and procedures

CHAPTER COMPETENCIES

LEARNING OBJECTIVES
Upon successfully completing this chapter, you will be able to:
1. Spell and define the key terms
2. Describe the various systems for scheduling patient office visits, including manual and computerized scheduling
3. Identify the factors that affect appointment scheduling
4. Explain guidelines for scheduling appointments for new patients and return visits
5. List three ways to remind patients about appointments
6. Describe how to triage patient emergencies, acutely ill patients, and walk-in patients
7. Describe how to handle late patients and patients who miss their appointments
8. Explain what to do if the physician is delayed
9. Describe how to handle appointment cancellations made by the office or by the patient
10. Schedule an appointment for a new patient
11. Schedule a return appointment
12. Schedule a referral following third-party guidelines

KEY TERMS

acute	constellation of symptoms	precertification	streaming
buffer	consultation	providers	tickler file
chronic	double booking	referral	wave scheduling system
clustering	matrix	STAT	

RESPONSIBILITY FOR SCHEDULING and managing the flow of patient care in a medical office or clinic is one of the most important duties assigned to a medical assistant. As appointment manager, you make the first, last, and most durable impression on the patient and **providers**. Depending on your demeanor and actions, that impression can be favorable or unfavorable. A properly used appointment system helps maintain an efficient office. If improperly used, it can mean confusion and chaos; more important, it can waste precious time for the patient, the provider, and the staff.

To use the office facilities and the physician's availability most efficiently, determine which patients will be seen, when they will be seen, and how much time to allot to each of them, depending on their problems. Of course, every practice will have occasional delays and emergencies. Your responsibility is to manage all of this while maintaining a calm, efficient, and polite attitude.

APPOINTMENT SCHEDULING SYSTEMS

There are two systems of appointment scheduling for outpatient medical facilities: the manual system, which uses an appointment book, and a computerized scheduling system. The choice of systems will depend on the size of the practice, how many providers' schedules must be managed, and the preferences of the staff responsible for the daily schedule. Whether a medical office uses a manual or computerized system, many of the guidelines for effectively scheduling the workday discussed in this chapter are the same.

Manual Appointment Scheduling

Medical offices may choose to use a manual appointment scheduling system even if the other administrative functions in the office are computerized.

The Appointment Book

If your medical office uses a manual system of scheduled appointments for patient office visits, you will need an appointment book. An appointment book provides space for noting appointments for an entire year. It may have a single sheet for each day and a separate page for each provider or show an entire week on two facing pages. Some offices prefer an appointment book with pages showing only one day at a time; others may want to see a whole week at a glance. A different color page for each day may also be desired.

The more information required for scheduling, the larger the pages should be. Make sure the book has enough space for all pertinent information (e.g., patient's name, telephone number, reason for visit), is divided into time units appropriate for your practice (e.g., 10- or 15-minute intervals), can open flat on the desk where it will be used, and fits easily into its storage place when not in use.

Establishing a Matrix

Before you begin using the appointment book, you will have to set up a **matrix**. A matrix is established by crossing out times that providers are unavailable for patient visits (Fig. 6-1). For example, the physician may have a breakfast meeting and not be in the office until 10:00 A.M. This is indicated by crossing out the blocks from 8:00 to 10:00 A.M. Write in the reason for crossing off the space (e.g., vacation, meeting, hospital rounds). Some practices reserve specific times or even days for certain activities, such as physical examinations and surgery. Also, it is advisable to block off 15 to 30 minutes each morning and afternoon to accommodate emergencies, late arrivals, and other delays. Some physicians want their professional or personal obligations noted on the appointment schedule so that patients are not booked immediately before these times.

Once you have acquired and prepared an appointment book, it is not enough to schedule a time and date for a patient visit and hope everything will run smoothly. Before actually making an appointment, you should review the schedule carefully, evaluating the needs of each patient and considering the physician's preferences and availability of the office facilities. At the beginning of each day, copies of the schedule should be distributed to all staff members. Along with the notations in a patient's chart, the pages of

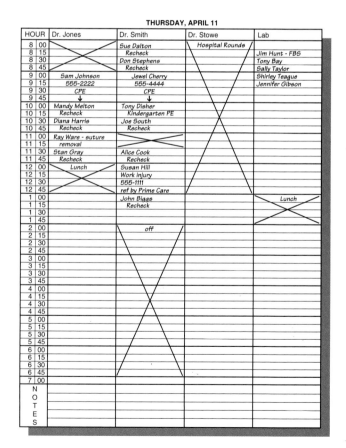

FIGURE 6–1. Sample page from manual appointment book.

```
Visual PRO/5                                    _|□|x
 Settings  Edit  Print  Help
PRINT APPOINTMENT SCHEDULES              DATE 06/17/03

ENTER:  99-CANCEL   CR-MORE

              <LEONARD H. MCCOY, MD - 18-Jun-03>
 Time  TOA  Patn# Patient Name        Phone#     Alt.ID#    STS.ID

09:00a OV   5020 JOHNSON, CARMEN L.    336/768-5348 []        .SS
09:00a
09:15a OV   5024 JENKINS, RHONDA L.    336/768-5348 []        .SS
09:30a OV   2030 MABE, DONNA NELSON    919/765-8912 [ ]       .SS
09:45a OV   2056 WRIGHT, HENRY SIMON   919/765-8574 [HMO - B1] .SS
10:00a WI   2235 SMITH, ASHLEY         003/456-7889 [345]     .SS
10:15a OV   5004 SMITH, WILLIAM        336/768-5348 []        .SS
10:30a NP   2776 SIMPSON, MARJORIE     336/768-5348 []        .SS
10:45a OV   5080 BUNNY, GREY           336/768-5348 []        .SS
11:00a
12:00p
01:30p NP   2777 COLTRANE, COURTNEY    336/768-5348 []        .SS
01:45p OV   2060 THOMAS, JEFFERY LEE   919/768-4110 [2060]    .SS
01:45p WI   5024 JENKINS, RHONDA L.    336/768-5348 []        .SS

-- MORE --
```

```
Visual PRO/5                                    _|□|x
 Settings  Edit  Print  Help
PRINT APPOINTMENT SCHEDULES              DATE 06/17/03

ENTER:  99-CANCEL   CR-MORE

              <LEONARD H. MCCOY, MD - 18-Jun-03>
 Time  TOA  Patn# Patient Name        Phone#     Alt.ID#    STS.ID

02:00p CPE  5006 EVANS, RUSSELL        336/768-5348 []        .SS
02:15p CPE  5006 EVANS, RUSSELL        336/768-5348 []        .SS
02:30p OV   2768 MORRISON, JAMES       336/768-5348 []        .SS
02:45p
03:00p OV   2496 BOWERS, MILLIE E      919/475-2401 [LEXNE]   .SS
03:15p NP   2778 SAMUEL, MICHAEL       336/768-5348 []        .SS
03:45p OV   2015 CARTER, ROY LEE       919/378-2589 [HMO/AMA - B1] .SS
04:00p RC   2518 CARPENTER, PETER      919/760-0408 []        .SS
04:10p RC   2545 ZUCKER, CELIA         910/765-8414 [12487]   .SS
04:15p
04:30p OV   2038 RAGEN, ARTHUR CHARLES 919/765-8524 [MCD - B5] .SS


-- END OF DAY --
```

FIGURE 6-2. A computer-generated appointment schedule with space for all providers of care. (Courtesy of MICA Information Systems, Winston-Salem, North Carolina.)

the appointment book provide documentation of a patient's visits and any changes, such as cancellations and rescheduled appointments. This provides further legal documentation to protect the physician and the patient in case of a dispute, as discussed in Chapter 2.

Computerized Appointment Scheduling

Medical management software designed to assist with administrative functions includes systems for appointment scheduling. Computerized scheduling often saves time. Information used to establish a matrix (e.g., hospital rounds 7:30–8:30, lunch 12:30–1:30) has to be entered only once.

Any medical office software will have an appointment toolbar that requires one click to add a patient, add to the waiting list, see a calendar, or search for available times. Many software packages offer an advanced search that defines the resources required for a certain type of appointment.

This quick method allows you to search for available appointment times. Typically, you enter the desired date, and the computer displays the schedule for that day, showing any available time slots. Another feature allows you to search the

appointment database for the next available time slot. For example, a patient is instructed to return in 3 months and has a preference for the time of day. You can search for the first available afternoon appointment with that particular provider.

Depending on the specific software, you can also print numerous documents, such as the daily or weekly appointment schedule, appointment reminders, or billing slips. Once the daily schedule is printed, this important document is referred to as the daily activity sheet or the day sheet and is the guide for everyone involved in the flow of patient care. Figure 6-2 shows a computer-generated daily activity sheet.

An important advantage to computerized appointment scheduling is the easy access to billing information. For example, a patient may call for an appointment, and the medical assistant can inform the patient that he needs to pay his balance due of $32 when he comes in to be seen. Credit and collections are discussed in Chapter 13.

 Checkpoint Question

1. Why is a matrix established?

TYPES OF SCHEDULING

Structured Appointments

Most medical offices use a system of structured or scheduled appointments for office visits. Each patient is assigned a time on the schedule and allotted a specific period for examination and treatment. Box 6-1 shows examples of time allotment. The advantages of this system include good time management and optimum use of the office facility. Additionally, a daily schedule may be developed and charts may be prepared in advance of patient arrival.

Box 6-1

HOW MUCH TIME DO I ALLOT?

Every outpatient medical facility has variables that determine the time allotted for each service. Factors like the number of providers, the number of examination rooms, and the size of the office must be considered when establishing the appointment scheduling guidelines. This partial list of typical outpatient services shows an estimate of the time needed for each.

Complete physical examination	1 hour
School physical	30 minutes
Recheck	15 minutes
Dressing change	10 minutes
Blood pressure check	5 minutes
Patient teaching	30 minutes–1 hour

A disadvantage of this system is that a patient may need more of the physician's time than you have scheduled. Therefore, it is important that you ask the proper questions at the time the appointment is made to anticipate the time needed. Such questions might include "Why do you need to see the doctor?" The patient's reply will tell you how many issues will be addressed. "Do you have a form to be completed for your physical?" The answer to this question will tell you whether this is a school physical or a complete physical.

The practice of adding **buffer** time to the schedule gives extra time to accommodate emergencies, walk-ins, and other demands on the provider's daily time schedule that are not considered direct patient care. Such tasks include returning phone calls, reviewing records, and transcribing reports. For example, you may cross off 30 minutes at the beginning and end of the daily schedule to be used as a buffer.

Methods of scheduling patients include clustering, wave, modified wave, stream, and double booking.

Clustering

Clustering is grouping patients with similar problems or needs. For example, an obstetrics and gynecology practice may see all pregnant patients in the morning and other patients in the afternoon. A pediatrician may schedule vaccinations on certain days of the week. Special tests like sigmoidoscopies may be scheduled one morning a week. Advantages to clustering include maximum use of special equipment, ease in maintaining control of the schedule, the ability to provide many patients with information about their particular situation at the same time, and efficient use of employees' time.

Wave and Modified Wave

Outpatient medical facilities may use the **wave scheduling system** or modify the wave system in ways that work for their particular specialty. With the wave system, several patients are scheduled the first 30 minutes of each hour. They are seen in the order that they arrive at the office. The second half of each hour is left open. This technique works well in large facilities with several departments giving medical care. For example, several patients may arrive for a 9:00 appointment, be seen by the physician, be sent to the laboratory for blood work, and return to the physician 20 minutes later. The physician has the second part of the hour to see these patients after their testing. That second half of each hour is used as a buffer or extra time that can be used for emergencies, walk-ins, returning phone calls, and tasks other than direct patient care. Modifications to this system may include seeing new patients who will have complete physical examinations on the hour with three or four rechecks scheduled on the half hour. For example, a 75-year-old man being seen for a complete physical would be scheduled at 9:00 A.M., with a 22-year-old being seen for a follow-up of strep throat and a 6-year-old being seen for recheck of an ear infection scheduled at 9:30 A.M.

Fixed Scheduling

Fixed scheduling is the most commonly used method. It divides each hour into increments of 15, 30, 45, or 60 minutes. The reason for each patient's visit will determine the length of time assigned. Patients who are late or do not report for their appointment can cause major problems in the flow of the day. It is helpful to schedule chronically late patients at the end of the day. Another tactic is to tell the patient to arrive 30 minutes prior to the time you schedule.

Streaming

Streaming is a method that helps minimize gaps in time and backups. Appointments are given based on the needs of the individual patient. If a patient is being seen for a complete physical, 1 hour may be allotted. The next patient seen may need a blood pressure recheck, which would be allotted a 15-minute slot. Although this method ensures a smooth work flow, the medical assistant scheduling the appointment must understand the procedures and guidelines for deciding the time that should be allotted. Box 6-1 outlines examples of services and their probable time allotments.

Double Booking

With **double booking** two patients are scheduled for the same period with the same physician. This works well when patients are being sent for diagnostic testing because it leaves time to see both patients without keeping either one waiting unnecessarily.

Flexible Hours

Offices that operate with flexible hours are open at different times throughout the week. For example, Monday, Wednesday, and Friday office hours might be from 8 A.M. to 5 P.M., and Tuesday and Thursday office hours might be from 8 A.M. to 8 P.M. Some offices may also be open on Saturdays for all or part of the day. Patients still have scheduled appointments, but this greater range of available appointment times better accommodates work and family schedules. Your main challenge with flexible hours is to determine which patients really need to be scheduled for these special times. For example, Saturday appointments may be reserved only for patients whose work schedules do not permit weekday appointments. Flexible hours are most often used by clinics, group practices, and family physicians.

Open Hours

A medical office that operates with open hours for patient visits is open for specified hours during the day or evening. Patients may arrive at any time during those hours to be seen by the physician in the order of their arrival; there are no scheduled appointments. This system is commonly seen in emergency walk-in clinics and eliminates patient complaints such as "I had an appointment at 2 P.M. but had to wait until 3 P.M. to be seen." Open-hour scheduling, however, has some clear disadvantages:

- Effective time management is almost impossible.
- The facilities may be overloaded at some times and empty at other times.
- Charts must be pulled and prepared as each patient arrives.

So that patients are seen in the order in which they arrive, some offices use sign-in sheets. Some sign-in sheets require that patient's record the reason for their visit. The use of sign-in sheets is prohibited under the Health Insurance Portability and Accountability Act of 1996 regulations, as discussed in Chapter 5. Effective April 2003, sign-in sheets are considered a breach of confidentiality, since patients signing the sheet can see the names and medical conditions of other patients.

Checkpoint Question

2. What are the three systems that can be used for scheduling patient office visits?

FACTORS THAT AFFECT SCHEDULING

Patients' Needs

People express their needs in varied ways. A patient might be feeling uncertainty, embarrassment, shyness, or fear. With a patient in an emotional state, even the slightest real or imagined miscommunication can lead to negative response from the patient. Be courteous and maintain your professionalism.

Before scheduling an appointment, you should determine:

- Why the patient wishes to see the physician
- How long the patient has had the symptoms
- Whether the problem is **acute** (abrupt onset) or **chronic** (longstanding)
- The most convenient time for the patient to come in (e.g., early morning or evenings)
- Any special transportation services the patient requires (community or hospital van services operate only during certain hours)
- Whether the patient needs to see other office staff
- Any third-party payers' constraints
- Receipt of necessary documentation for referrals when the patient is enrolled in a program that requires such documentation (third-party payers are discussed further in Chapter 16)

Control of the appointment schedule is your responsibility. Strive to accommodate a patient's requests whenever possible, but not if it will overload the schedule. For example, if a patient requests a 2 P.M. appointment this Tuesday and you already have patients in that time slot, politely explain that you cannot schedule the appointment then unless you have a cancellation. You might offer a later time on Tuesday or on another day at 2 P.M.. You can also ask if the patient wishes to be put on a move-up list to be notified if an earlier appointment opens up. In other words, you control the schedule. Do not let it control you.

Providers' Preferences and Needs

The management of the practice depends on the desires and requirements of the providers working in it. Providers in a medical practice may include the physician, nurse practitioner, or physician's assistant. Some providers often run behind schedule; others are extremely punctual. Recognize your providers' habits and communicate any problems to a supervisor. The physician may allow you to adjust the schedule to accommodate his or her habits. If you are employed to assist the physician with clinical duties (e.g., removing sutures, performing electrocardiograms, giving injections), the schedule can be adjusted to accommodate a larger number of patients while still allowing the provider enough time to give each patient personal attention.

As discussed earlier, the physician also needs time to receive and return telephone calls, review laboratory and pathology reports, dictate chart notes or correspondence, and so on. If your physician is on the staff of a teaching hospital, you may also have to block off time for clinic conferences and other teaching duties.

The physician will need time to meet with unscheduled office visitors other than patients. Such visitors might include other physicians and sales representatives from medical supply or pharmaceutical companies. You should determine in advance how the physician wants you to handle these visitors. For example, the physician may want to be notified immediately if another physician comes to the office. With salespersons or pharmaceutical representatives, however, the physician may have another staff member meet with them or may request that an appointment be scheduled for a more convenient time.

Physical Facilities

The physical facilities available in the medical office will affect the management of the appointment schedule. Consider these points: How many providers use the facility? How many examination rooms are there? Is it necessary to resterilize instruments between procedures, or is more than one set of instruments available? You would not want to schedule two sigmoidoscopies at the same time, for example, if the office has only one appropriately equipped examination room. You must thoroughly understand the requirements for procedures to be performed in the office to schedule appointments accurately.

Checkpoint Question

3. What are three factors that can affect appointment scheduling?

SCHEDULING GUIDELINES

Whether the patient is making an appointment by telephone or in person, be pleasant and maintain a helpful attitude. Always write the patient's telephone number on the schedule when making appointments. Emergencies and delays are unavoidable, and schedule corrections can be made quickly if the telephone number is handy. Leave some time slots open during each day, perhaps 15 to 20 minutes in the morning and in the afternoon. Invariably problems will arise (e.g., late patients, emergencies) and disrupt the regular appointment schedule. These open blocks can allow the schedule to catch up. Also, patients calling for appointments will not appreciate being told that no time is available for 2 or 3 weeks. Open slots can be used to schedule brief appointments as needed. Procedure 6-1 describes the steps for scheduling appointments for new patients.

New Patients

Most appointments for new patients are made by telephone. The information you exchange at this encounter is crucial, and entering the patient's data accurately is imperative. The first encounter with a new patient is discussed in Procedure 6-1.

Procedure 6-1

Making an Appointment for a New Patient

Steps	Reason
1. Obtain as much information as possible from the patient, such as: • Full name and correct spelling • Mailing address (not all offices require this) • Day and evening telephone numbers • Reason for the visit • Name of the referring person	To stay on schedule, you must allow enough time for the appointment. This information will help determine appointment needs and save time at the first visit.
2. Explain the payment policy of the practice. Most offices require payment at the time of an initial visit. Instruct patients to bring all pertinent insurance information.	Patients must understand this policy if they are to follow it.
3. Be sure patients know your office location; give concise directions if needed. You may also want to give patients an idea of how long they can expect to be at the office.	Helps patients arrive on time and lets them budget their time.
4. To avoid violating confidentiality, ask the patient if it is permissible to call at home or at work.	Some patients are sensitive about messages left on an answering machine or given to a coworker.
5. Before ending the call, confirm the time and date of the appointment. Say, "Thank you for calling, Mr. Brown. We look forward to seeing you on Tuesday, December 10, at 2 P.M."	Repeating the appointment time will ensure that effective communication has taken place and increase the likelihood that the patient will be there on time.
6. Always check your appointment book to be sure that you have placed the appointment on the correct day in the right time slot.	Failure to record every appointment in the proper location can cause overbooking, frustrated physicians and staff, and irate patients.
7. If the patient was referred by another physician, you may have to call that physician's office before the appointment for copies of laboratory work, radiology and pathology reports, and so on. Remember, the patient must give authorization to release medical documents (see Chapter 8). Give this information to the physician prior to the patient's appointment.	Having the necessary information will eliminate ordering of tests that have already been done and will give the physician the tools to care for the patient.

An office brochure can be mailed to the patient in advance of the appointment. Some offices send new-patient forms to be filled out and brought in at the appointment. When scheduling an appointment for a new patient, follow these guidelines:

1. Allow an adequate amount of time for the appointment. To do so, obtain as much information as possible from the patient:
   • Full name and correct spelling
   • Mailing address
   • Day and evening telephone numbers
   • Reason for the visit
   • Name of the referring physician or individual
   • Responsible party and third party payer (insurance plan)
2. Explain the office's payment policy. Most offices require full or partial payment at the time of an initial visit, and patients must understand this policy. Instruct patients to bring all pertinent insurance information.
3. Be sure patients know your office location; if needed, give them concise directions. You may also want to tell patients how long they can expect to be at the office.
4. Some patients are sensitive about messages left on an answering machine or given to a coworker. To avoid violating confidentiality, ask the patient if it is permissible to call at home or at work and include this information in the patient's chart.
5. Before ending the call, confirm the time and date of the appointment. You might say, "Thank you for calling Mr. Brown. We look forward to seeing you on Tuesday, December 10, at 2 P.M."
6. Always check your appointment system or book to be sure that you have placed the appointment on the correct day in the right time slot.
7. If the patient was referred by another physician, you may need to call that physician's office in advance of the appointment for copies of laboratory work, radiology and pathology reports, and so on. Remember, the patient must give authorization to release medical documents (see Chapter 8). Give these reports to the physician prior to the patient's appointment.

Established Patients

Established patients will be given return appointments when necessary. Most return appointments are made before the patient leaves the office. Procedure 6-2 describes the steps for scheduling a return appointment.

Procedure 6-2

Making an Appointment for an Established Patient

Steps	Reason
1. Determine what will be done at the return visit. Check your appointment book or computer system before offering an appointment.	If a specific examination, test, or scan is to be performed, you will want to avoid scheduling two patients for the same examination at the same time.
2. Offer the patient a specific time and date. Avoid asking the patient when he or she would like to return, as this can cause indecision.	Give the patient a choice, and if neither time is convenient, offer another specific time and date. Giving a patient a choice is good practice. "Mrs. Chang, we can see you next Tuesday, the 15th, at 3:30 P.M. or Wednesday, the 16th, at 9:00 A.M."
3. Write the patient's name and telephone number in the appointment book or enter it in the computer.	Writing the phone number in the appointment book or making a notation in the computer will give you a quick reference if you need to call the patient to change the appointment.
4. Transfer the pertinent information to an appointment card and give it to the patient. Repeat aloud the appointment day, date, and time to the patient as you hand over the card (Fig. 6-4).	Repeating the information reinforces the patient's memory and helps ensure that the appointment will be kept.
5. Double-check your book or computer to be sure you have not made an error.	Errors in appointments waste the patient's, staff's, and physician's time.
6. Whether in person or on the phone, end your conversation with a pleasant word and a smile.	A smile always feels good to a patient who may be apprehensive about needing to return to the doctor.

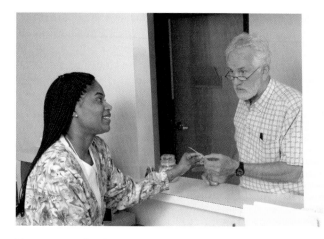

F IGURE 6 – 3. Photograph of a medical assistant handing a patient an appointment card.

When making a return appointment, follow these guidelines:

1. Carefully check your appointment book or screen before offering an appointment time. If a specific examination, test, or x-ray is to be performed on the return visit, avoid scheduling two patients for the same examination at the same time.
2. Offer the patient a specific time and date. For example, you might say, "Mrs. Hernandez, I have next Tuesday, the 15th, available at 3:30 P.M." (Avoid asking the patient when he or she would like to return, as this can elicit indecision.) If the offered appointment is not convenient, offer another specific time and date.
3. Write the patient's name and telephone number in the appointment book or enter in the information on the appointment screen.
4. Transfer the pertinent information to an appointment card and give it to the patient. Computerized systems print an appointment card. Repeat aloud the appointment day, date, and time to the patient as you hand over the card (Fig. 6-3).
5. Double-check your book or screen to be sure you have not made an error.
6. End your conversation with a pleasant word and a smile.

PREPARING A DAILY OR WEEKLY SCHEDULE

In most offices, as medical assistant you are responsible for preparing a daily and weekly schedule of appointments. Make a copy for the providers and other office staff members. When there are changes in the schedule, ensure that corrections are made on all copies. Place the next day's schedule on the physician's desk before he or she leaves for the day. Give the next week's schedule to the physician before he or she leaves on Friday. Schedules should include not only patients' appointments but also hospital rounds, surgeries, meetings, and any personal engagements on the schedule. Computer systems print a daily or weekly schedule, but you must remember to make changes manually as the day progresses.

PATIENT REMINDERS

Offices use various kinds of reminders to tell a patient about an appointment that should be made or to remind them that an appointment has been made on a specific date and time. These reminders are the appointment card, the telephone call, and the mailed card.

Appointment Cards

An appointment card is given to the patient when he or she leaves the office. It should have the following information:

- Patient's name
- Day, date, and time of the return visit
- Physician's name and telephone number

If the patient requires a series of appointments, try to make them on the same day of the week and at the same time of day. This will make it easier for the patient to remember the appointments. Unless your appointment card allows you to list the complete series of appointments, however, give the patient a card for the next appointment only and repeat this procedure after each subsequent visit. When the patient has to save several cards, they can easily be lost or cause confusion. If using a manual system, write on the card with ink so that it cannot be altered. Computer appointment scheduling software provides appointment cards that can be printed on special perforated paper.

Telephone Reminders

All new patients and patients with appointments scheduled in advance should receive a telephone reminder the day before their appointment. Computer systems can place the call to the programmed number and remind the patient of the appointment with a prerecorded message. Remember, do not call a patient at work or leave a message unless you have been given permission to do so. Make the telephone reminder simple. Identify your office, yourself, and state the date and time of the appointment. For example, you might say, "This is Ms. Palmer from Dr. Reid's office. I'm calling to confirm your appointment for tomorrow, Thursday, February 10, at 3:30 P.M." Unless the patient has a question, then say, "Thank you and good-bye." This reminder helps jog the patient's memory, and if the patient must cancel or reschedule an appointment, you will have time to fill the slot. Keep a list with the names and phone numbers of patients who have asked to be called or who need to be seen sooner than their next appointment. This list may be called a cancellation list, a waiting list, or a move-up list. Make a notation on the

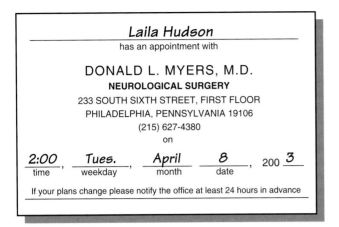

FIGURE 6-4. Sample reminder postcard.

appointment schedule, such as confirmed, left message, or no answer.

Mailed Reminder Cards

Some offices send reminder cards instead of making phone calls. Reminder cards are also used to remind patients who could not be reached by phone that it is time to keep an upcoming scheduled appointment. These should be mailed at least a week before the date of the appointment. In addition, reminder cards are sent after a set period since a patient's last appointment. Reminder cards are often used to alert patients to the need for annual examinations (e.g., Pap smears, mammograms, prostate examinations).

To handle this kind of reminder, keep a supply of preprinted postcards in the office (Fig. 6-4). The cards should have a simple one- or two-sentence message, such as,

---

Box 6-2

A TICKLER FILE CAN TICKLE YOUR MEMORY

A **tickler file** helps remind you to do something by a certain time in the future. It can be something as simple as a card file box (like a recipe box) or an accordion folder with insert guides in chronological order. The guides may be in weekly or monthly divisions. Put patient appointment reminder cards in the appropriate location in the file. Check the file each week or month, depending on the divisions, then mail the reminders.

Medical office computer software often offers help with patient reminders. With a search of the database, a report of every female patient over age 50, for example, could be generated. Some systems even generate patient reminders based on preprogrammed criteria.

"According to our records, you are due for your annual physical. If you would kindly call the office, we will be glad to arrange an appointment for you." The physician's name, address, and telephone number should be printed on the card. Place the card in a tickler file (Box 6-2) and mail it at the appropriate time. Some medical management software packages produce a list that can be used to alert patients of necessary services.

Checkpoint Question

4. What are the three types of patient reminders?

ADAPTING THE SCHEDULE

Emergencies

When a patient calls with an emergency (Fig. 6-5), your first responsibility is to determine whether the problem can be treated in the office. The office should have a policy for evaluation of the situation. The word **STAT** is used in the medical field to indicate that something should be done immediately (Box 6-3). You also should have a list of appropriate questions to ask the patient, such as "Are you having chest pain? Are you having difficulty breathing? How long have you had the symptoms?" (Box 6-4). When several symptoms occur together, they may indicate a particular problem. This group of complaints is referred to as a **constellation of symptoms**. One group of symptoms found to indicate a certain disorder is severe right lower quadrant pain, nausea, and fever. A physician who sees this constellation of symptoms considers appendicitis.

Patients Who Are Acutely Ill

Patients who are acutely ill often have serious though not life-threatening conditions. These patients need to be seen as soon as possible but not necessarily on that same day.

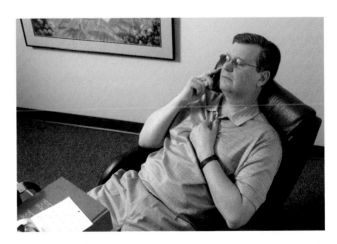

FIGURE 6-5. Patient at home making an emergency call.

Box 6-3

WHEN DOES THE PATIENT NEED TO BE SEEN NOW?

When the patient calls with any of the following complaints:

- Shortness of breath
- Severe chest pain
- Uncontrollable bleeding
- Large open wounds
- Potential accidental poisoning
- Bleeding in a pregnant patient
- Injury to a pregnant patient
- Shock
- Serious burns
- Severe bleeding
- Any symptoms of internal bleeding (dark, tarry stools; discoloration of the skin)

Note: Remember to check with the physician for proper procedures concerning triage.

Obtain as much information about the patient's medical problem as you can so your message to the physician will allow him or her to decide how soon the patient should be seen. Place the chart with a note in the location selected by the physician, and tell the patient you will call back as soon as the physician makes a decision.

Walk-in Patients

Walk-in patients are those who arrive at the office without a scheduled appointment and expect to see the physician that day. Typically, the physician will have a set protocol, or prescribed list of steps, for handling such situations. In general, you must first determine the reason for the walk-in. Patients with medical emergencies need to be seen immediately. Other patients can be asked to have a seat in the waiting room while you inform the physician of the patient's pres-

Box 6-4

COULD IT BE A HEART ATTACK?

When a patient calls complaining of the following constellation of symptoms, you should assume that this is a potential heart attack:

- Shortness of breath
- Chest pain
- Arm or neck pain
- Nausea and/or vomiting

Studies have shown that in women, early symptoms of a heart attack are different from those in men. These symptoms include jaw, neck, and back pain and severe fatigue. Keep this in mind when questioning the patient.

Call 911 and stay on the line with the patient. Do not advise the patient to drive to the hospital. Follow office policies for such an emergency.

ence. The physician can then make the decision to see the patient or not.

If the patient is to be seen, explain that you will work him or her into the schedule as soon as possible for a brief examination. When the patient leaves the office, you might apologize for the delay, then ask the patient to schedule an appointment for the next visit.

If the physician decides not to see a walk-in patient, you will have to ask the patient to schedule an appointment and to return later.

Late Patients

Patients who are late cause problems in the schedule. You should gently but firmly apologize for any delay but tell the patient, "You were late and Dr. Wooten is seeing another patient now. The doctor should be able to see you in about 15 minutes." Patients who are routinely late should be politely advised that "according to our office policy, patients who are more than 15 minutes late will have to be rescheduled." Some offices have found that scheduling the habitually late patient at the end of the day is helpful. In addition, ask patients to call the office if they know ahead of time they are going to be late.

Physician Delays

Of course, sometimes the physician calls in to say he or she has been delayed and will be in the office later. If office hours have not yet begun, call patients with appointments scheduled early, and give them the option of coming in later in the day or rescheduling the appointment for another day. If patients are waiting in the office, inform them immediately if the physician will be delayed. For example, you might say, "Dr. Franklin has been delayed and will probably be 20 to 30 minutes late. Would you like to wait, or would you prefer to reschedule for another time?" Always keep your patients informed; most people will understand if they know you have not ignored or forgotten them. Most patients appreciate the fact that the physician would also be available to them in an emergency. If you reschedule an appointment, note in the patient's chart the reason for the cancellation or rescheduling.

Missed Appointments

A missed appointment, or no-show, occurs when a patient neglects to keep an appointment and does not notify the office. When this happens, call the patient to try to determine why the appointment was missed and to reschedule for another time. If you are unable to reach the patient by telephone, send a card asking the patient to call the office to reschedule. Note in the patient's chart the missed appointment and that you have either rescheduled the appointment or mailed a card to schedule another appointment. Even if the facility does not routinely remind patients of appointments, be sure to call and remind habitually late patients the day before the appointment.

Box 6-5

CHARTING EXAMPLE

05/12/03–1530

Mrs. Parrish was called regarding missing scheduled appointment for today at 9:30A.M. Patient said she forgot about the appointment. Appointment was rescheduled for 05/14/03 at 10:00A.M. Patient was advised of the need to have regular prenatal checkups. Patient verbalized understanding. Dr. Wong was notified that appointment was missed and rescheduled.—Norreen Brooks, CMA

Continued failure to keep appointments should be brought to the attention of the physician, who may want to call the patient personally (particularly if the patient is seriously ill) or send a letter expressing concern for the patient's welfare. In extreme cases, the physician may choose to terminate the physician–patient relationship. See Chapter 2 for the proper procedure for this action. Notations of all actions and copies of any letters sent to the patient should become a permanent part of the individual's medical record. Box 6-5 is a sample of a chart note.

CANCELLATIONS

Cancellations by the Office

You may have to cancel a patient's appointment if the physician is ill, has an emergency, or has personal time off. Patients who must be rescheduled need not be told the specific reason for the physician's absence. These cancellations should be noted in the patient's medical record.

When you have advance notice, write a letter to patients with appointments you must cancel, indicating that the physician will be away from the office but will return by a certain date. Patients should be alerted to cancellations a week before their appointments. Ask the patient to call the office to reschedule. If you have to cancel on the day of the appointment, call the patient and explain. For example, you might say, "Dr. Flora has been called out of the office unexpectedly. Would it be convenient to reschedule your appointment for sometime next week?" If the patient arrives at the office before you can contact him or her, apologize and politely explain the situation. Most patients will be understanding. When a physician is unavailable for an extended period, another physician must cover the practice or be on call. Everyone in the office should have a list of names and addresses of on-call physicians, and you should give this information to your patients, according to your office policy. When a locum tenens, or substitute physician, is employed, the office appointments will not be interrupted (see Chapter 2).

Cancellations by the Patient

When a patient cancels an appointment, ask the reason for the cancellation and mark it on your appointment schedule and in the patient's chart. Offer to reschedule at another time. If the patient is being seen for a continuing problem, be sure he or she understands the necessity for the follow-up visit. If the patient wants to call back for an appointment, make a note to yourself to check on the call-back in a few days. If a patient cancels appointments frequently, bring this to the physician's attention.

If a patient cancels an appointment and you have a full schedule, no action is needed. If your schedule is light, however, refer to your move-up list to try to fill the vacancy.

MAKING APPOINTMENTS FOR PATIENTS IN OTHER FACILITIES

Referrals and Consultations

When the provider requests assistance from another physician in **consultation** or makes a **referral** to another physician for the patient, make certain that the referral meets the requirements of any third-party payers. Managed care companies like HMOs have strict requirements regarding **precertification** and documentation for referrals to specialists and other facilities. (See Chapter 16.) Be sure the physician you are calling is on the preferred provider list for the patient's insurance company. Patients should be given a choice when being referred to a specialist.

When calling another physician's office for an appointment for your patient (Procedure 6-3), provide the following information:

- Physician's name and telephone number
- Patient's name, address, and telephone number
- Reason for the referral
- Degree of urgency
- Whether the patient is being sent for consultation or referral (see Box 6-6 for an explanation of the terms referral and consultation)

Record in the patient's chart the time and date of the call and the person who received your call. Tell the person you are calling that you wish to be notified if your patient does not keep the appointment. If this occurs, be sure to tell the physician and enter this information in the patient's record.

Write the name, address, and telephone number of the referral doctor on your office stationery and include the date and time of the appointment. Give or mail this information to your patient. The patient may call the referring physician to make his or her own appointment. If this is the situation, ask the patient to call you with the appointment date and document it in the chart.

Procedure 6-3

Making an Appointment for a Referral to Another Provider

Steps	Reason
1. Make certain that the requirements of any third-party payers are met.	Some third-party payers require that referrals be precertified. Preexisting conditions may not be covered for referral. Most companies require that only the patient's primary care physician (PCP) or gatekeeper make referrals. It is important to research each situation. Telephone numbers for precertification and questions will be printed on the back of the insurance card.
2. Refer to the preferred provider list for the patient's insurance company. Allow the patient to choose a provider from the list.	Managed care companies have strict requirements for precertification and documentation for referrals (see Chapter 16). If there is more than one provider with the same qualifications, the patient should always be given a choice.
3. Have the following information available when you make the call: • Physician's name and telephone number • Patient's name, address, and telephone number • Reason for the call • Degree of urgency • Whether the patient is being sent for consultation or referral	The referred or consulting physician's office needs to know these things to serve the patient well.
4. Record in the patient's chart the time and date of the call and the name of the person who received your call.	This is necessary for proper documentation of the patient's care.
5. Tell the person you are calling that you wish to be notified if your patient does not keep the appointment. If this occurs, be sure to tell your physician and enter this information in the patient's record.	This is necessary for proper documentation of the patient's care.
6. Write down the name, address, and telephone number of the doctor you are referring your patient to and include the date and time of the appointment. Give or mail this information to your patient.	It is important that the patient have a reminder so the appointment will be kept.
7. If the patient is to call the referring physician to make the appointment, ask the patient to call you with the appointment date, then document this in the chart.	Recording the appointment information in the patient's chart completes the transaction and proves that the physician's order was carried out.

Diagnostic Testing

Sometimes, patients are sent for diagnostic testing or treatment at another facility. Such testing includes laboratory tests, radiology, computed tomography, magnetic resonance imaging, and nuclear medicine studies. These appointments are usually made while the patient is still in the office. Before scheduling, determine the exact test or tests the physician requires and how soon the results are needed. (Be sure to indicate to the facility if the results are needed immedi-

Box 6-6

REFERRAL OR CONSULTATION?

It is important to know the difference between a referral and a consultation. According to the coding guidelines in the *Current Procedural Coding Terminology*, a consultation is a request for the opinion of a colleague. A letter is provided to the referring physician by the consultant and contains the consulting physician's impression and recommendations for the patient, but the patient returns to the referring physician for treatment. For example, an orthopedist may send a patient with rheumatoid arthritis to a rheumatologist for medication management, but the orthopedist will continue the patient's care based on the rheumatologist's recommendations.

A referral usually involves a specialist and requires that the patient's care be transferred to that specialist. For example, a patient may see a physician for an ingrown toenail but be referred to a podiatrist for care.

ately, or STAT.) Also, check with the patient for any time restrictions he or she may have. Give the facility the patient's name, address, telephone number, the exact test or tests required, and any other special instructions from the physician. Give the patient a laboratory or x-ray referral slip with the time and date of the appointment and the name, address, and telephone number of the outside facility.

Some laboratory studies or x-ray tests require advance preparation by the patient. Give your patient a written and verbal explanation of the required preparation, and be sure he or she understands the importance of following the instructions. On the patient's chart, note the name of the outside facility and the date and time of the appointment. Also place a reminder in your tickler file or on your appointment schedule to be sure the test results are received as requested.

Surgery

You also assist with the scheduling of procedures in a hospital operating room or an outpatient surgical facility. Determine the patient's need for precertification with the insurance carrier. You may have to call the number on the back

ñ Spanish Terminology

¿A qué se debe su visita?	Why do you need to see the doctor?
¿Desde cuándo se siente mal?	How long has this being going on?
¿Prefiere la cita en la mañana o en la tarde?	Would you prefer morning or afternoon?
Llamo para recordarle su cita.	I am calling to remind you of your appointment.
Le daré una cita para que vea al Doctor nuevamente.	I will give you an appointment to return to see the doctor.
Para su próxima visita, por favor traiga su tarjeta del seguro y todas las medicinas que esté tomando.	Please bring your insurance card and medicine bottles with you for your appointment.

Días de la semana	Days of the week	Horas del día	Times of the Day
Domingo	Sunday	A la una	One o'clock
Lunes	Monday	El medio pasado uno	1:30
Martes	Tuesday	Dos en punto	2:00
Miércoles	Wednesday	Son las dos y media	2:30
Jueves	Thursday	Tres en punto	3:00
Viernes	Friday	Son las tres y media	3:30
Sábado	Saturday	Siete en punto	7:00
		Son las siete y media	7:30
		Ocho en punto	8:00
		Son las ocho y media	8:30
		Nueve en punto	9:00
		Son las nueve y media	9:30

of the patient's insurance card for a precertification number. Call the participating facility chosen by the patient and specify the time and date the physician has requested. The operating facility will need to know the exact procedure, the amount of time needed, the type of anesthesia required, and any other special instructions your physician may have. The facility will also need the patient's name, age, address, telephone number, insurance information, and the precertification number if required.

If the hospital has supplied your office with preadmission forms, give a copy to the patient and make sure he or she understands the need to complete and return the form in a timely manner. Follow the policies of the surgical facility regarding preadmission testing, which may include laboratory studies, x-rays, or autologous blood donation (donation of a person's own blood in advance). Write down all appointment dates, times, and locations for the patient and be certain he or she understands where to go and when.

Finally, note in the patient's record the name of the operating facility and the date and time the surgery is scheduled. You may also need to arrange for hospital admission by providing the same information to the hospital admitting department.

Checkpoint Question

5. What information should be readily available when calling to schedule a patient for surgery in another facility?

WHEN THE APPOINTMENT SCHEDULE DOES NOT WORK

No appointment schedule runs smoothly all the time, and an occasional glitch is to be expected. If, however, you find that your schedule is chaotic nearly every day, you should determine the cause. Evaluate the schedule over time, generally 2 to 3 months. For example, make a list of all patients seen, their arrival times, the amount of time they spent with the physician, the time they left, and the amount of time needed to perform each examination or treatment. Since the work flow of the office affects every staff member, involve all employees in your study.

Office meetings are an ideal way to identify scheduling problems. Your evaluation may reveal that many of your patients are arriving late or that you have not allotted enough time for certain procedures. Sometimes, a habitually delayed physician is the problem. You may find that too many staff people are making appointments. If this is the case, you can assign only one staff person to handle all scheduling. Some problems may never be completely solved. If they are identified, however, you can often make adjustments to avoid causing frustration for both patients and office personnel.

CHAPTER SUMMARY

The outpatient medical facility can be chaos without an efficient appointment system. Moving patients through the facility while treating each person equally and thoroughly is one of the biggest challenges in the medical office. It is difficult for a busy practice to run smoothly all of the time. You need structure, but you must be flexible. Available times, equipment and room usage, and personnel coverage must be considered when finding just the right formula for a well-run and efficient office.

The goals of the outpatient medical facility are to provide quality patient care and maintain financial stability. To reach those goals, an office must have a plan for the efficient scheduling and carrying out of the daily activities. Appointment scheduling systems include manual systems using appointment books and computerized systems that render helpful reports and daily activity sheets. The size of a practice, the number of physicians, the types of services, and so on are considered when establishing an appointment scheduling system. Sick patients calling to make appointments should be given priority, and there are established guidelines for determining the urgency of a patient's problem. Other functions, such as phone calls, reviewing records, and lunch breaks, are also scheduled into the daily activities of the office. An established protocol or list of steps should be in place to handle pharmaceutical representatives and other visitors to the office. As the medical assistant at the front desk, you will be one of the most important factors in the daily operation of the outpatient medical facility. As a medical assistant, you will make appointments, document encounters with patients that deal with appointments, and make referrals to other health care facilities. Learning the issues involved in successful appointment scheduling will help you make sure your facility runs smoothly.

Critical Thinking Challenges

1. Assume that you are the office manager in a physician's office. Create a policy and procedure for scheduling patients.
2. Sign-in sheets can cause a breach in patient confidentiality. What other methods could you use that would limit the potential for invasion of patient privacy?
3. You notice that patients typically wait 30 to 45 minutes past their scheduled appointment times because of the physician. How would you approach a physician who chronically runs late?

Answers to Checkpoint Questions

1. A matrix is established to indicate times of each day that are not available for patient appointments.

2. The three systems that can be used for patient office visits include scheduled appointments, flexible hours, and open hours.

3. The three factors that can affect scheduling are patients' needs, physicians' preferences, and the physical facilities.

4. The three types of reminders are appointment cards, telephone reminders, and mailed reminder cards.

5. When scheduling a patient for surgery, the following information is needed: demographic and insurance information, the patient's name, age, address, telephone number, precertification number (if required), diagnosis, surgery planned, and any special instructions.

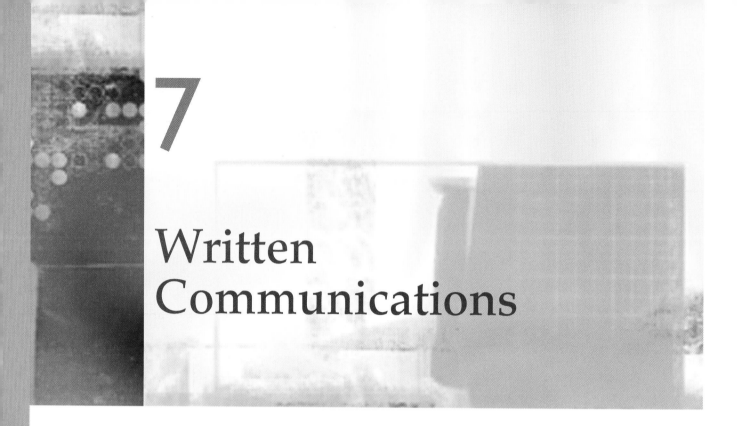

7

Written Communications

CHAPTER OUTLINE

PROFESSIONAL WRITING
Basic Grammar and Punctuation
Guidelines
Basic Spelling Guidelines
Guidelines for Medical Writing

LETTER DEVELOPMENT
Components of a Letter
Letter Formats
Writing a Business Letter
Types of Business Letters

MEMORANDUM DEVELOPMENT
Components of a Memorandum

**SENDING WRITTEN
COMMUNICATION**
Facsimile Machines
Electronic Mail
United States Postal Service
Other Delivery Options

**RECEIVING AND HANDLING
INCOMING MAIL**
Types of Incoming Mail
Opening and Sorting Mail
Annotation

**COMPOSING AGENDAS AND
MINUTES**

ROLE DELINEATION COMPONENTS

GENERAL: Communication Skills
- Adapt communications to individual's ability to understand
- Recognize and respond effectively to verbal, nonverbal, and written communications
- Utilize electronic technology to receive, organize, prioritize, and transmit information

GENERAL: Legal Concepts
- Perform within legal and ethical boundaries

ADMINISTRATIVE: Administrative Procedures
- Perform basic administrative medical assisting functions

CHAPTER COMPETENCIES

LEARNING OBJECTIVES
Upon successfully completing this chapter, you will be able to:
1. Spell and define the key terms
2. Discuss the basic guidelines for grammar, punctuation, and spelling
3. Describe six key guidelines for medical writing
4. Discuss the eleven key components of a business letter
5. Describe the three steps to writing a business letter
6. Describe the process of writing a memorandum
7. Discuss the various mailing options
8. Identify the types of incoming written communication seen in a physician's office
9. List the items that must be included in an agenda
10. Identify the items that must be included when typing minutes

PERFORMANCE OBJECTIVES
Upon completing this chapter, you will be able to:
1. Write a business letter
2. Write a memorandum
3. Address and send written communication
4. Open and sort mail

KEY TERMS

agenda	enclosure	margin	salutation
annotation	font	memorandum	semiblock
BiCaps	full block	proofread	template
block	intercaps		

THE ABILITY TO WRITE WELL IS an important skill for medical assistants. Your written communication must be clear, concise, and correct. Poorly written documents reflect negatively both on the physician's practice and on you. You will be responsible for creating and handling many types of written communication. Examples of written communication include letters, consultation reports, agendas, and minutes from meetings. Written communication may be sent or received through the postal service, facsimile machines, or electronic mail. This chapter discusses guidelines for professional writing, letter development, memorandum writing, sending written communication, handling incoming mail, and composing agendas and minutes.

PROFESSIONAL WRITING

Professional writing is different from writing letters to your friends or family members. The goal of professional writing is get information communicated in a concise, accurate, and comprehensible manner. Slang or idiomatic terms that are commonly used in writing letters to friends are not appropriate for business letters. For example, "Drop by and say hi" is not suitable for a professional letter, even if you know the recipient personally.

Basic Grammar and Punctuation Guidelines

Grammatical rules seem to be an endless maze of twists and turns! And each rule comes with numerous exceptions. You must be familiar with these rules and be able to apply them to your writing. Key rules of punctuation and grammar are listed in Box 7-1.

Basic Spelling Guidelines

Good spelling skills take time to acquire. Box 7-2 gives you basic tips for spelling. Many words sound exactly alike but are spelled differently and have different meanings. Be very careful with these words. Which of the following sentences has a spelling error?

* Wound cultures were taken from the left lower leg site.
* Wound cultures were taken from the left lower leg cite.

The first sentence is correct. Site and cite sound alike, and both are spelled correctly, but in the second sentence, the wrong word was used. These types of errors occur as a result of poor word usage and poor spelling. Appendix E lists words that are most likely to be misused or misspelled.

Guidelines for Medical Writing

Writing letters to medical professionals follows many of the standard guidelines. There are, however, some specific guidelines about which you need to be aware. They are discussed next.

Box 7-1

BASIC GRAMMAR AND PUNCTUATION TIPS

Punctuation

* Period (.)—Used at end of sentences and following abbreviations.
* Comma (,)—Used to separate words or phrases that are part of a series of three or more. The final comma before the "and" may be omitted. A comma can also be used after a long introductory clause or to separate independent clauses joined by and, but, yet, or, and nor.
* Semicolon (;)—Used to separate a long list of items in a series and to separate independent clauses not joined by a conjunction (e.g., and, but, or).
* Colon (:)—Used to introduce a series of items, to follow formal salutations, and to separate the hours from minutes indicating time.
* Apostrophe (')—Used to denote omissions of letters and to denote the possessive case of nouns.
* Quotation marks (" ")—Used to set off spoken dialogue, some titles (e.g., journal articles, newspaper articles, television and radio program episodes), and words used in a special way.
* Parentheses [( )]—Used to indicate a part of a sentence that is not part of the main sentence but is essential for the meaning of the sentence. Also used to enclose a number, for confirmation, that is spelled out in a sentence.
* Ellipsis (. . .)—Used in place of a period to indicate a prolonged continuation of a conversation or list. Also used to display individual items or to connect phrases that are loosely connected.
* Diagonal (/)—Used in abbreviations (c/o), dates (2003/2004), fractions (3/4), and to indicate two or more options (AM/FM).

Sentence Structure

* Avoid long, run-on sentences.
* A verb must always agree with its subject in number and person.
* Ensure that the proper pronoun (he or she) is used.
* Adjectives should be used when they add an important message. Don't overuse adjectives or adverbs. Remember, double negatives used in one sentence make the sentence positive.

Capitalization

* Capitalize the first word in a sentence, proper nouns, the pronoun "I," book titles, and known geographical names.
* Names of persons, holidays, and trademark items should be capitalized.
* Expressions of time (a.m. and p.m.) should not be capitalized.

BASIC SPELLING TIPS

When in doubt about the spelling of a word, always use a dictionary or a spell check. Keep in mind that a computer spell check will check for spelling but will not alert you to inappropriate word usage.

- Remember this rhyme: I comes before e, except after c, or when sounded like a as in neighbor and weigh. Examples: achieve, receive. (The exceptions are either, neither, weird, leisure, and conscience.)
- Words ending in -ie drop the e and change the i to y before adding -ing. Examples: die, dying; lie, lying.
- Words ending in -o that are preceded by a vowel are made plural by adding s. Example: studio, studios; trio, trios. Words ending in o that are preceded by a consonant form the plural by adding es. Examples: potato, potatoes; hero, heroes.
- Words ending in -y preceded by a vowel form the plural by adding s. Examples: attorney, attorneys; day, days. Words ending in -y that are preceded by a consonant change the y to i and add es. Examples: berry, berries; lady, ladies.
- The final consonant of a one-syllable word is doubled before adding a suffix beginning with a vowel. Examples: run, running; pin, pinning. If the final consonant is preceded by another consonant or by two vowels, do not double the consonant. Examples: look, looked; act, acting.
- Words ending in a silent -e generally drop the e before adding a suffix beginning with a vowel. Examples: ice, icing; judge, judging. The exceptions are dye, eye, shoe, and toe. The e is not dropped, however, in suffixes beginning with a consonant unless another vowel precedes the final e. Examples: pale, paleness; argue, argument.
- For all words ending in -c, insert a k before adding a suffix beginning with e, i, or y. Examples: picnic, picnicking; traffic, trafficker.

Accuracy

Many of the medical documents or letters that you will write contain information that requires precision, accuracy, and careful attention to details. Inaccurate information in some letters can lead to injury of a patient and lawsuits and can harm the physician's practice. Some of your letters will be placed in the patient's permanent medical record. Most letters will start with the physician asking you to draft a letter. He may or may not give you some notes to follow. Either way, your responsibility in typing the letter is to be as accurate as possible and to question anything about which you are unsure. Here are some examples of inaccuracy:

- You wrote, "The patient was started on the MVP chemotherapy regimen." The physician, however, had written "MVPP." These are two completely different regimens. MVP is used for treating lung cancer, and MVPP is used for Hodgkin's lymphoma.
- The physician wrote, "Patient was told to take Dristan Cold tablets." You rearranged the sentence, however, and wrote "The patient had a cold and was told to take Dristan tablets." Dristan Cold contains an antihistamine medication that plain Dristan does not. Never edit a physician's sentence unless you are sure that it will not affect the meaning.
- The physician wrote, "There is no reason for him to start radiation therapy at this time." You wrote, however, "There is reason for him to start radiation therapy at this time." The simple elimination of the word "no" completely changes the meaning of the sentence and can lead to errors in patient care.
- The physician wrote, "Hospitalization is needed because the patient continues to be violent." You typed, however, "Hospitalization is needed because the patient continues to be violet." The meaning of the sentence has been changed by the elimination of one "n" in violent.

Checkpoint Question

1. What are three consequences that could arise from inaccurate information in a business letter?

Spelling

Spell check in word processing programs can be a great asset, but it has limitations. Medical terminology spell check software should be added to your computer and be updated frequently.

You can add medical terms into your computer's spell check dictionary, but make sure that any word you add is spelled correctly! Spell checks can never be 100% stocked with all the needed terms, especially in the medical profession, as new technologies, medications, and treatments arise daily. Remember, spell check will not recognize words that are spelled correctly but misused. Which of the following sentences has a spelling error?

- The patient's mucus was yellow.
- The patient's mucous was yellow.

Mucus (noun) refers to a sticky secretion. Mucous is a type of membrane that secretes mucus. The second sentence is wrong. Here is another example:

- The physician received a plague.
- The physician received a plaque.

There is a big difference between plaque (commemorative item) and plague (bacterial disease)! Box 7-3 lists some commonly used medical words that can easily be misspelled or misused.

BOX 7-3

COMMONLY MISUSED OR MISSPELLED MEDICAL TERMS

- anoxia and anorexia
- aphagia and aphasia
- bowl and bowel
- emphysema and empyema
- fundus and fungus
- lactose and lactase
- metatarsals and metacarpals
- mucus and mucous
- parental and parenteral
- postnatal and postnasal
- pubic and pubis
- rubella and rubeola
- serum and sebum
- uvula and vulva

Capitalization

Pay particular attention to how words, names, and abbreviations are capitalized. Words or phrases with unusual capitalization are called **intercaps** or **BiCaps**. Never change how a word is capitalized unless directed to do so. Ask for clarification and mark the proof letter with a question mark for the physician to answer. For example m-BACOD is a very different medication regimen from M-BACOD. Here are some other common medical intercaps: pH, RhoGam, rPA, ReoPro, aVR.

Abbreviations and Symbols

Abbreviations and symbols can save time in long handwriting and with typing. Use abbreviations sparingly. When typing professional letters, you should spell out all abbreviations that are not universally accepted (e.g., P.M.). Become familiar with the abbreviations and symbols that are used where you work. Most offices have a policy listing their approved ones. Appendix D lists the most common abbreviations. Following are some ways abbreviations can be misinterpreted:

- The physician wrote, "The patient had good BS." You assumed that BS meant bowel sounds, so you typed "The patient had good bowel sounds," but the physician meant the abbreviation BS to mean breath sounds.
- Do not change < or > signs to *less than* or *greater than* unless you are sure of what the statement is saying. For example, "The patient will not be admitted to the hospital until her hemoglobin is less than 13." If you made a mistake and typed "greater than 13," confusion could occur.
- The symbols for male (♂) and female (♀) are commonly used in handwritten notes, but you should re-

place these symbols with words when writing a business or professional letter.

Plural and Possessive

Converting words to plural or possessive form can be tricky in English. Refer to your medical terminology book or a dictionary when you are unsure. Which of the following sentences is correct?

- The patient had multiple bullas.
- The patient had multiple bullae.

The second sentence is correct. *Bullae* means multiple blisters; *bulla* is one blister.

Numbers

In general, numbers one to ten should be spelled out, except when used with units of measurement (e.g., 5 mg), and those over 10 may be expressed as a numeral. Here are some important tips you will need to remember about numbers:

- Numbers referring to an obstetrical patient's medical history are not written out: "The patient is a gravida 3, para 2." Do not convert these numbers.
- Watch decimal point placement. There is a huge difference in medication between 12.5 mg and 1.25 mg.
- Double-check that you have not transposed numbers. For example, you typed, "The patient's red blood cell count was 5.1," but it was actually 1.5. A red blood cell count of 1.5 is incompatible with life.

WHAT IF

You are writing a letter and can't find out how to spell a word. What should you do?

Begin with your computer's spell check software. Spell check is generally under the heading Tools at the top of the screen. Most programs offer suggestions for the misspelled word. Be very careful that you do not select the wrong word on the suggestion list. You may also either look up the word in a dictionary or use an online dictionary. Two Web addresses that offer online dictionaries are given in this chapter. You may ask a colleague for spelling assistance. An option is to exchange the word for another word from a thesaurus. Be sure that the meaning of the sentence does not change if you use a different word. If these steps do not work, print the letter, mark the word with a question mark, and leave it for the physician. Never mail a letter with a spelling error.

- Roman numerals should never be changed to words. For example, "lead II of the patient's electrocardiogram" should never be changed to "lead two of the patient's electrocardiogram."
- Many health care professionals use military time. Time that is written in military style does not have to be changed if the recipient of the letter is familiar with it (doctors, nurses). If the letter is going to a patient or other person who may not be able to interpret it, however, either convert the time or express the standard time in parenthesis; for example, "The patient's next appointment is at 1430 hours (2:30 P.M.)." No colons are used in military time.
- Temperatures must always have the correct symbol for Celsius or Fahrenheit included (98.6°F or 37°C).
- Telephone numbers should include the area code in parentheses or followed by a hyphen, then the number with a hyphen. Add extensions to the number by placing a comma after the last digit of the number, then type Ext. and the number: (800) 555-0000, Ext. 6480. Periods may replace hyphens and parentheses: 800.555.0000.

LETTER DEVELOPMENT

Writing effective business letters is a skill that requires practice and careful attention to detail. To write a professional business letter, you must:

- Understand the components of a letter
- Use the correct letter format
- Ensure that the message is clear, concise, and accurate

These skills are described in the following sections.

Components of a Letter

A typical business letter has 11 components. We will explore each one, beginning at the top of the page. For easy reference, Figure 7-1 displays a sample business letter with these components marked.

1. *Letterhead.* The letterhead consists of the name of the practice or physician, address, telephone number, fax number, and sometimes the company logo. The letterhead is often embossed in color and centered on the top of the page. The letterhead may also be preset into a **template**. (Templates are discussed later in the chapter).
2. *Date.* The date includes the month, day, and year. It should be positioned two to four spaces below the letterhead. The date must be typed on only one line and abbreviations should not be used.
3. *Inside address.* The inside address refers to the name and address of the person to whom the letter is being sent. A nine-digit zip code should be used if available. The inside address is placed four spaces

down from the date unless the letter is being mailed with a window envelope and it will not be aligned correctly. Never abbreviate city or town names. States can be abbreviated. (See Appendix C for a list of abbreviations approved by the postal service.) Never abbreviate business titles (e.g., President, Chief Executive Officer). Here are some other points to remember:
- If the letter is going to a business, type the name of the addressee, followed by his or her title, name of the business on the next line, then the address.
- If the letter is being addressed to two or more people at different addresses, type the individual address block one line space under the other or place the addresses side by side.
- If the letter is going to two people at the same address but with different last names, type the woman's name on the first line, man's name on the second line, then the address. If the sexes are the same, do them in alphabetical order, followed by the address.
4. *Subject line.* The subject line, an optional component, is used to state the intent of a letter or to indicate what the letter is regarding. It is placed on the third line below the inside address and is written as Re: (an abbreviation for regarding) followed by the subject. For example, Re: Blood tests.
5. *Salutation.* The **salutation** is the greeting of the letter. It is placed two spaces down from the inside address or the subject line. Capitalize the first letter of each word in the phrase and end the phrase with a colon. It is permissible to eliminate the salutation if the letter is informal or if a subject line has been used. When writing to a physician, write out the word doctor. Here are some recommendations when writing salutations:
- If the letter is going to one person and the gender is known write, Dear Mr. Rogers.
- If the letter is going to one person and the gender is *not* known, write, Dear Pat Smith (use the person's first name).
- If the letter is going to a woman and a man with different last names, always address the woman first: Dear Ms. Ray and Mr. Oscar.
- If the letter is going to several people, place them in alphabetical order: Dear Mr. Andersen, Mr. Cats, Ms. Dart, and Mr. Raymond.
- To Whom It May Concern, Dear Sir, or Dear Madam should not be used.
6. *Body of the letter.* The body of the letter contains the message. It should be single-spaced with double spacing between the paragraphs. Here are some guidelines for writing the body of the letter:
- If the letter is more than one page long, try to avoid dividing a paragraph at the end of a page. If you must, leave at least two sentences at the bot-

Benjamin Matthews, M.D.
999 Oak Road, Suite 313
Middletown, Connecticut 06457
860-344-6000   ①

February 2, 2003   ②

Dr. Adam Meza
Medical Director   ③
Family Practice Associates
134 N. Tater Drive
West Hartford, Connecticut 06157

Re: Ms. Beatrice Suess ④

Dear Doctor Meza: ⑤

Thank you for asking me to evaluate Ms. Suess. I agree with your diagnosis of rheumatoid arthritis.
Her prodromal symptoms include vague articular pain and stiffness, weight loss and general malaise.
Ms. Suess states that the joint discomfort is most prominent in the mornings, gradually improving
throughout the day.

My physical examination shows a 40-year-old female patient in good health. Heart sounds normal,
no murmurs or gallops noted. Lung sounds clear. Enlarged lymph nodes were noted. Abdomen
soft, bowel sounds present, and the spleen was not enlarged. Extremities showed subcutaneous
nodules and flexion contractures on both hands.

⑥

Laboratory findings were indicative of rheumatoid arthritis. See attached laboratory data. I do
not feel x-rays are warranted at this time.

My recommendations are to continue Ms. Suess on salicylate therapy, rest and physical therapy.
I suggest that you have Ms. Suess attend physical therapy at the American Rehabilitation Center
on Main Street.

Thank you for this interesting consultation.

Yours truly,   ⑦

Benjamin Matthews, MD
                            ⑧
Benjamin Matthews, MD

BM/es ⑨

Enc. (2) ⑩

cc: Dr. Samuel Adams ⑪

FIGURE 7–1.   Components of a business letter. This letter is done in full block format and contains these elements: (1) letterhead, (2) date, (3) inside address, (4) subject line, (5) salutation, (6) body, (7) closing, (8) signature and typed name, (9) identification line, (10) enclosure, (11) copy.

tom of the first page. Use the widow and orphan control feature of your word processor program to prevent orphan lines from appearing.

- Tables and graphs should not be broken. They should appear on one page only.
- Web addresses and e-mail addresses should fit on one line and never be continued to another page.
- If the letter is more than one page long, page numbers should be used.
- Use a bulleted format to highlight key points for the reader. For example, "The possible side effects of this medication are:" (then list them vertically with a bullet symbol).
- Letterhead is used only on the first page of the letter. The second page should be the same quality paper as the letterhead. Start the second page with a continuation line (name of person the letter is going to and the date of the letter). Continue the letter two lines down from the continuation line. Your margins must be the same as those on page 1. Most templates type the continuation line for you.

7. *Closing.* The closing concludes the letter. Some common closings are: Sincerely, Yours truly, Regards, Respectfully, and Cordially yours. Only the first word is capitalized and a comma follows the phrase. Closings are placed two spaces down from the end of the letter. Never put the closing alone on a page.

8. *Signature and typed name.* The name of the person sending the document is typed four spaces below the closing, with the person's title typed directly below. The physician will read and sign the letter above the typed name. If you are instructed to sign the letter, sign the physician's name followed by a slash mark and your name, e.g., Susan James, MD/Raymond Smith, RMA.

9. *Identification line.* The identification line, an optional component, indicates who dictated the letter and who wrote it. It consists of abbreviations only. The initials of the person who dictated the letter are capitalized (generally the physician); the initials of the writer of the letter are in lower case (generally these will be yours). The identification line can also be called the reference line.

10. *Enclosure.* An **enclosure** is something that is included with a letter. It is abbreviated Enc. and is placed two spaces down from the identification line. The number of documents included is placed in parentheses; if only one document is included, just the abbreviation Enc. is used.

11. *Copy.* The abbreviation c is used to indicate that a duplicate letter has been sent. It is typed two spaces below the enclosure line. Usually, letters are copied to managers, supervisors, or to the physician who requested that the given information be dispersed.

Checkpoint Question

2. Whose address is typed as the inside address? What is the purpose of the salutation? What is the purpose of the identification line?

Letter Formats

There are three basic types of letter formats: *full block*, *semiblock*, and *block*. Office policy or the physician preference's will dictate which format you use.

Full Block

In **full block** format, each line is flush left. Full block is the most formal format and is most commonly used for professional letters. Figure 7-1 shows a letter in full block format.

Block

In **block** format, the date, subject line, closing, and signatures are flush right. All other lines are flush left (Fig. 7-2).

Semiblock

In **semiblock** format, the first sentence of each paragraph is indented five spaces, if done on a typewriter, or is tabbed, if done on a computer (Fig. 7-3). Semiblock is also referred to as modified block.

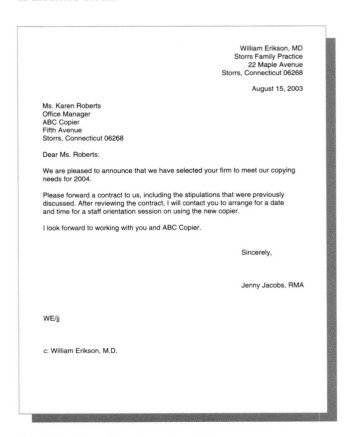

FIGURE 7-2. Sample block letter.

Elizabeth Jones, M.D.
750 East Street, Suite 205
Hialeah, Florida 33013
305-311-2666

June 12, 2003

Margaret Trent
18 Cambridge Street
Hialeah, Florida 33013

Dear Ms. Trent:

    As per our phone conversation, your blood glucose level remains elevated.
It is essential that we stabilize your blood sugar level.

    In order to achieve normal blood sugar levels, you must follow the enclosed
diet. A meeting with a Registered Dietitian can be arranged for you to discuss
any dietary concerns you may have.

    I am also enclosing patient education instructions for the use of a glucometer.
You must test your blood sugar every morning and keep a diary of your results.
Glucometers can be purchased from any pharmacy. If you need assistance in
using the glucometer, please contact Raymond Smith, CMA, at 555-6423.

    Presently, I do not wish to prescribe any medications. If we are unable to
get your blood sugar under control, I will prescribe an oral diabetic medication.

    Please call my office and schedule an appointment for the week of June 20
for a blood draw and a follow-up visit.

Sincerely,

Elizabeth Jones, M.D.

EJ/rs

enc. (2)

F I G U R E 7 – 3 .   *Sample semiblock letter.*

Writing a Business Letter

To create a professional business letter, follow these three steps: preparation, composition, and editing. Box 7-4 gives you some guidelines for starting to write a letter.

Preparation

Good preparation is a key element in writing professional business letters. Preparation consists of planning the content and the mechanics of the letter.

Mental Preparation. Before you begin to compose a letter, mentally prepare your message. You might start formulating the message by envisioning yourself talking to the person to whom you are sending the letter. Preparation offers three benefits:

1. It helps eliminate writer's block.
2. It gets you to focus on the message, not the mechanics (e.g., spelling, grammar, punctuation).
3. It enhances your organization.

Using cue cards or note cards will help ensure all the necessary information is covered in the letter.

Mechanics of the Letter. Before you begin to type the letter, select the appropriate *template*, *margin*, and *font*. A template

---

B o x   7 - 4

HOW TO START WRITING A LETTER

By determining the answers to these four questions, you can better prepare the message of your letter.

1. Who is my reader?

   It is very important that you use proper gender identification. Be especially careful with names that can be used for males or females (eg, Sam, Kelly, Ronnie, Alex, Tracy). Determine the reader's comprehension level. Letters to physicians will be more technical and will use medical terminology. Letters to patients will be less technical and use medical terminology sparingly.

2. What do I want my reader to do?

   This is your call to action; make it clear and specific. For example, you might write, "Please complete the enclosed insurance form (2 pages). Be sure to include all necessary information and sign your name. Place the form in the enclosed envelope and return it to our office by June 15, 2003." Avoid using "at your earliest convenience"; include a date for the required action. If possible, include a response mechanism, such as a self-addressed, stamped envelope.

3. What do I want to say?

   Briefly list the necessary information. To help you remember all of the necessary information, ask yourself who, what, where, when, why, and how.

4. How will I organize my message?

   Here are three basic ways that you can organize your message:

   - *Chronological:* Discuss items in a sequential manner, beginning with the earliest date and proceeding to the most recent date. For example, when discussing the physician's career, list his or her earlier experiences before the most recent career achievements.
   - *Problem oriented:* Let the reader know about a specific problem and provide instructions for correcting the problem. For example, if a patient's blood work came back with abnormal findings, a letter would be sent, identifying the problem (e.g., low hematocrit) and advising the patient on the possible causes, treatments, and follow-up procedures.
   - *Comparison:* Evaluate the effectiveness of two or more items. For example, as an office manager, you may have to write to the physician comparing two service contracts or two sample computer software packages.

Box 7-5

FONTS

Here are fonts that would be suitable for a business letter:
- This is 12-point Times New Roman.
- This is 10-point Times New Roman.
- This is 12-point Garamond.
- **This is 12-point Arial.**

Here are fonts and sizes that would not be appropriate:
- This is 8-point Times New Roman.
- **This is 12-point Colossalis Black.**
- **THIS IS 12-POINT COTTONWOOD.**
- This is 12-point Tekton.
- **This is 12-point impact.**

provides you with the skeleton of the letter. The key elements are already set and spaced correctly, so you just type in the pertinent information. Most computers have numerous letter templates or a letter wizard. These programs will make the process of letter writing easy, fast, and professional. You may use macros in your template to make repetitive tasks faster.

The **margin** is the blank space around the letter. A 1-inch margin is used for both left and right sides of the letter and the bottom. Margins are used to center the components of the letter in a standarized manner. If you select a template, your margins will be set for you.

Next, select the font. A **font** is the typeface; it affects the way words look and how easy it will be to read the letter. Choose a font that is easy to read and that is appropriate in size. Avoid cute or elegant fonts that can be difficult to read or see. The most common fonts used in business letters are Times New Roman, Garamond, and Arial. Box 7-5 gives you some examples of fonts and their sizes.

 Checkpoint Question

3. Before you begin to type a letter, name three mechanics that you need to select.

Composition

The goal of composition is to ensure that your message is transmitted clearly, concisely, and accurately to your reader. As you did during preparation, focus on the message, not on the mechanics.

A clear message ensures that your reader knows precisely what is expected; an unclear message leaves room for doubt.

Unclear: Please contact me.
Clear: Please contact me by Thursday, October 1.
Unclear: You need to make an appointment for blood work.

Clear: Call Temple Hospital laboratories (555-4010) and make an appointment for a blood glucose test on March 13.

A concise message is short and to the point. Wordy phrases with many adjectives should not be used.

Not concise: Please enclose a check in an envelope for exactly $50.
Concise: Please enclose a $50 check.

An accurate message includes the correct date, time, figures, and information. Inaccurate messages cause delays and confusion and can lead to poor public relations.

Editing

After you have composed the letter, edit it for both grammatical errors and factual information. Editing is a key step in making your letter a success. Editing entails two steps: proofreading and corrections.

Proofreading. Whenever possible, have a colleague **proofread** (read text and check for accuracy) your letter and provide constructive criticism. Be sure to maintain confidentiality. If you are using a computer, consider printing out a hard copy of your document for proofreading; some individuals find it difficult to proofread a document on the computer screen. Check for the following items:

- Accuracy of all information
- Clarity and conciseness
- Grammar
- Spelling
- Punctuation
- Paragraphs appropriate in length and limited to one subject
- Capitalization
- Logical organization and flow

Use proofreaders marks (Box 7-6) to speed up the editing process. These are standard marks used to indicate corrections. You should become familiar with the basic marks.

 Checkpoint Question

4. What is the purpose of proofreading?

Corrections. After making corrections, print a final copy of the letter. As discussed earlier in the chapter, a computer spell check should be used with caution, as it highlights misspelled words but not incorrectly used words.

Types of Business Letters

You will be asked to create and type various letters. Letters that you write will be sent to patients, insurance companies, other health care providers, pharmaceutical companies, and

Box 7-6

STANDARD PROOFREADER MARKS

ℱ or ℬ or ℐ   delete; take it out

◡   close up; print as one word

ℬ   delete and close up

∧ or > or ∧   caret; insert here ⟞ (something

insert a space

eq #   space evenly where indicated

stet   let marked text stand as set

tr   transpose; change order the

/   used to separate two or more marks and often as a concluding stroke at the end of an insertion

[set farther to the left

]   set farther to the right

⌒   set æ or fl as ligatures æ or fl

⸗   straighten alignment

‖   straighten or align

✗   imperfect or broken character

☐   indent or insert em quad space

ᑫ   begin a new paragraph

ⓢⓟ   spell out (set 5 lbs. as five pounds)

cap   set in capitals (CAPITALS)

sm cap or s.c.   set in small capitals (SMALL CAPITALS)

ℓc   set in lowercase (lowercase)

ital   set in italic (*italic*)

rom   set in roman (roman)

bf   set in boldface (**boldface**)

= or -/ or ⌒ or |H/   hyphen

$\frac{1}{N}$ or en or |N/   en dash (1965–72)

$\frac{1}{M}$ or em or |M/   em—or long—dash

∨   superscript or superior ($\overset{2}{\vee}$ as in πr^2)

∧   subscript or inferior ($\overset{2}{\wedge}$ as in H_2O)

◇ or ✗   centered ($\overset{\cdot}{\diamond}$ for a centered dot in $p \cdot q$)

⌃   comma

⌄   apostrophe

⊙   period

; or ;/   semicolon

: or ⊡   colon

∨∨ or ⌄⌄   quotation marks

(/)   parentheses

[/]   brackets

OK/?   query to author: has this been set as intended

⌐ or ⅃[1]   push down a work-up

⊘[1]   turn over an inverted letter

wf[1]   wrong font; a character of the wrong size or esp. style

[1] The last three symbols are unlikely to be needed in making proofs of photocomposed matter.

various businesses. Here are some common types of letters that you may write:

- Letters welcoming new patients to the practice
- Letters to patients regarding their test results
- Consultation reports to other health care professionals
- Workers' compensation letters verifying the patient's injury or treatment
- Justification or explanation of treatments to insurance companies
- Cover letters for transferring patients' records to another practice
- Clarification or explanation to patients regarding fees or billing concerns
- Thank you letters to sales representatives
- Physician changes for on-call schedules (generally sent to the hospital and covering physicians)
- Announcements of new services, hours, or office location changes.

MEMORANDUM DEVELOPMENT

A **memorandum** (often called a memo) is for communication within the office or with another department only; it is never sent to patients. It is less formal than a letter and is generally used for brief announcements.

Components of a Memorandum

A memorandum contains the standard elements in the following list. Use these guidelines to complete each element. Figure 7-4 shows a sample memorandum.

1. *Heading.* The word Memorandum is typed across the top of the page.
2. *Date.* Use the same rules for letters when typing the date for memorandums.
3. *To.* List the names of all recipients in either alphabetic or hierarchic order. If the memorandum is going to a particular group (e.g., all department managers, all employees), it can be addressed to the group.
4. *From.* List the name and title of the person sending the memorandum.
5. *Subject.* Insert a brief phrase describing the purpose of the memorandum.
6. *Body.* Write the message of the memorandum here.
7. *Copy (c).* Use the same rules as for letters when sending duplicate copies of memorandums.

Salutations and closings are not used in memorandums. All lines in a memorandum are justified left, and 1-inch margins are used. Writing a memorandum entails the same steps (preparation, composition, editing) as writing a business letter. The memorandum should be read and initialed by the physician before it is distributed. Your computer software will have a memorandum template.

Franklin Dermatology Center
123 Main Street
Rockfall, Kansas
913-755-2600

Memorandum

To: All Medical Assistants
From: Patty Stricker, Office Manager
Date: 12/03/03
Re: Holiday time

Please notify me by December 10 of any requests you have for taking time off during Christmas or New Year's. Remember that holiday requests will be based on seniority. The office will be closed at noon on December 24. The office will be closed on the 25th and reopen on the 26th. The office will also close on December 31st at noon. The office will be closed on January 1, reopening on the 2nd.

If you have any questions, please e-mail me.

F I G U R E 7 – 4 . Sample memorandum.

Checkpoint Question

5. What are memorandums used for?

SENDING WRITTEN COMMUNICATION

After the document has been written, proofread, and signed, it is ready for you to send it to its receiver. Fold the letter in thirds and place it in an envelope. Procedure 7-1 explains how to do this. Procedure 7-2 shows you how to fold a letter into a envelope with a window. Most professional letters are sent through the postal service. Other types of written communications are sent through facsimile machines or by electronic mail. Here are two key steps to remember when sending any type of written communication:

- All attempts must be made to ensure patient confidentiality. The outside of envelopes should be marked confidential when the correspondence contains information about a patient. Send letters only to known or confirmed addresses.
- Return addresses must be used so that mail can be returned if the recipient is no longer at the given address.

Facsimile Machines

Facsimile, or fax, machines allow the medical office to send and receive printed material over a phone line. These machines offer a convenient and cost-effective way to transmit records, orders, prescriptions, test results, and other materials that require quick receipt. Always use a cover sheet (Fig. 7-5) when sending papers through a fax machine. At minimum a cover sheet should have the following information:

- Name, address, telephone, and fax number of the physician's practice
- Name of the intended receiver of the fax
- Number of pages being sent, counting the cover sheet
- Telephone number of the fax machine of the intended recipient

---

Procedure 7-1

How to Fold a Letter for a No. 10 Envelope

Equipment/Supplies

- Letter, 8.5 × 11
- Envelope, no. 10

Steps	Purpose
1. Place the letter right side up and flat on a table.	Ensures that the letter will be folded correctly and neatly.
2. Bring the bottom third of the letter up and make a solid crease line.	Divides the letter into equal thirds. Solid crease displays a professional look.
3. Fold the top third of the letter down to within three eighths of an inch of the first fold. Make a solid crease.	Ensures that the second fold does not interfere with the first fold. A solid crease displays a professional look.
4. Place the letter in the envelope with the last fold at the top of the envelope.	Allows the recipient to open the letter easily. Ensures that the letterhead is seen first.

Procedure 7-2

How to Fold a Letter for an Envelope With a Window

Equipment/Supplies

- Letter, 8.5 × 11
- Envelope, no. 10 with a window

Steps	Purpose
1. Place the letter face down on a flat surface.	Ensures that the letter will be folded correctly and neatly.
2. Bring the bottom third of the letter up. Make a solid crease line.	Divides the letter into equal thirds. Solid crease displays a professional look.
3. Fold the top third of the letter down to within three eighths of an inch of the first fold. Make a solid crease.	Ensures that the second fold does not interfere with the first fold. A solid crease displays a professional look.
4. Place the letter in the envelope. Turn the envelope over and look at the window.	Makes sure the letter is correctly seated in the envelope and the address can be read.

Cardiology Associates
Maria Sefferin, MD
897 Bayou Drive
Philadelphia, PA
215-112-9999

facsimile transmittal

To: _____ Fax: _____

From: _____ Date: _____

Re: _____ Pages: _____

CC: _____

☐ Urgent ☐ For Review ☐ Please Comment ☐ Please Reply ☐ Please Recycle

Comments:

CONFIDENTIAL INFORMATION

The information in the facsimile message and any accompanying documents is confidential. This information is intended only for use by the individual or entity name above. If you are not the intended recipient of this information you are hereby notified that any disclosure, copying or distribution of this information is strictly prohibited. Please notify the sender immediately by telephone.

FIGURE 7-5. Sample fax cover sheet.

- Date and time the fax was sent
- Confidentiality statement (e.g., "The information in the facsimile message and any accompanying documents is confidential. This information is intended only for use by the individual or entity name above. If you are not the intended recipient of this information you are hereby notified that any disclosure, copying or distribution of this information is strictly prohibited. Please notify the sender immediately by telephone").

When you receive a fax, photocopy it if it is printed on thermal paper (text printed on thermal paper fades quickly), then forward it to the appropriate person. The fax machine should be checked regularly throughout the day, and all items should be sorted quickly.

Sometimes when you fax a given letter, the fax machine may be busy or the number dialed may be busy. If the number is busy, it is not acceptable to leave the fax papers in the machine for redial unless you are sure that no one else will have access to that document. Never leave documents unattended.

Electronic Mail

Electronic mail, or e-mail, allows computer-to-computer communication, whether within the same facility or anywhere throughout the world. The communication occurs through a modem. Each computer must be linked to an on-line service provider. Chapter 10 discusses electronic mail in more detail. Here are a few things you should remember about sending letters via electronic mail:

- Confidentiality cannot be guaranteed.
- Follow the usual steps of preparation, composition, and editing.
- You can attach letters to an e-mail by clicking on the file attachment icon, locating the letter, and inserting it. It is always a good idea to open the attachment to make sure that you are attaching the correct letter or version.

United States Postal Service

Written communication is commonly sent via the United States Postal Service (USPS). Envelopes must be correctly prepared so that the optical character readers (OCR) used by the USPS can sort the mail quickly and efficiently. The OCR reads the envelope, scanning for information. The OCR scans all envelopes using these margins: $\frac{1}{2}$ inch on either side and $\frac{5}{8}$ inch from the top or bottom of the envelope. Addresses or notations outside of these margins will not be read.

Addressing Envelopes

The standard business envelope is no. 10. USPS regulations state that the minimal size of an envelope is $3\frac{1}{2} \times 5$ inches. It must be rectangular and no less than 0.007 inch thick. The standard no. 10 business envelope is $4\frac{1}{8} \times 9\frac{1}{2}$ inches.

The return address is placed in the upper left hand corner. It should not exceed five lines. The return address is typed with the same guidelines as for letters and is single spaced. Often, medical offices have the return address preprinted on the envelope.

The recipient's address is typed 12 spaces down from the top and centered on the face of the envelope. All words of the address should begin with a capital letter. Only postal abbreviations for states should be used, and no punctuation is used between the postal abbreviation and the zip code. All addresses must include the five-digit zip code; whenever possible, the four-digit expanded zip code should also be used. The expanded zip code allows the USPS to sort and route the mail faster and more accurately. Envelopes should not be handwritten, as this does not portray a professional image. The entire address should not exceed five lines. Your software may allow you to insert a USPS PostNet bar code. This is generally inserted two to three lines below the address. This bar code accelerates USPS sorting. Always check your software to make sure it is certified by the USPS.

Special notations such as "confidential" or "personal" are placed on the left-hand side of the envelope two lines below the return address. Notations for hand canceling and special delivery are made in the upper right-hand corner of the envelope below the postage. Nothing should be printed in the right lower corner of the envelope, because the USPS uses that space for its bar codes. Figure 7-6 displays a properly addressed envelope.

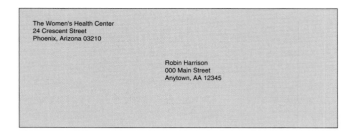

FIGURE 7-6. Properly addressed envelope.

Here are some additional things to remember regarding envelopes:

- Be sure that graphics or logos do not impede the OCR's ability to read the address.
- Do not use fancy fonts that may impede the OCR's ability to read the address.
- A minimum of eight-point type is recommended by the USPS.
- Do not use dark envelopes.
- White or tan envelope with black type is preferred.
- Do not use the # sign; if it cannot be avoided, leave one space between the # sign and the number (this is a USPS recommendation).
- If you are using an envelope with a window frame, there should be an eighth-inch clearance around the address.

 Checkpoint Question

6. What does an optical character reader do?

Affixing Postage

Proper postage must be affixed to the envelope by a stamp, permit imprint, or a postage meter machine. Postal meter machines are in-house machines that are regulated by the USPS. They contain a prepaid amount of postage and can imprint the postage stamp either directly on the envelope or onto an adhesive tape that is applied to the envelope. Some machines weigh, stuff, and seal the envelopes. The date on the postal machine must be changed daily, and the ink roller must be kept full.

The physician may opt to use the USPS permit imprint program. In this case, you take the mail, sealed and ready to be sent, to the post office. The postal clerk passes your letters through the USPS machine, and a permit stamp is placed on the envelope. The postal clerk deducts the postage charges from your prepaid account. The advantages to this system are that is saves time and does not require the office to care for the postal meter machine.

USPS Mailing Options

Mail can be sent in a variety of ways based on its urgency and value. The following is a brief description of the services offered by the USPS:

Spanish Terminology

¿Donde está la oficina de correos?	Where is the post office?
Tengo que enviar esta carta.	I need to mail this letter.
¿Cuanto cuesta el franqueo?	How much does the postage cost?

- Express mail, the fastest service, ensures delivery of your package by the next day (by noon in most areas). Express mail is delivered 7 days a week. The rate starts at $13.65, and fees increase by weight and destination. Express mail is automatically insured for $500. Additional insurance is available.
- Priority mail, the second fastest service, offers 2-day delivery to most destinations. The maximum weight is 70 pounds, and the maximum size is 108 inches combined length and girth. The rate is based on the weight of the package. You can purchase up to $5,000 of insurance for packages.
- First-class mail is the service used for sending standard mail (letters and postcards) weighing up to 13 ounces. Mail weighing more than 13 ounces will be considered priority mail.
- Standard mail (A) is used by companies to mail books and catalogs. Standard mail (B) is used to mail packages weighing more than 1 pound. The maximum weight is 70 pounds, and the maximum measurement is 130 inches combined length and girth.
- Postal rates, fees, and services are subject to change. You must stay abreast of the latest information. Use the USPS website for additional information and updates.

USPS Special Services

A certificate of mailing is used to prove that a document was mailed. No record is kept at the post office. It does not provide proof that the letter was received by the addressee.

Certified mail provides a mailing receipt and a record of the mailing at the local post office (Fig. 7-7). This service is available only for first-class and priority mail. Return receipts can be purchased in conjunction with this. Return receipts are used to prove that the recipient received the document (Fig. 7-8).

Registered mail provides the most protection for valuables. It is available only for priority and first-class mail. The maximum insurance that can be obtained is $25,000. This service can be combined with return receipts.

International rates are available from your local post office. Type the address as discussed earlier, and type the name of the country on the last line without abbreviations (Japan, Korea), All physician offices should have a supply of express and priority mail envelopes along with a current fee schedule.

Other Delivery Options

Many other companies specialize in document and package delivery, particularly with next-day or second-day delivery services. Examples of these companies include Airborne Express, Federal Express, and United Parcel Service (UPS). Use the company with which the physician has an account. Fees vary, so you may have to contact each company for prices and available services. These companies offer services such as tracking, pick-up services, money back guarantees, and proof of delivery. The tracking service can be done through their websites.

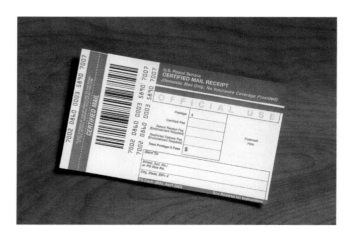

FIGURE 7–7. Certified mail receipt.

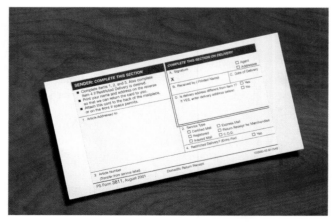

FIGURE 7–8. Return receipt.

RECEIVING AND HANDLING INCOMING MAIL

Part of the daily routine for a medical assistant is handling the incoming mail. Sort the mail quickly and promptly to ensure efficient functioning of the office.

Types of Incoming Mail

Many types of mail are received daily in a physician's office:

- Advertisements
- Bills for office services
- Consultation letters
- Hospital communications and newsletters
- Laboratory and radiographic reports
- Office supply magazines
- Patient correspondence
- Payments from insurance companies and patients
- Professional journals
- Literature from professional organizations
- Samples (drugs, laboratory test kits)
- Waiting room magazines

Opening and Sorting Mail

Each physician will have an individual policy on which mail you should open and how you should process it. Any mail marked urgent should be handled first, followed by mail about patient-related issues. Promotional materials should be handled last. Some physicians will have you sort, file, and respond to mail without their review. In some practices, however, all mail is placed in a special file folder and handled only by the physician or office manager. Box 7-7 lists general guidelines for opening and sorting the mail. Most physicians will open and handle their own e-mail. If the physician is on vacation, he or she will apply an auto reply response to his or her e-mail address.

When the physician is away, personal mail is placed on his or her desk and left for the physician to handle. Mail that pertains to patient care issues should be opened and handled appropriately. Ask your supervisor if you are unsure which pieces of mail you should open. If the mail requires an urgent response, the covering physician should be contacted unless otherwise directed. Mail should never be allowed to accumulate in outside mailboxes because patient information is confidential.

Checkpoint Question

7. What mail must be opened first?

Annotation

Some physicians request that letters be annotated. **Annotation** involves reading a document and highlighting the key points. If the letter is very detailed, a summary of the key

---

Box 7-7

OPENING AND SORTING MAIL

1. Gather the necessary equipment: a letter opener, paper clips, and a date stamp.
2. Open all letters and check for enclosures; paper clip these to the letter. If the letter states that enclosures were sent but they are not in the envelope, contact the sender and request them. Indicate on the letter that the enclosures were missing and the name of the person you contacted.
3. Date-stamp each item.
4. Sort the mail into categories and deal with it appropriately. Generally, you should handle the following types of mail as noted:
   - Use a paper clip to attach test results to the patient's chart; place the chart in a pile for the physician to review.
   - Record promptly all insurance payments and checks and deposit them according to office policy.
   - Account for all drug samples and appropriately log them into the sample book.
   - Dispose of miscellaneous advertisements unless otherwise directed.
5. Distribute the mail to the appropriate staff members. For example, mail can be for the physician, nurse manager, office manager, billing clerk, or other personnel.

---

points should be written in the margins. The summary should be factual and not editorialized.

COMPOSING AGENDAS AND MINUTES

Two other forms of written communication are agendas and minutes. The purpose of an **agenda** (Figure 7-9) is to outline briefly the topics to be discussed at a meeting.

It allows the meeting participants to prepare any necessary reports before the meeting and to anticipate questions. Agendas usually begin with a call to order, followed by a review of previous meeting minutes, old business updates, then new business. Adjournment is the last item on the agenda.

You should type the minutes of a meeting as soon as possible, including the following:

- List of members present
- List of members absent
- Date and time the meeting was called to order
- Statement regarding the acceptance of the previous minutes
- Brief description of discussions

Quality Improvement Committee
February 15, 2003
Agenda

   I.   Call to order
  II. Review and acceptance of the minutes from
       January 10, 2003
 III. Old business
       A. Copy machine updates
       B. Insurance updates for overdue accounts
 IV. New business
       A. New contract for laboratory supplies
       B. Scheduling guidelines for summer vacations
  V. Adjournment

F IGURE 7–9.   Agenda.

- List of reports that were submitted
- Date and time of the next meeting
- Adjournment time
- Signature of the person who prepared the minutes and the chairperson's signature

CHAPTER SUMMARY

As a medical assistant, you need excellent written communication skills. Careful attention to detail is essential. Good grammar, punctuation, and spelling are key skills. Be careful when you use your computer spell check. It will not recognize words that are misused. You will use these skills to write letters, memorandums, and other correspondence. These letters will be sent to patients, physicians, and businesses. After writing these documents, you must be able to select the appropriate service for mailing your letters. Your primary goal with all written communication is to get your message across in a clear, concise, and accurate manner.

Critical Thinking Challenges

1. Create a business letter. Include all the components and use the full block format. Print your unedited copy and, using proofreaders marks, indicate your corrections. Make the corrections and reprint a final copy. Ask your instructor to review both copies.

2. Write 10 sentences using terms from Box 7-3. Use some terms correctly and others incorrectly. Exchange your sentences with another student. Correct your peer's sentences.

3. Collect five pieces of mail that you have received at home. What method of affixing postage did they use? Go to your local USPS office. Obtain either a priority mail or express mail envelope. Correctly address the envelope.

4. Suppose the physician told you to read his e-mails while he was on vacation. In doing so, you come across a personal piece of information that you know he would not want you to see. How would you handle it? Would you tell anyone that you saw it? Would you question the physician about it?

Answers to Checkpoint Questions

1. Inaccurate information in a business letter can lead to injuries to the patient and lawsuits and can harm the physician's practice.

2. The inside address is the address of the person to whom the letter is going. The salutation is the greeting. The identification line shows the initials of the person who dictated the letters and the initials of the person who typed the letter.

3. Before you begin to type a letter, select the template, font, and margins that you will use.

4. Proofreading allows you to check the accuracy and content of the letter.

5. Memorandums are used for communication within the office and with other departments.

6. The USPS uses optical character readers to quickly and efficiently sort the mail.

7. Any mail marked urgent must be opened first.

 Websites

Here are some Web addresses that may help you:
Airborne Express
    www.airborne.com
Medical dictionary
    www.medical-dictionary.com
Merriam-Webster's Dictionary
    www.m-w.com
United Parcel Service
    www.ups.com
United States Postal Service
    www.usps.com

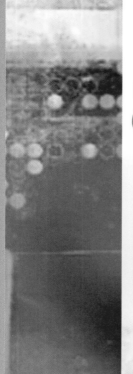

8

Medical Records and Record Management

CHAPTER OUTLINE

STANDARD MEDICAL RECORDS
Contents of the Medical Record

ELECTRONIC MEDICAL RECORDS
Electronic Medical Record Security
Other Technologies for Medical Record Maintenance

MEDICAL RECORD ORGANIZATION
Provider Encounters

DOCUMENTATION FORMS
Medical History Forms
Flow Sheets
Progress Notes

MEDICAL RECORD ENTRIES
Charting Communications With Patients
Additions to Medical Records

WORKERS' COMPENSATION RECORDS

MEDICAL RECORD PREPARATION

FILING PROCEDURES

FILING SYSTEMS
Alphabetic Filing
Numeric Filing
Other Filing Systems

CLASSIFYING MEDICAL RECORDS

INACTIVE RECORD STORAGE

STORING ACTIVE MEDICAL RECORDS
Record Retention

RELEASING MEDICAL RECORDS
Releasing Records to Patients
Reporting Obligations

ROLE DELINEATION COMPONENTS

GENERAL: Legal Concepts
- Perform within legal and ethical boundaries
- Prepare and maintain medical records
- Document accurately
- Implement and maintain federal and state health care legislation and regulations

ADMINISTRATIVE: Administrative Procedures
- Perform basic administrative medical assisting functions

CHAPTER COMPETENCIES

LEARNING OBJECTIVES

Upon successfully completing this chapter, you will be able to:

1. Spell and define the key terms
2. Describe standard and electronic medical record systems
3. Explain the process for releasing medical records to third-party payers and individual patients
4. List and explain the EMR guidelines established to protect computerized records
5. List the standard information included in medical records
6. Identify and describe the types of formats used for documenting patient information in outpatient settings
7. Explain how to make an entry in a patient's medical record, using abbreviations when appropriate
8. Explain how to make a correction in a standard and electronic medical record
9. Identify the various ways medical records can be stored
10. Compare and contrast the differences between alphabetic and numeric filing systems and give an example of each
11. Explain the purpose of the Health Insurance Portability and Accountability Act

PERFORMANCE OBJECTIVE

Upon successfully completing this chapter, you will be able to:

1. Prepare and file a medical record file folder

KEY TERMS

alphabetic filing	electronic medical records	microfilm	reverse chronological order
chief complaint	(EMR)	narrative	SOAP
chronological order	flow sheet	numeric filing	subject filing
cross-reference	medical history forms	present illness	workers' compensation
demographic data	microfiche	problem-oriented medical	
		record (POMR)	

MEDICAL RECORDS HAVE A VITAL role in ensuring quality patient care. Proper medical records management requires adherence to certain legal, moral, and ethical standards. If these standards are disregarded, a breach of contract between patient and physician may occur, exposing the patient to potential embarrassment and making the physician vulnerable to lawsuits. (See Chapter 2.)

Medical records have many uses, including research, quality assurance, and patient education. Information gathered from medical records aids the government in planning for future health care needs and protecting the health of the public.

A thorough and accurate medical record furnishes documented evidence of the patient's evaluation, treatment, change in condition, and communication with the physician and staff.

STANDARD MEDICAL RECORDS

The standard practice of recording and filing patient information in a folder and labeling it with the patient's name or a number is gradually being replaced by the use of **electronic medical records (EMR)**, but in the meantime, a physician accumulates mounds of paper every day. A medical facility has a variety of options for record keeping. The best systems are those that have been tried, revised, and revised again. No matter how the records are stored, make sure that the information is:

- Easily retrievable
- Kept in an orderly manner
- Complete
- Legible
- Accurate
- Brief

Whether a record is on paper or a computer disk, all medical records have the same contents.

Contents of the Record

A medical record in an outpatient facility, often called a chart or a file, contains confidential clinical information about the patient's health and treatment in addition to the billing and insurance information discussed in Chapter 13.

General information such as name, address, telephone number, date of birth, social security number, credit history, and next of kin is vital to a complete chart but should never be intermingled with the clinical information. Metal fasteners can be used to keep certain pages on one side of the chart. For a thorough discussion and samples of typical medical reports found in the medical record, see Chapter 9.

The following information is typically found in the clinical section of the medical chart:

- *Chief complaint*—A description of the symptoms that led the patient to seek the physician's care. This information is supplied by the patient during the interview at the beginning of the visit. It is usually stated in the patient's own words in quotation marks. For example, the patient complains of "something stuck in my throat."
- *Present illness*—A more specific account of the chief complaint, including time frames and characteristics. For example, the patient says it started 2 days ago. She describes the pain as severe and stabbing and reports taking Tylenol with no relief.
- *Family and personal history*—A review of any major illnesses of family members, including grandparents, parents, siblings, aunts, and uncles. Any previous major illnesses and surgeries of the patient are listed under personal history.
- *Review of systems*—A systematic review of the body's ten systems to detect problems not yet identified. For example, problems with the integumentary system (skin) may be identified if the patient reports a rash, areas of discoloration, or change in a mole.
- *Progress notes*—Documentation of each patient encounter, including information obtained in phone calls and refills of prescriptions.
- *Radiographic reports*— Reports of any x-ray studies performed in the office. If patients are sent to other facilities for radiographs, a report of that study is placed in the chart.
- *Laboratory results*—A copy of the results of any laboratory work done in the office or a report from an outside facility.
- *Consultation reports*—Any reports from other physicians regarding consultations with the patient.
- *Medication administration*—Some facilities use a separate sheet to log medications given in the office. If an opioid is given, still another form is completed, as discussed in Chapter 2.
- *Diagnosis or medical impression*—The most recent entry on the progress note will contain the provider's opinion of the patient's problems.
- *Physician's and/or medical assistant's identification and signature*—Experts have suggested that you sign your entire name instead of initials, with your credentials written after the name, e.g., Susan Jones, CMA.
- *Documented advance directives, such as living will and power of attorney for medical care*—A copy of any instructions from the patient regarding end-of-life decisions or the appointment of another person who can give consent for treatment for the patient.
- *All correspondence pertaining to the patient*—Any letters or memos generated in the facility and sent out are copied and placed in the chart. Correspondence from other physicians is also included in the chart.

 Checkpoint Question

1. What is the chief complaint?

ELECTRONIC MEDICAL RECORDS

Outpatient medical facilities often use computers for storing patient **demographic data** (e.g., address, phone number), insurance billing, printing statements, managing appointments, and word processing. Data are saved, backed up, and stored electronically. In addition to accounting and tracking, computer charting in the clinical area is becoming more common in physician offices. Such systems often use a touch screen, making it easy to store a patient's history, vital signs, and any other information. Documents such as letters from other providers are scanned and become a part of the permanent electronic record. Computer record keeping has many advantages, including legibility, easy storage and retrieval, and improved documentation. Documentation is improved because the computer will require that specific information be inserted. For example, when completing a patient history form, the computer will ask, "Is this patient male or female?" The question must be answered before you can move to the next screen, which prevents missed documentation. A paperless system eliminates the need for paper and storage space, and the possibility of losing a chart is nonexistent. Computer charting takes less time than handwriting notes. Medical record software will continue to expand and integrate data in ways that will further revolutionize medical documentation.

Computers do have some disadvantages, however, including downtime, cost, security issues, equipment failure, and the need for more in-depth staff training. In the medical office, the setup may consist of a mainframe with various terminals placed throughout the office.

Electronic Medical Record Security

With computer records, confidential health information is at risk for being seen by unauthorized persons. The Health Insurance Portability and Accountability Act of 1996 (HIPAA) was passed to ensure the privacy of patients' records without creating problems transferring information between health professionals, which might harm the quality of care. HIPAA's privacy rule applies to health insurance plans, insurance clearinghouses, and health care providers who perform administrative transactions electronically (e.g., electronic billing, electronic claims submission). After review and some changes, HIPAA's final rule took effect in April 2003.

The American Medical Association (AMA) and many risk management companies have published guidelines for the EMR. Following are suggestions and guidelines based on HIPAA's requirements for practices using computers to transfer or store patient information. Experts advise physicians and office managers considering software programs to look for the following capabilities:

- User friendly commands that allow users to move easily within the system.
- Spell check, free text fields for inserting corrections and late entries. The electronic record is corrected by

using the same rules as in the standard record. Entries are not deleted but corrected, with an explanation to avoid the appearance of hiding information.
- Security levels to limit entry to all functions. For example, a receptionist does not need access to the physician's personal taxes.
- A system to repel hackers. Evidence shows that persons with access to technology can invade patients' records stored on computer databases. This is a gross breach of confidentiality and is illegal.

To maintain security, facilities are urged to do the following:

- Keep all computer backup disks in a safe place away from the practice.
- Store disks in a bank safe-deposit box.
- Use passwords with characters other than letters and encrypt the passwords.
- Change log-in codes and passwords every 30 days.
- Prepare a backup plan for use when the computer system is down.
- Turn terminals away from areas where information may be seen by patients.
- Keep the fax machines and printers that receive personal medical information in a private place.
- Ensure that each user is restricted to the information needed to do his or her job.
- Train employees on confidentiality and each person's responsibility. With HIPAA's final rule, effective April 2003, training is available from vendors of medical software.
- Design a written confidentiality policy that employees sign.
- Conduct routine audits that produce a trail of each employee's movement through the EMR system.
- Include disciplinary measures for breaches of confidentiality.

In this era of paperless medical offices, care must be taken to protect the privacy of the patient as carefully as in the world of paper.

Other Technologies for Medical Record Maintenance

Providers may use a handheld personal data device (PDA), laptop, or personal computer (PC) in central areas or examination rooms. The same security measures apply to these items. Patients should not have access to computer screens in the examination room. The physician should take care in keeping a personal data system, just as he or she protects the prescription pad. The personal data device may contain the entire *Physicians' Desk Record*, giving the provider information needed for prescribing drugs at the fingertips. Other applications of the PDA include downloading patient education materials and documenting and transferring information about patient encounters when the office is closed.

MEDICAL RECORD ORGANIZATION

Information in the paper medical record is usually organized in a standard chart order and placed in a specially designed folder. The order in which documents are placed in the medical record depends on the physician's preference. As mentioned earlier, the demographic information is kept separate from the clinical information. The clinical portion of the medical record is organized in either a source-oriented or a problem-oriented format. In source-oriented medical records, all similar categories or sources of information are grouped together. The typical groupings:

- Billing and insurance information
- Physician orders
- Progress notes
- Laboratory results
- Radiographic results (magnetic resonance imaging, computed tomography, ultrasound)
- Patient education

All documentation in these categories is placed in **reverse chronological order**; that is, the most recent documents are placed on top of previous sheets.

Provider Encounters

Whether the patient is seen by a physician assistant, nurse practitioner, or physician, the visit is documented.

Narrative Format

Some providers document visits in the narrative form. **Narrative** is the oldest documentation form and the least structured. It is simply a paragraph indicating the contact with the patient, what was done for the patient, and the outcome of any action. In the sample page shown in Figure 8-1, the chart entries made by the CMA are in narrative format.

Some offices record new patients' encounters in the history and physical format, which is discussed in Chapter 9. Visits of established patients returning for follow-up are documented in a different format. Although some offices use the same format for new and established patients, the most common formats used to document each established patient encounter are narrative, SOAP, and POMR.

SOAP Format

The **SOAP** (subjective-objective-assessment-plan) format is one of the most common methods for documenting patient visits. The *subjective* component is a statement of what the patient says. Whenever possible, actual quotations by the patient should be used. The *objective* component is what is observed about the patient when the medical assistant begins the assessment and when the provider does the examination. The *assessment* portion is a phrase stating the impression of

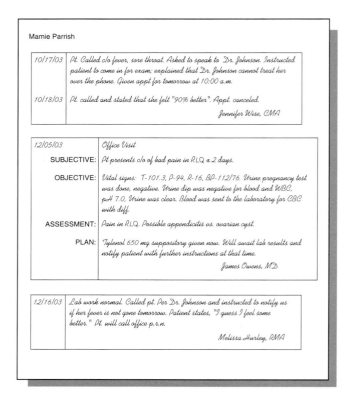

FIGURE 8-1. Sample page from patient's progress record.

what is wrong or the patient's diagnosis. If a final diagnosis cannot be made yet, the provider lists possible disorders to be ruled out, called the differential diagnosis. The *plan* is a list of interventions that are to be carried out. In Box 8-1, the note is written in the SOAP format.

POMR Format

The **problem-oriented medical record (POMR)** lists each problem of the patient, usually at the beginning of the folder, and references each problem with a number throughout the folder. This method was developed by Dr. Lawrence Week and is a common method of compiling information because of its logical flow and the ease with which information can be reviewed. In group practices where patients may be seen by more than one physician, the POMR format makes it easier to track the patient's treatment and progress. For instance, if Mr. Jones has hypertension and hyperglycemia, each diagnosis will be assigned a problem number as soon as the diagnosis is made:

2/4/9 #1. Hypertension
2/4/9 #2. Hyperglycemia

At each subsequent visit made by Mr. Jones, these problems will be referenced by these numbers. If a problem develops and is resolved, the problem number will be terminated by a single strike-through with a date beside it or by adding an X to a heading that indicates resolution of problems. Chronic problems, such as hypertension and hyperglycemia, will be retained by number for as long as the patient remains with the practice. These may be divided by headings of acute and chronic or short-term and long-term for convenience.

POMR documents are divided into four components:

1. *Database.* This contains the following:
   - Chief complaint (Fig. 8-2 shows charting for a chief complaint and history of present illness)
   - Present illness
   - Patient profile
   - Review of systems
   - Physical examination
   - Laboratory reports
2. *Problem list.* This includes every problem the patient has that requires evaluation, including social, demographic, medical, and surgical problems. (Demographic problems relate to statistical characteristics of certain populations.)

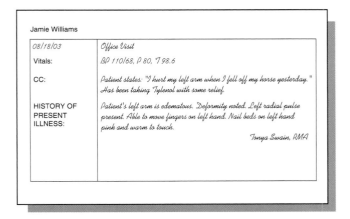

Jamie Williams

08/18/03	*Office Visit*
Vitals:	*BP 110/68, P 80, T 98.6*
CC:	*Patient states: "I hurt my left arm when I fell off my horse yesterday." Has been taking Tylenol with some relief.*
HISTORY OF PRESENT ILLNESS:	*Patient's left arm is edematous. Deformity noted. Left radial pulse present. Able to move fingers on left hand. Nail beds on left hand pink and warm to touch.* *Tonya Swain, RMA*

FIGURE 8–2. Charting a chief complaint and history of present illness.

3. *Treatment plan.* This includes management, additional workups that may be necessary, and therapy.
4. *Progress notes.* These are structured notes corresponding to each problem.

Checkpoint Question

2. What are three common formats used to document patient–provider encounters?

DOCUMENTATION FORMS

Using printed forms and flowcharts in the medical record saves space and time and allows for easy retrieval of information. They are usually customized to meet the needs of the individual practice. Some forms, like vaccination records, are required by federal law. In the paperless office, these forms are completed by the patient and transferred to the patient's electronic record by data entry, and then the completed form is shredded.

Medical History Forms

Medical history forms are commonly used to gather information from the patient before the visit with the physician. Many medical offices mail these forms to new patients and have them bring the completed form to their visit. This gives the patient the opportunity to concentrate on the questions, gather information about the family history, and give a more complete history. Whether the patient brings the completed form or fills out the history form in the office, you will review the information with the patient to clarify any questions and add additional information gathered in the interview. Specialty practices use forms designed to gather the type of information they will need to manage the patient's care. For example, an orthopedist's history form might include fields for prior orthopedic injuries, accident information, and flow sheets for physical therapy visits.

Flow Sheets

The **flow sheet** is designed to limit the need for long, hand-written care notes by allowing information to be recorded in either graphic or table form. Generally, flow sheets are designed for a given task. Color-coded sheets for medication administration, vital signs, pediatric growth charts, and so on eliminate the need to read through the pages of a chart to retrieve information. For example, if the physician asks you what the baby weighed 3 months ago, you find the pink growth chart, which saves time and frustration. An advantage of using electronic medical records is the capability of converting such information to charts, graphs, and flow sheets. In a computer medical record, clicking an icon for a growth chart takes you to a screen that allows you to enter the information. The software transfers the numbers to a graph. Figure 8-3 shows the growth chart that appears on the screen. When you refill a patient's daily blood pressure medication, you enter the information into the computer record, and it is transferred to the medication record. The record of all entries related to the patient's medications can then be easily retrieved by clicking on the medication icon. Figure 8-4 is an example of a medication flow chart from a fictitious patient's electronic chart.

Progress Notes

Progress notes are written statements about various aspects of patient care. Some facilities use a lined piece of paper with two columns. The left column is used to document the date and time, and the right column is used to write the note. Oth-ers use a plain or lined piece of paper without columns. The progress notes will reflect each encounter with the patient chronologically, whether by phone, by e-mail, or in person. No matter what form is used for documenting, you must always include the date, time, your signature, and credential.

 Checkpoint Question

3. List three advantages of using flow sheets in a medical chart.

MEDICAL RECORD ENTRIES

Proper medical record entries are necessary for efficient communication and for legal considerations. The medical record allows health care practitioners to communicate among themselves and therefore provide the best care possible for the patient. Good communication fosters continuity of patient care.

The medical record is a legal document that can be subpoenaed in a malpractice suit. If the documentation is accurate, timely, and legible, it can help win a lawsuit or prevent one altogether. If the documentation is messy, inaccurate, or improperly done, however, it can raise questions that might cause the practice to lose a malpractice suit. Figure 8-5 shows the difference between a well-written chart note and one that leaves in question what really happened. The golden rule in documentation is that if it is not documented, it was not done. Therefore, all patient procedures, assessments, interventions, evaluations, teachings, and communications must be documented.

Follow these guidelines for documenting in patients' medical records:

1. Make sure you know the office policy regarding charting. Find out who is allowed to write in the chart and the procedures for doing so.
2. Make sure you have the correct patient chart. If the patient's name is common, ask for a birth date or social security number as a double check.
3. Always document in ink.
4. Always sign your complete name and credential.
5. Always record the date of each entry. Some outpatient facilities record the time as well. Using military time will eliminate the need to use A.M. and P.M. (Fig. 8-6).
6. Write legibly. Printing is more legible than cursive writing.
7. Check spelling, especially medical terms, before entering them into the chart. Chapter 7 offers help with spelling.
8. Use only abbreviations that are accepted by your facility. Abbreviations can cause confusion and errors in patient care if they are overused, used incorrectly, or open to interpretation. For instance, the abbreviation BS might stand for bowel sounds,

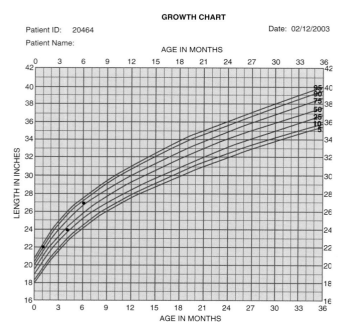

F I G U R E   8 – 3 .   Growth chart from electronic medical record.

Ardmore Family Practice, P.A.
2805 Lyndhurst Avenue
Winston-Salem, NC 27103
PHONE: 336-659-0076
FAX: 336-659-0272

Patient: MICHAEL FIELDS   **Date:** 02-12-2003 9:06 AM

MEDICATIONS

Date	Drug Name	Strength/Form	Dispense	Refill	Sig	Last Dose/ Disc Date	Status
1/28/03	SINGULAIR	10 MG TABS	5	0	1 PO BID		NEW
1/28/03	ZITHROMAX	200 MG/5ML SUSR	5	0	1 P.O Q DAY		NEW
1/22/03	ACCUPRIL	10 MG TABS	34	4	1 PO QD	1/28/03	CONTINUE
1/22/03	ADVIL	200 MG TABS	1	1	1/2 Q A.M.	1/25/03	NEW
1/22/03	ALTACE	5 MG CAPS	60	5	ONE TWICE DAILY	1/28/03	CONTINUE
1/22/03	MACROBID	100 MG CAPS	14	0	1 PO BID	1/28/03	CONTINUE
8/26/02	ALTACE	5 MG CAPS	60	5	ONE TWICE DAILY		CONTINUE
8/7/02	PRECOSE	25 MG CAPS	60	0	1/2 B.I.D.	10/5/02	NEW
5/2/01	ACCUPRIL	10 MG TABS	34	4	1 PO QD		NEW
5/2/01	ACCUPRIL	20 MG TABS	30	0	1 PO QD		NEW
5/2/01	ACCUPRIL	40 MG TABS	30	5	1 PO QD		NEW
4/25/01	ACCUPRIL	20 MG TABS	30	0	1 PO QD	4/25/01	NEW
4/25/01	ACCUPRIL	40 MG TABS	30	5	1 PO QD		NEW
4/25/01	MACROBID	100 MG TABS	14	0	1 PO BID	5/1/01	NEW
3/2/01	ACIPHEX 20 MG	TABS	30	6	1 PO QD		NEW
3/2/01	ACTOS 30 MG	TABS	30	2	1 PO QD		NEW
1/23/01	ENTEX PSE	120-600 MG TB12	45	0	1 PO BID		NEW
1/23/01	NASONEX	50 MCG/ACT SUSP	1	3	2 SPRAYS EACH NOSTRIL QD		NEW
8/24/99	ADALAT CC	60 MG TBCR	34	5	1 PO QD	8/24/99	NEW
7/8/99	NITROGLYCERIN	0.4 MG/DOSE AERS	100	1	1 TAB SL Q 5 MIN X 3, IF CHEST PAIN PERS	7/8/99	NEW
6/26/99	CLARITIN	10 MG TABS	30	5	ONE EVERY MORNING		NEW
6/23/99	CELEBREX 100 MG	CAPS	90	3	1 PO Q AM AND 2 PO Q PM		NEW
6/3/99	GLUCOPHAGE	850 MG TABS	90	6	ONE 3 TIMES DAILY	6/3/99	NEW
6/3/99	HYTRIN	5 MG CAPS	30	6	ONE EVERY DAY	6/3/99	NEW

FIGURE 8–4. Medication administration flow sheet.

Correct

| 9-15-03 | Pt. Called to cancel appt. for recheck of UTI on 9-16-03. States she is feeling better. Advised to keep appointment, since Dr. Smith wants to repeat a urinalysis to see if her bladder infection has cleared up. Pt. states, "I don't see any sense in that; I'm not coming". Advised Dr. Smith. |
| | Fred Lane, CMA |

Incorrect

| 9-15-03 | Pt. Called to cancel appt. | Fred Lane, CMA |

FIGURE 8–5. Right and wrong chart entries.

breath sounds, or blood sugar. Box 8-2 shows abbreviations used in charting, and Appendix D has a general list of commonly used abbreviations. Chapter 9 fully explains the use of abbreviations in medical documentation.

9. When charting the patient's statements, use quotation marks to signify the patient's own words.

10. Do not attempt to make a diagnosis. For example, if the patient says, "My throat is sore," do not write pharyngitis. It is not within the scope of your training to diagnose.

11. Document as soon as possible after completing a task to promote accuracy.

12. Document missed appointments in the patient's chart. Chart your attempts to reach the patient to remind him or her of the appointment.

13. Document any telephone conversations with the patient in the chart.

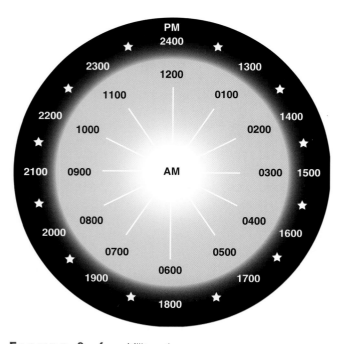

FIGURE 8–6. Military time.

Box 8-2

ABBREVIATIONS USED IN CHARTING

In office charting, use these common abbreviations to save time and space.

Abbreviation	Meaning
ā	before
abd	abdomen
ant.	anterior
AP	anteroposterior
Ax	axillary
b.i.d.	twice a day
BP	blood pressure
C	Celsius
c̄	with
CC	chief complaint
C/o	complains of
CPX	complete physical examination
Cx	canceled
D/C	discontinue
F	Fahrenheit
Fx	fracture
h.s.	bedtime, hour of sleep
Hx	history
L	left
LLE	left lower extremity
LLQ	left lower quadrant
LUE	left upper extremity
LUQ	left upper quadrant
NKDA	no known drug allergies
noct.	nocturnal
p̄	after
p.c.	after a meal
PE	physical examination
p.r.n.	as needed
pt.	patient
q.i.d.	4 times a day
R	right
R/O	rule out
RLE	right lower extremity
RUE	right upper extremity
RLQ	right lower quadrant
RUQ	right upper quadrant
R/s	rescheduled
s̄	without
SOB	shortness of breath
spec	specimen
s/p	status post
STAT	immediately
t.i.d.	3 times a day
TPR	temperature, pulse, respiration

When correcting a charting error, draw a single line through the error, initial it, date it, and document the correct information.

left 05/15/03 TW

05/15/03 Patient presents today complaining of pain in ~~right~~ eye. Tracy Wiles, CMA

FIGURE 8–7.   Correcting an error.

14. Be honest. If you have given a wrong medication or performed the wrong procedure, as soon as the appropriate supervisor is notified, document it, then complete an incident report (see Chapter 11). State only the facts; do not draw any conclusions or place blame.
15. Never document for someone else, and never ask someone else to document for you.
16. Never document false information.
17. Never delete, erase, scribble over, or white-out information in the medical record because this can be construed as attempting to cover the truth and tampering with a legal document. If you do make an error, draw a single line through it, initial it, and date it. Then write the word "correction" and document the correct information (Fig. 8-7). You can click on an icon to make a correction in the electronic chart, but the original information is not deleted. For example, if you discover that you have entered the wrong date of birth after the patient's information has been saved, you can correct it, but most systems allow only certain users to make changes in the saved database.

Charting Communications With Patients

In addition to documenting patient visits to the facility, other encounters and communications may occur and should become a part of the permanent record. To ensure continuity of care and patient safety, charts should contain a progress sheet or some sort of tool to record each communication with a patient. Actions taken by the physician or employees as directed by the physician on behalf of the patient should be charted. For example, when a prescription is phoned to a pharmacy, the action is recorded. The physician may give instructions to be carried out regarding a patient, such as calling the patient with normal test results. This should be concisely explained in the chart. These entries should appear in **chronological order**. Dates that are out of order and gaps between entries may confuse the reader and give the appearance of poor service. For this reason, entries should be made immediately after communications with the patient.

Telephone communications with patients are typically recorded in a narrative manner. When a patient calls or e-mails the office, the conversation must be documented in the chart immediately. Phone calls should be documented with the time and date of the call, patient's problem or request, and actions taken by the person making the entry. If special telephone message pads are used, a copy should be placed in the patient's chart. E-mails from patients should be printed and kept in the chart. Replies to a patient's e-mail should be printed out and included with the progress sheet. Remember, care must be taken to protect the patient's privacy when using electronic means to communicate.

Additions to Medical Records

Any additions to a medical record, such as laboratory results, that are smaller than the standard 8.5 × 11 inches should be transcribed onto a full sheet of paper or shingled and placed in the appropriate area of the chart. Shingling is taping the paper across the top to a regular-size sheet. Each sheet is then added under the current one with a piece of tape across the top. Each sheet can be lifted to view the entire document. Most laboratory reports are computer generated and will come ready to insert into the chart. All additions to the medical record (e.g., laboratory results, radiographic reports, consultation reports) should be read and initialed by the physician before you put them in the chart.

Checkpoint Question

4. What is the golden rule in documentation?

WORKERS' COMPENSATION RECORDS

From time to time, a patient who is active in your practice may seek treatment for a **workers' compensation** case or an injury or illness related to employment. The government requires employers to provide insurance for care when an injury occurs at work. Workers' compensation is discussed in Chapter 17. When this occurs, do not simply add the information to the patient's medical record. Instead, start a new record. A workers' compensation medical record actually belongs to the employer, so the data in that record can be reviewed by the employer's insurance carrier. No information about the patient's previous health or family history that is not pertinent to the workplace incident should be made available to the insurance carrier.

Before treating a patient for a possible workers' compensation case, you must first obtain verification from the employer unless the situation is life-threatening. Be sure to document the name of the person who authorizes treatment as well as any other information that becomes available during the verification process.

Workers' compensation cases are kept open for 2 years after the last date of treatment for any follow-up care that may be required. After that time, care may not be covered under the same case. Even after the care is complete, the separate record is kept with the patient's other record, and information is incorporated into the original record as needed.

MEDICAL RECORD PREPARATION

To start filing, you need folders, labels, and any other appropriate supplies. Keep these supplies on hand and follow the same steps every time you put together and file a medical record. Procedure 8-1 outlines the steps for preparing a medical record file. Over the course of many years, you may have to replace worn-out folders or peeling labels and stickers. Do so before the folder tears or the labels fall off.

After preparing the folders, you may also want to prepare several out guides, that is, plastic sheets with a tab (projection) and a pocket for index cards. Type "Out guide" on the tabbed edge of the sheet. Then, when you remove a chart, write the date, name of the patient, your initials, and where the chart can be found on an index card. Place the card inside the out guide, and put the out guide in the spot in the file cabinet where the chart was. An out guide indicates that the chart has been removed and where it can be found. Hospitals and larger clinics often use a wand to keep track of charts and radiographs. When a chart arrives in a certain location, a wand is passed over a bar code. When the patient's number is entered into the computer, the screen shows the location of the patient's chart at the moment. If it is in the file cabinet, that is also indicated.

Procedure 8-1

Preparing a Medical File

Equipment/Supplies

- File folder
- Title, year, and alphabetic or numeric labels

Step	Reason
1. Decide the name of the file (a patient's name, company name, or name of the type of information to be stored).	Properly naming a file allows for easy retrieval.
2. Type a label with the title *in unit order* (e.g., Lynn, Laila S., *not* Laila S. Lynn).	Typing the label in unit order helps avoid filing errors.
3. Place the label along the tabbed edge of the folder so that the title extends out beyond the folder itself. (Tabs can be either the length of the folder or tabbed in various positions, such as left, center, and right.)	This ensures easy readability.
4. Place a year label along the top edge of the tab before the label with the title. This will be changed each year the patient has been seen. *Note:* Do not automatically replace these labels at the start of a new year; remove the old year and replace with a new one only when the patient comes in for the first visit of the new year.	Doing this makes removing inactive files more time efficient. At the beginning of each new year, you can easily spot the records that are years beyond your storage time limit in the active file area. Doing this also can help you locate inactive files if patients return years later. (By determining the last year the patient was seen, you can narrow your search to files with a matching year label.)
5. Place the appropriate alphabetic or numeric labels below the title.	This aids in accurate filing and retrieval.
6. Apply any additional labels that your office may decide to use.	Labels noting special information (e.g., insurance, drug allergies, advanced directives) act as quick and easy reminders.

FILING PROCEDURES

Every day in the medical office, information is added to a patient's chart. It is best to keep this information filed on a daily basis. Pieces of paper to be added can be kept in a central location until filed so that employees can retrieve it if needed before the patient's next visit. This holding area should be used only until the daily filing can be done. In a paperless office, these additions to the medical record are scanned into the system and the original paper is shredded.

To ensure efficient and speedy filing and document retrieval, follow these four steps:

1. *Condition.* Prepare items by removing loose pieces of tape or paper clips. Make sure each sheet of paper includes the patient's name in case a second page gets separated from the first page.
2. *Index.* Separate business records from patient records.
3. *Sort.* Put each group of records in proper order to be filed on shelves, either alphabetic or numeric. This makes actual filing go much faster because you are not moving up and down and back and forth to find the proper letter area; you will just move down in order.
4. *Store.* Place each record in the proper storage area, as described next.

Checkpoint Question

5. Why is it necessary to make a new chart for an established patient who is being seen for an injury sustained at work?

FILING SYSTEMS

The two main filing systems are alphabetic and numeric. In some practices you may use both systems, each for different types of files.

Alphabetic Filing

As the name implies, **alphabetic filing** is a system using letters. Begin alphabetic filing by distinguishing the first, second, and third unit as described in Box 8-3. (A unit is each part of a name or title that is used in indexing.) Using the first letter of the first unit, place your records in small groups in order from A to Z. After that, take each small group and gradually work through the second and consecutive letters to put the small groups in order. Using this process allows you to work in a progressive order as you add records to existing files.

If the entire first unit is the same, move onto the second unit. If the second unit is still the same, move onto the third unit. Occasionally, you will have records whose units one, two, and three are identical. In such cases, it does not matter which one is filed first; use extreme caution, however, when retrieving records with identical units to prevent errors. Ask-

---

Box 8-3

INDEXING RULES FOR ALPHABETIC FILING

When filing records alphabetically, use these indexing rules to help you decide the placement of each record. Indexing rules apply whether you use the title of the record's contents or a person's name.

File by name according to last name, first name, and middle initial, and treat each letter in the name as a separate unit. For example, Jamey L. Crowell should be filed as Crowell, Jamey L. and should come before Crowell, Jamie L.

- Make sure professional initials are placed after a full name. John P. Bonnet, D.O., should be filed as Bonnet, John P., D.O.
- Treat hyphenated names as one unit. Bernadette M. Ryan-Nardone should be filed as Ryan-Nardone, Bernadette M. not as Nardone, Bernadette M. Ryan.
- File abbreviated names as if they were spelled out. Finnigan, Wm. should be filed as Finnigan, William, and St. James should be filed as Saint James.
- File last names beginning with Mac and Mc in regular order or grouped together, depending on your preference, but be consistent with either approach.
- File a married woman's record by using her own first name. Helen Johnston (Mrs. Kevin Johnston) should be filed as Johnston, Helen, not as Johnston, Kevin Mrs.
- Jr. and Sr. should be used in indexing and labeling the record. Many times a father and son are patients at the same facility.
- When names are identical, use the next unit, such as birth dates or the mother's maiden name. Use Durham, Iran (2-4-94) and Durham, Iran (4-5-45).
- Disregard apostrophes.
- Disregard articles (a, the), conjunctions (and, or), and prepositions (in, of) in filing. File *The Cat in the Hat* under Cat in Hat.
- Treat letters in a company name as separate units. For ASM, Inc., "A" is the first unit, "S" is the second unit, and "M" is the third unit.

---

ing the patient to provide his or her birthday will ensure that you have the right patient and avoid confusion.

With alphabetic filing, color coding may also be used. Letters of the alphabet are color-coded and affixed to each folder, or a color-coded bar is placed next to the label with the patient's name. For example, names beginning with A to F may be blue; G to L, green; M to T, yellow; and U to Z, purple. Using this system, Michele Beals would have a blue strip, Laurie Palmer would have a yellow strip, Lauren

Kayser's would be green, and Dana Warbeck would have purple. Finding misfiled charts is easier. With one glance at the cabinet, for example, you can spot one purple tab in the middle of the green ones.

Numeric Filing

Numeric filing uses digits, usually six. The digits are typically run together but read as three groups of two digits. For example, the record filed as 324478 is read as 32, 44, 78. Commas are not placed or any separation used when applying the labels to the tabbed edge of the file folder. The records are placed in numeric order without concern for duplication, which may sometimes happen with the alphabetic system. If you use this technique, it is called straight digit filing because you are reading the number straight out from left to right.

Sometimes, the file label will look the same, 324478, but will be read in the reverse order: 78, 44, 32. This technique is called terminal digit filing; that is, the groups of numbers are read in pairs from right to left. Be careful not to mix the two filing systems. If using both techniques within your office, be sure to keep them separate by changing the folder color or some other means to prevent errors. The chart is filed by using the last pairs of digits.

Box 8-4

ALPHABETIC FILING EXAMPLES

The following patient records are to be filed alphabetically:

Mary P. Martin
Floyd Pigg, Sr.
Susan Bailey
Ellen Eisel-Parrish
Anita Putrosky
Susan R. Hill
Sister Mary Catherine
Cher
Stephen Dorsky, MD
Mrs. John Moser (Donna)

The proper order is:

Susan Bailey
Cher
Stephen Dorsky
Ellen Eisel-Parrish
Susan R. Hill
Mary P. Martin
Donna Moser
Floyd D. Pigg
Anita Putrosky
Sister Mary Catherine

Box 8-5

NUMERIC FILING EXAMPLES

The following patient records are to be filed numerically:

LeRoy Flora   213456
Ramsey Curtis   334387
Sharon Moore   979779
Cathy King   321138

In straight digit filing, the proper order is:

213456
321138
334387
979779

In terminal digit filing, the proper order is:

321138
213456
979779
334387

With files in which one or two groups of numbers are the same numbers, you refer to the second or third groups or numbers. For example, in straight digit filing (reading from left to right) the number 003491 comes before 004592. The first group of numbers (00) is the same for both files, so you determine the order of filing by the second group of numbers; in this case, 34 comes before 45.

In terminal digit filing (reading from right to left), 456128 would come before 926128. The first two groups of numbers (28 and 61) are the same for both files, so you go to the third group of numbers; in this case, 45 comes before 92.

Numeric filing plays an important role in the medical office. With tests for human immunodeficiency virus (HIV) and acquired immunodeficiency syndrome (AIDS) and their results being held in strict confidence, the use of numeric filing is becoming even more popular. When this technique is used, it is important to keep a **cross-reference** in a secure area, away from patient areas, listing the numeric code and the name of the patient. Such a reference is called a master patient index. This way limited numbers of people know who the patient is, which maintains privacy. Boxes 8-4 and 8-5 show how to file patient records alphabetically or numerically.

Other Filing Systems

The medical office keeps files other than patient records. An office manager keeps files on employees, insurance policies, accounts payable, and so on. For this type of filing, systems include **subject filing**, in which documents are arranged alphabetically according to subject (e.g., insurance, medications, referrals); geographic filing, in which documents are grouped alphabetically according to locations, such as state, county, or city; and chronological filing, in which documents are grouped in the order of their date.

Checkpoint Question

6. What are the two main filing systems? Briefly describe each.

CLASSIFYING MEDICAL RECORDS

Records are classified in three categories: active, inactive, or closed. Active records are those of patients who have been seen within the past few years. The exact amount of time is designated within each practice; it usually ranges from 1 to 5 years. Keep these records in the most accessible storage spot available because you will be using them regularly.

Inactive records are those of patients who have not been seen in more than the designated time set aside for active records. You will still keep these records in the office, but they do not have to be as accessible as the active files. Usually, they are placed on bottom shelves to eliminate constant bending when reaching for active files, or they may be stored in another room within the office. "Inactive" patients have not formally terminated their contact with the physician, but they have either not needed the physician's services or have not informed the office regarding a move, change in physician, or death.

Closed records are those of patients who have terminated their relationship with the physician. Reasons for such termination might include the patient moving, termination of physician–patient relationship by letter, no further treatment necessary, or death of the patient.

INACTIVE RECORD STORAGE

Inactive records can be stored in the office in an out-of-the-way area, such as a basement or attic. They may even be kept in the physician's home. This practice is permitted because the records belong to the physician, but it is not recommended because at any time the office staff may need access to these records. Many practices use **microfilm** or **microfiche** to store closed records. Microfilm and microfiche are ways to photograph documents and store them in a reduced form. Microfilm, a popular method for storing large volumes of records, particularly in hospitals and clinics, uses a photographic process that develops medical records in miniature on film. Information is stored on cards holding single film frames or in reels or strips for projection on compact electric viewers placed at convenient office locations. The cost of the equipment is declining, making this a more practical method for storing and retrieving inactive files.

Microfiche is a miniature photographic system that stores rows of images in reduced size on cards with clear plastic sleeves rather than on film strips. Information can be handled manually, examined on a viewer that enlarges the record, or reproduced as hard copy on a high-speed photocopier. A standard microfiche card holds more than 60 pages of information. The microfiche process allows 3,200 papers to be reduced to fit on a single 4 × 6-inch transparency.

Checkpoint Question

7. What are the three classifications of medical records? Describe each.

STORING ACTIVE MEDICAL RECORDS

Medical offices use a variety of storage methods for active files that are used on a daily basis. Shelf files are stationary shelves. Shelving units are stacked on each other or placed side by side. These shelves may also be custom-ordered to the width you need. Records are stored horizontally, and labels are read from the side. Figure 8-8 shows such shelving units.

Drawer files are a type of filing cabinet. The drawer pulls out for easy access and visibility of all records. This type of filing system allows you easier access to all sides of files, which can help in searches for missing files that may have been pushed to the back or behind other files. Drawer files also allow easier filing because you can read from above the files, rather than squatting to read the labels from the sides as you work your way down to the lower shelves. A disadvantage is that these files take up a great deal of space.

Rotary circular or lateral files allow records to be stored in units that either spin in a circle or stack one behind the other, enabling you to rotate different units to the front. This system allows for maximum use of office space and is suggested for a medical office with large quantities of records to be stored. With shelf or drawer units, more wall space is needed to spread out each unit, but with rotary files, less wall space is needed.

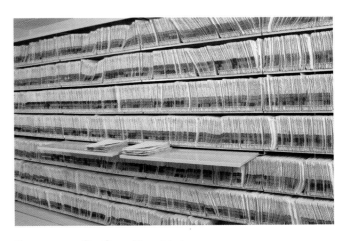

FIGURE 8-8. File cabinets.

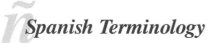
Spanish Terminology

Por firmar aquí, usted nos da permiso de compartir su información medical con su compañía de seguro.	By signing here, you are giving us permission to share your medical information with your insurance company.
Necesitaremos copias de su historia medical de los archivos de su médico anterior.	We will need copies of your medical records from your previous doctor.

Even the paperless medical office must consider storage because backup copies of computerized records must be made daily and stored in a safe, fireproof location. Security experts advise storing backup disks off-site.

Record Retention

As discussed in Chapter 2, the statute of limitations is the legal time limit set for filing suit against an alleged wrongdoer. The time limit varies from state to state. You must observe the statute of limitations in your particular state to know how long medical and business records should be kept in storage.

It is recommended that medical records be stored permanently, because in some states malpractice lawsuits can be filed within 2 years of the date of discovery of the alleged malpractice. The statute of limitations for minors is extended until the child reaches legal age in every state; the time given past the legal age varies, however.

Tax records and liability plans, including old and new policies, should be permanently stored in a fireproof cabinet. Older liability plans may provide coverage should a mal-

practice lawsuit be filed later, after that policy expires and a new policy takes effect.

Insurance policies should also be stored in a fireproof cabinet. You can keep the newest policy and discard the older one.

Canceled checks should be kept in fireproof storage for at least 3 years. After that, keep them indefinitely in regular storage.

Receipts for equipment should be kept until each item listed on the receipt is no longer being used.

Checkpoint Question

8. How long should medical records be kept?

RELEASING MEDICAL RECORDS

Although the physical medical record legally belongs to the physician, the information belongs to the patient. Any release of records must first be authorized by the patient or the patient's legal guardian. When releasing a medical record, provide a copy only. *Never* release the original medical record except in limited circumstances (see the Legal Tip nearby).

Insurance companies, lawyers, other health care practitioners, and patients themselves may request copies of medical records. All requests should be made in writing, stating the patient's name, address, and social security number, and must contain the patient's *original* signature authorizing the release of records. Never release information over the telephone. You will have no way of verifying that the person with whom you are speaking is actually the person who has authorization.

Unless the request is made by the patient, state laws allow facilities to charge a fee for copying the medical record. The AMA published guidelines for physicians to ensure ethical business practices. They recommend a reasonable fee for reproduction of records to be no more than $1 per page or $100 for the entire record, whichever is less. If the record is less than 10 pages, the office may charge up to $10 to cover postage and miscellaneous costs associated with the retrieval process. Laws may vary from state to state.

You must follow certain guidelines even with a signed authorization release form (Fig. 8-9). The authorization form must give the patient the opportunity to limit the information to be released. Patients may release only information relating

LEGAL TIP

The only time an original record should be released is when it is subpoenaed by a court of law. In such situations, the physician may wish to have the judge sign a document stating that he or she will temporarily take charge of the medical record. This signed document should be filed in the medical office until the record is returned. To further ensure the record's safety, a staff member can transport the original record to court on the day it is requested, then return the record at the end of the court session that day. As soon as it is known that a record will be part of a court case, the record should be kept in a locked cabinet. When the court orders that a record be submitted to the court at a given date and time, the legal order is termed *subpoena duces tecum*.

I,_____Harold Eisner_____ , (patient or legal guardian) give
          (patient's name)

permission to___Dr. June Clark_____ to release my medical records
              (physician's name)

from _05/01/2002_ through __02/01/2003_ to
    (date)   (date)

Prime Health Group, 555 Elm Road, Greenwich, CT 05611_____
           (organization's name and address)

_Harold Eisner_____ _2/15/03_ _Lisa Smith_____ _2-15-03_
Patient's signature   Date   Witness signature   Date

F I G U R E   8 – 9 . Sample authorization to release information.

to a specific disorder, or they may specify a time limit. They may not, however, ask that the physician leave out information pertinent to the situation. References to mental health diagnosis or treatments, drug or alcohol abuse, HIV, AIDS, or any other sexually transmitted disease may not be released without specific mention on the signed authorization form. If it is not specifically requested, when you are copying the record, place a piece of blank white paper over any such areas of information. Never white-out these areas on the original document or mention what these blank areas are.

Releasing Records to Patients

For a thorough discussion of releasing medical records, see Chapter 2. When patients request copies of their own records, the doctor makes the decision about what to copy. Patients aged 17 and under cannot get copies of their own medical records without a signed consent from a parent or legal guardian, except for emancipated minors. They may obtain certain services independently (check your state's law regarding treatment of minors), however; in such cases, under the law, you are not permitted to contact the parent or guardian. Some states allow minors to seek treatment for sexually transmitted diseases and birth control without parental knowledge or consent. Sometimes, the parent or guardian may still be billed for these services without the bill being itemized. The billing statement should include only the treatment dates and amount due.

Checkpoint Question

9. What is required for a legal disclosure of a patient's HIV status?

Reporting Obligations

Although patients' records are confidential, in certain situations concerning the public's health and safety, the law requires reporting information to particular authorities. Re-

quirements for reporting vary among states. Generally, the following types of items must be reported: vital statistics, communicable diseases, child and elderly abuse or maltreatment, and certain violent injuries (see Chapter 2).

CHAPTER SUMMARY

Medical records not only are a means of communication among health care providers but also are legal documents depicting the quality of patient care. Preparing and maintaining medical records is an important responsibility. To ensure efficient recording and retrieval, you must be familiar with the varied documentation forms as well as the different kinds of filing systems. In addition, you must adhere to strict guidelines when releasing any information in patients' medical records. Electronic medical records are giving rise to new issues in protecting medical records. The patient's privacy must be protected at all times. The quality, use, and care of the medical record are reflections of the quality of the outpatient facility itself.

Critical Thinking Challenges

1. Interview a fellow student with a hypothetical injury. Document the incident with the chief complaint and the present illness.
2. Compare and contrast alphabetic filing with numeric filling. Which system do you think works better? Explain your response.
3. Instruct a fellow student in the requirements of your office regarding the release of medical records.
4. Write an office policy for maintaining confidentiality with electronic modalities, such as fax machines, printers, laptops, and computer screens.

Answers to Checkpoint Questions

1. The patient's chief complaint is the reason the patient is seeing the physician.
2. Narrative, SOAP, and POMR are three common formats for recording patient–provider encounters.
3. The advantages of using flow sheets in the medical chart are that they limit the need for long handwritten notes, save time and space, and make it easier to locate information.
4. The golden rule in documenting is that if it is not documented, it was not done.
5. The chart of the patient injured on the job has information that should not be available to the employer,

who has access only to the information about the worker's injury.

6. The two main filing systems are alphabetic (using letters to file records) and numeric (using digits to file records).

7. The three classifications of medical records are active (seen within the past few years), inactive (not cur-rently being seen but still patients), and closed (relationship is terminated because of death, patient moved, or change in physician).

8. Medical records should be kept forever.

9. Permission to release information about a patient's HIV status must be specifically given on the release form that is signed by the patient.

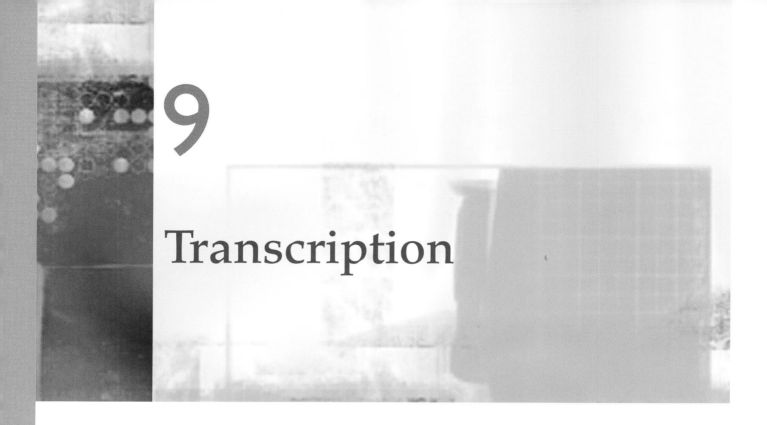

9

Transcription

CHAPTER OUTLINE

ROLE DELINEATION COMPONENTS

GENERAL: Communication Skills
- Recognize and respond effectively to verbal, nonverbal, and written communications
- Use electronic technology to receive, organize, prioritize, and transmit information

GENERAL: Legal Concepts
- Prepare and maintain medical records
- Document accurately

ADMINISTRATIVE: Administrative Procedures
- Perform basic administrative medical assisting functions

CHAPTER COMPETENCIES

LEARNING OBJECTIVES
Upon successfully completing the chapter, you will be able to:
1. Explain the role of the medical assistant in performing medical transcription
2. Explain the roles of the JCAHO and HIPAA on medical transcription
3. List the various reports generated in inpatient and outpatient medical facilities
4. List the rules of medical transcription as outlined by the AAMT
5. Discuss the various medical transcription systems

PERFORMANCE OBJECTIVES
Upon successfully completing the chapter, you will be able to:
1. Transcribe various medical reports from taped dictation
2. Use proper punctuation, grammar, and spelling

KEY TERMS

analogue   digital   transcription

MEDICAL TRANSCRIPTION

Transcription is the process of typing a dictated message. The word *transcript* is from Latin and translates literally to "across writing," meaning to change the spoken word to written word. In the medical office, certified medical assistants (CMAs) often use the skills taught in this chapter. The role delineation chart by the American Association of Medical Assistants (AAMA) discussed in Chapter 1 reveals that medical transcription is a function of the practicing medical assistant (Fig. 9-1). Therefore, as with all topics covered in this text, accrediting agencies require that this skill be taught in accredited medical assisting educational programs.

Those who choose to focus their education on medical transcription are trained to transcribe both inpatient and outpatient reports. The types of reports you will transcribe in a physician's office are different from those seen in the inpatient or hospital facility. The transcription training you receive as a medical assistant focuses on outpatient documents. Most hospitals employ certified medical transcriptionists. Some physicians' offices use outside medical transcription companies, and this is another employment opportunity for the trained medical assistant. In today's computerized world, with a modem and sound privacy protection practices, a transcriptionist could conceivably generate and transmit reports from anywhere in the world.

To transcribe well, you must

- Be a fast and accurate typist
- Have a strong vocabulary in medical terminology
- Have a thorough knowledge of grammar, spelling, and punctuation rules
- Have excellent listening skills
- Have good editing skills

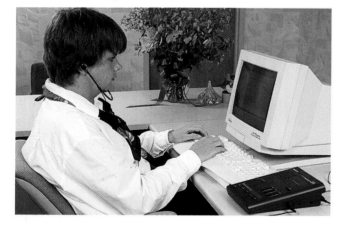

FIGURE 9-1. A transcriptionist must have good communications and computer skills.

The Transcription Process

When a patient visits a physician's office, the provider either writes the findings or dictates a report into a handheld microphone. The provider places the cassette tape and the charts from that day in a designated area. The employee responsible for transcription listens to the tape on a machine called a transcriber. A foot pedal controls play, rewind, and fast forward. The words are typed into a word processor, proofread, and printed. The printed copy is placed on the chart and given to the provider for review. Corrections are made and a final copy is printed and given to the provider for final review and signature. Copies of the report are distributed to anyone the provider names to receive a copy, and a copy is placed in the chart. As tapes are transcribed, they are erased and given back to the provider to use again.

When an office is paperless, the process is the same, but the document is entered into the record instead of being printed. A visual signal can alert the provider as reports become ready for edit. The provider accesses the report and makes edits or marks errors. When the provider is ready to authenticate the report, the stroke of a key "signs" the report. The software allows the provider to check the status of a report at any time.

Off-site Transcription

Many medical offices outsource their transcription through various types of services. Individuals or companies offer services to physicians ranging from picking up tapes and delivering the work on hard copy to transmitting the documents through e-mail.

Several large transcription companies operate solely on the Internet. These websites can be found at the end of the chapter. You can log on, and after passing an online examination, you may begin receiving dictation via modem. The report is transmitted back to the company, which sends it to the provider. Usually, the transcriptionist must buy the necessary equipment. The new regulations of the HIPAA (Health Insurance Portability and Accountability Act) discussed in earlier chapters will require changes in practices for transmission of confidential information via modem.

REPORT FORMATTING

There is no set format for each type of medical document. Every facility has its own format and design, but any professional document should be well balanced and attractive, with single spacing, double spacing between headings, and 1-inch margins. Being familiar with the logical sequence and proper sorting of information for each type of document will help you adapt to any prescribed format. Headings and subheadings are used to report the information gathered in the course of a patient encounter. These general headings are seen in the sample reports in Figures 9-2 to 9-9.

Transcribing a Medical Document

Steps	Purpose
1. Prepare the equipment: transcribing machine, headphones, transcription (dictation) tapes, computer or typewriter, paper, letterhead, and envelopes.	Having everything ready will cut down on interruptions and will help you focus. Concentration is key to being productive.
2. Select a transcription tape with the oldest date, unless there are special requests for priority reports.	Most dictation systems have the capability of *marking* a document for priority status. This alerts you to complete marked dictation first.
3. Turn on the transcriber, and insert and rewind the tape.	Always rewind the tape so that the document starts in the beginning.
4. Put on the headset and position the foot pedal in a comfortable location.	The foot pedal is operated by pressing a certain area for a certain function. In some machines, pressing the left side of the pedal rewinds the tape, pressing the right side fast-forwards it, and pressing the center plays the tape.
5. Play a sample of the tape. Adjust the volume, speed, and tone dials to your comfort.	This promotes efficiency and speed.
6. Select the appropriate format and place proper patient identification on the page.	Proper patient identification is essential for legal and ethical reasons.
7. Play a short segment of the tape by pressing the foot pedal, stop the tape, and type the message.	As your speed and skills progress, you will not need to stop the tape as often.
8. If you come across an unfamiliar term, leave enough blank space for the provider to write it in and continue transcribing. When you have finished the document, contact the physician or colleague or use a reference book to fill in the blank.	A thorough knowledge of medical terminology will minimize time spent looking up words.
9. When you are finished, place the initials of the provider, followed by a slash and your initials, on the bottom of the page. The date that each was done should be added.	The reader must know who dictated the report and who transcribed the document and the dates each was carried out.
10. Spell check the document by using medical spell check software.	The spell checker of standard word processing programs does not recognize most medical terms. Medical spell check software is available to ensure accuracy.
11. Print and proofread the document.	Spell checkers mark only misspelled words, not errors. You need to proofread the hard copy for other errors. After typing a lengthy report, it is common to overlook errors. It is helpful to have a coworker also proofread.
12. Leave the document, along with the tape, in a designated area for review.	After reviewing the document, the provider will sign it, indicating that the report is accurate. If corrections are necessary later, a revised copy must be placed with the original report. The final copy should include a notation to identify it as a revised copy.
13. After the provider has reviewed and approved the document, make a copy of the report for the patient's chart.	Reports can be mailed, faxed, or e-mailed. Be careful to follow the guidelines for protecting patients' privacy outlined in Chapter 8.
14. Send the report to the recipient.	This allows the report to be filed.
15. Erase the tape and return it to the dictation area.	Tapes that are not erased cause confusion to the provider when they are recording and may infringe on a patient's right to privacy.

TYPES OF MEDICAL REPORTS

Hospital (inpatient) documents and medical office (outpatient) documents are different. The most common documents transcribed in a medical office are history and physical examination (H&P) reports, consultation reports, and progress reports. Practices that offer diagnostic tests are required to generate a report of the findings. For example, a neurologist's practice may perform electroencephalography (EEG) to measure the electrical activity in the brain. The medical assistant transcribes a dictated report of the findings. Other types of documents in outpatient facilities are reports of minor surgical procedures, legal abstracts, and general office correspondence.

Documents that are seen in the hospital setting include H&Ps, consultation reports, radiology and pathology reports, transfer summaries, discharge and death summaries, and autopsies. Many radiologists who work in hospitals also have a private practices and will dictate a report for each radiology procedure done in the office. You need to become familiar with the reports generated in a hospital because they become a part of the office chart and are used for insurance. Figures 9-6 to 9-9 are samples of typical reports generated in a hospital or inpatient setting.

History and Physical Examination Reports

In the inpatient setting, the H&P is a vital part of the quality of patient care. The JCAHO (Joint Commission on Accreditation of Healthcare Organizations) accredits and regulates every aspect of the policies and practices of hospitals and physician offices owned by hospital organizations.

The JCAHO guidelines require hospitals to provide a H&P on a patient's chart within 24 hours of admission in a facility. This report is dictated by the admitting physician and must be signed or authenticated electronically within a specified time. Many times the patient is seen in the office, and the physician makes the decision to admit. The examination takes place in the office, but the report is dictated to the hospital, which is responsible for transcription. Many physicians use the H&P format to record a patient's annual physical examination in the office as well.

The H&P is divided into two sections: the history, which gives an overview of the patient's medical, family, and social history; and the report on the physical examination, which reviews the results of the examination. Figure 9-2 is a sample history and physical examination report.

Consultation Reports

When one provider refers a patient to another, usually a specialist, the consulting physician prepares a consultation report to report the findings of the encounter. A consultation report contains a detailed account of the consulting physician's findings and recommendations regarding the

CENTRAL MEDICAL GROUP, INC.

Department of Internal Medicine

201 Medical Center Drive • Central City, US 90000-1234 • PHONE: (012) 125-8888 • FAX: (012) 125-3434

PATIENT: COHEN, SARA E.   DATE: April 8, 20xx

HISTORY

CHIEF COMPLAINT: Epigastric distress

HISTORY OF PRESENT ILLNESS: This 33-year-old Caucasian female comes in because of excessive burping, epigastric distress and nausea for several weeks. Coffee makes it worse. She complains that it is worse at night when lying down. She gets an acid-like taste in her mouth. She has tried antacids, to no avail.

PAST MEDICAL HISTORY: The patient states that she had the usual childhood diseases. She has had no serious medical illnesses and has been involved in no accidents. Family History: There is some diabetes on her mother's side. Her mother is 52 and has hypertension. Her father, age 56, is living and well. She has a sister who is anemic and a brother who has ulcers. Social History: The patient discontinued smoking ten years ago. Drinks alcohol socially. Allergies: NKDA. Current Medications: Medications at this time consist of Entex, Guaifed, birth control pills, iron and vitamin supplements.

REVIEW OF SYSTEMS: HEENT: Chronic sinusitis. She sees an ENT specialist and an allergist. Respiratory: Negative. Cardiac: Occasional flutters. Gastrointestinal: As stated above. Genitourinary: Occasional infections. Pap smear is up-to-date and negative. She has had no mammogram at this point. Neuromuscular: Negative.

PHYSICAL EXAMINATION

GENERAL APPEARANCE: Reveals a well-developed, well-nourished female in no acute distress.

VITAL SIGNS: Blood Pressure: 120/80. Pulse: 76 and regular.

HEENT: Head normocephalic. Eyes: Pupils are equal, round, and reactive to light and accommodation. Fundi are benign. Ears, nose and throat are negative. NECK: No thyromegaly. No carotid bruits.

CHEST: Clear to percussion and auscultation. BREASTS: Reveal no masses. HEART: Normal sinus rhythm. No murmurs.

ABDOMEN: Liver, spleen and kidneys could not be felt. Femorals pulsate well, no bruits.

EXTREMITIES: No edema. Pulses are good and equal.

PELVIC & RECTAL EXAMS: Deferred to gynecologist.

NEUROLOGIC EXAM: Physiologic.

IMPRESSION: 1. PROBABLE PEPTIC ULCER DISEASE WITH GASTROESOPHAGEAL REFLUX.
                2. POSSIBLE GALLBLADDER DISEASE.

PLAN: Patient started on Pepcid 40 mg, 1 at night. She is given Gaviscon tablets so she can carry them with her. Schedule routine lab work and upper GI series. If negative, schedule ultrasound of the gallbladder.

D. Everley, M.D.

DE:mc
D: 4/8/20xx
T: 4/9/20xx

F I G U R E 9 – 2 . Sample history and physical examination report. (Reprinted with permission from Willis MC. Medical Terminology: The Language of Health Care, 1st ed. Baltimore: Williams & Wilkins, 1996.)

patient. These reports are often written in the format of the H&P but are structured as a letter to the physician who referred the patient. Chapter 6 discusses the use of the terms *referral* and *consultation*. Figure 9-3 is a sample consultation report.

Progress Reports

In the outpatient medical facility, the patient's progress is recorded on an ongoing sheet in the chart (see Chapter 8). When the notes are transcribed, they are printed either directly on this sheet or on special paper with perforations and adhesive backing. The reports are separated and stuck on the progress sheet. Remember, the entries in the medical record must be consecutive. This presents a problem if the transcription is not on the chart when the next entry is made. Entries that are out of order give the appearance of disorganization, improper record keeping, or even an attempt to cover up negligence.

Progress notes are formatted in several ways. These are discussed in Chapter 8. The SOAP (subjective, objective, assessment, plan) method of reporting a patient's visit is the most common format used in medical offices. The report is dictated in narrative form using general headings. In the outpatient medical facility, you will transcribe this information. Refer to Figure 9-4 as we examine each part of the report.

SOAP Notes

Subjective. The subjective portion of the report includes information that cannot be detected or measured. This information can only be provided by the patient. Pain and nausea are examples of subjective information. This heading also includes the *chief complaint* (CC), the reason the patient is at the facility. In the subjective section, the provider explains the chief complaint in detail, including how long the symptoms have been present and what remedies the patient has tried, along with their results. This is sometimes called the *history of present illness* (HPI). A subheading titled *Medication* may be included in this section to report medications that the patient is taking.

Objective. The objective information in this section comes from the physical examination, laboratory data, diagnostic test results, and other data that can be measured or observed. The patient's appearance, vital signs, any rash, and results of laboratory tests are examples of objective information. For example, the narrative report might say, "EEG is normal."

Assessment. As discussed earlier, the assessment portion of the report refers to the established or possible diagnosis based on the subjective and objective information provided and gathered. Other subheading titles include *Diagnosis*, *Evaluation*, *Impression*, and *Differential Diagnoses*.

Plan. The plan is the steps the physician intends to take. They are usually typed in a numbered list. Medications pre-

scribed, diagnostic tests ordered, referrals to other physicians, and return appointments are included in this section.

Checkpoint Question

3. Compare subjective and objective information. Give two examples of each.

Hospital Reports

H&Ps, consultation reports, operative reports, pathology reports, radiology reports, discharge summaries, and death summaries are generated primarily in inpatient facilities. Every document generated by a hospital transcription department is "copied to," that is, copied and sent to the physician who dictated it. These documents are kept in the physician's office chart.

Operative Report

Each surgical procedure performed in a hospital is documented. Physicians dictate an operative note immediately after the procedure. It is typed and put on the chart as soon as possible so that others caring for the patient have access to the information. When physicians perform surgery in their outpatient offices, the operative report is transcribed in the physician's office. The terms used in operative reports are often difficult. Many sutures and instruments are named for the person who developed them. A reference book for surgical terms is essential for transcribing. Information included in the operative reports includes the patient's preoperative and postoperative diagnoses, the type of anesthesia used, step-by-step details of the procedure, estimated blood loss, results of sponge and instrument counts, and the condition of the patient at the end of the procedure. The subheadings usually follow that format. Figure 9-5 is a sample operative report.

Pathology Report

Any organ or tissue removed from a patient in the operating room is examined by a pathologist. A pathology report outlines the findings of gross and microscopic examinations performed on organs, lesions, and tissue samples removed in surgery. Figure 9-6 is an example of a typical pathology report on a specimen.

Autopsy Report

Pathologists also dictate autopsy reports. An autopsy report, also called necropsy report or medical examiner report, is generated as the autopsy is performed. Autopsies are done to find the cause of death of a patient or to find or confirm diseases present. As discussed in Chapter 2, the law requires that autopsies be performed in certain situations. The autopsy report includes a preliminary diagnosis, a brief history of the
(text continues on page 168)

CENTRAL MEDICAL GROUP, INC.
Department of Otorhinolaryngology
201 Medical Center Drive • Central City, US 90000-1234 • PHONE: (012) 125-8888 • FAX: (012) 125-3434

Patient: Perron, Carleen   DATE: February 17, 20xx

Referring Physician: C. Camarillo, M.D.

CONSULTATION

REASON FOR CONSULTATION: This 28-year-old white female presents with a one week history of upper respiratory infection (URI), sinusitis, and some periorbital headaches in recent weeks. She also has expectorated yellow-green mucus occasionally and has had a history of tonsillitis.

MEDICATIONS: None. **ALLERGIES:** No known allergies (NKA). **SURGERIES:** None. **HOSPITALIZATIONS:** None.

PAST MEDICAL HISTORY/REVIEW OF SYSTEMS: Cardiopulmonary: There is no history of angina, dyspnea, hemoptysis, emphysema, asthma, chronic obstructive pulmonary disease (COPD), hypertension, or heart murmurs. Cardiovascular: There is no history of high blood pressure. Renal: There is no history of dysuria, polyuria, nocturia, hematuria, or cystoliths. Gastrointestinal: There is no history of gallbladder disease, hepatitis, pancreatitis, or colitis. Musculoskeletal: There is no history of arthritis. Endocrine: There is no history of diabetes. Hematologic: There is no history of anemia, blood transfusion, or easy bruising. Gynecological: The patient states her menses are regular, and the start of her last menstrual cycle occurred 15 days ago.

FAMILY HISTORY: The patient states her maternal grandmother has diabetes.

SOCIAL HISTORY: The patient is single and has no children. She denies smoking tobacco. She denies drinking alcoholic beverages. She denies taking drugs.

CHILDHOOD DISEASES: The patient has had the usual childhood diseases.

OTOLARYNGOLOGIC EXAMINATION: Otoscopy: Tympanic membranes (TMs) are dull and slightly congested. Sinuses: There is maxillary fullness. Rhinoscopic examination reveals mild nasoseptal deviation (NSD). Pharynx: There is moderate inflammation; no exudates. Oropharynx: No masses. Nasopharynx: No masses. Larynx: Clear. Neck: Supple. Cervical Adenopathy: There is mild adenopathy.

IMPRESSION:
1. MAXILLARY SINUSITIS.
2. PHARYNGITIS.
3. CHRONIC TONSILLITIS.

DISPOSITION:
1. Warm salt water gargle (WSWG).
2. Ery-Tab 333, #24, 1 t.i.d. p.c.
3. Robitussin.
4. Return to office (RTO) in one week.

P. Rodden MD

PATRICK RODDEN, M.D.

JR:ti
D: 2/17/20xx
T: 2/18/20xx

FIGURE 9–3. Sample consultation report. (Reprinted with permission from Willis MC. Medical Terminology: The Language of Health Care, 1st ed. Baltimore: Williams & Wilkins, 1996.)

CENTRAL MEDICAL GROUP, INC.
Department of Otorhinolaryngology

201 Medical Center Drive • Central City, US 90000-1234 • PHONE: (012) 125-8888 • FAX: (012) 125-3434

PROGRESS NOTES

Patient: PERRON, CARLEEN

03/30/20xx

S: The patient presents with a sore throat x 2 weeks.

O: Sinus exam: Maxillary and frontal congestion. Hypopharynx/adenoids: No inflammation.

A: Recurrent pharyngitis/sinusitis x 2 weeks.

P: 1) Ceftin 250 mg, #21, 1 t.i.d. p.o. p.c.

2) Entex LA, #30, 1 b.i.d. p.o.

3) Warm salt water gargle.

P Rodden MD
PATRICK RODDEN, M.D.

05/25/20xx

S: Recurrent sore throat every month.

O: Recurrent tonsillitis, cryptic tonsillitis. Sinus exam: Maxillary and frontal congestion. Neck: Supple; no masses. Hypopharynx/Adenoids: No inflammation. Paranasal Sinus X-ray: Bilateral frontal and maxillary sinusitis.

A: Recurrent tonsillitis, 8-10 times per year. Chronic maxillary and frontal sinusitis.

P: 1) Tonsillectomy discussed with the patient. The risks of general and local anesthesia, as well as the surgical procedure, were discussed with the patient. The consent form was signed.

2) An admitting order was given to the patient for CBC, UA, and BCP-7 to be done one day prior to being admitted.

3) Ceftin 250 mg, #21, 1 t.i.d. p.o. p.c.

4) Entex LA, #30, 1 b.i.d. p.o.

5) Beconase nasal inhaler, 2 sprays each nostril b.i.d.

6) Warm salt water gargle.

P Rodden MD
PATRICK RODDEN, M.D.

FIGURE 9-4. Sample progress report. (Reprinted with permission from Willis MC. Medical Terminology: The Language of Health Care, 1st ed. Baltimore: Williams & Wilkins, 1996.)

CENTRAL MEDICAL CENTER

211 Medical Center Drive • Central City, US 90000-1234 • PHONE: (012) 125-6784 • FAX: (012) 125-9999

OPERATIVE REPORT

DATE OF OPERATION: June 3, 20xx

PREOPERATIVE DIAGNOSIS: Chronic tonsillitis.

POSTOPERATIVE DIAGNOSIS: Frequent, recurrent tonsillitis.

SURGEON: Patrick Rodden, M.D.

ASSISTANT SURGEON: None

ANESTHESIOLOGIST: Robert Jung, M.D.

ANESTHESIA: General.

SURGERY PERFORMED: Tonsillectomy.

DESCRIPTION OF OPERATION: After general anesthesia induction, with intubation, the McGivor mouth gag and tongue retractor were utilized for exposure of the oropharynx. Local anesthetic consisting of 6 cc of 0.5% Xylocaine with 1:100,000 epinephrine was utilized. Tonsillectomy was carried out using dissection and air technique. The right tonsillectomy electrocoagulation Bovie suction was utilized for hemostasis. Examination of the nasopharynx was normal.

The patient tolerated the procedure well and went to the recovery room in good condition.

P. Rodden MD

PATRICK RODDEN, M.D.

JR:as
D: 6/3/20xx
T: 6/4/20xx

OPERATIVE REPORT	PT. NAME:	PERRON, CARLEEN
	ID NO:	672894017
	ROOM NO:	312
	ATT. PHYS:	PATRICK RODDEN, M.D.

FIGURE 9–5. Sample operative report. (Reprinted with permission from Willis MC. *Medical Terminology: A Programmed Learning Approach to the Language of Health Care*, 1st ed. Baltimore: Lippincott Williams & Wilkins, 2002.)

CENTRAL MEDICAL CENTER

211 Medical Center Drive • Central City, US 90000-1234 • PHONE: (012) 125-6784 • FAX: (012) 125-9999

PATHOLOGY REPORT

PATIENT: PERRON, CARLEEN
            28 Y (FEMALE)

DATE RECEIVED: June 3, 20xx   DATE REPORTED: June 4, 20xx

GROSS:

Received are two tonsils each 2.5 cm in greatest diameter.

MICROSCOPIC:

The sections show deep tonsillar crypts associated with follicular lymphoid hyperplasia. No bacterial granules are seen.

DIAGNOSIS:

CHRONIC LYMPHOID HYPERPLASIA OF RIGHT AND LEFT TONSILS.

Mary Needham MD
MARY NEEDHAM, M.D.

MN:gds

D: 6/4/20xx
T: 6/5/20xx

F IGURE 9 – 6 .   Sample pathology report. (Reprinted with permission from Willis MC. Medical Terminology: A Programmed Learning Approach to the Language of Health Care, 1st ed. Baltimore: Lippincott Williams & Wilkins, 2002.)

patient, findings from the examination of the gross anatomy of the body and its organs, findings of the microscopic examination of the cells, and a determination of cause of death.

Radiology Report

Each radiograph must be interpreted by a radiologist. Even when radiological procedures are performed in an emergency room or walk-in clinic, a radiologist must read the film and dictate a formal report. Radiology reports include

the title of the procedure, any contrast medium or nuclear medicine given, and an interpretation of the film (Fig. 9-7).

Discharge Summary

The discharge summary is a chronological account of the patient's hospital stay. If the patient is being transferred to another facility, this report may be titled *Transfer Summary*. It is a concise report of the reason for the patient's admission, tests performed, treatments given, results of those tests and treat-

CENTRAL MEDICAL CENTER

211 Medical Center Drive • Central City, US 90000-1234 • PHONE: (012) 125-6784 • FAX: (012) 125-9999

X-RAY REPORT

LUMBOSACRAL SPINE:
Multiple views reveal no evidence of fracture. There is slight lumbar spondylosis with slight lipping and minimal bridging. The disc spaces appear maintained except for slight narrowing at L4-L5 and L5-S1. There is also a Grade I spondylolisthesis of L5 on S1 and evidence of spondylolysis at L5 on the left. There is also slight dextroscoliosis in the lumbar region and slight increased lordosis in the lumbosacral region. The bony architecture is unremarkable except for eburnation between the articulating facets at L5-S1. The SI joints appear unremarkable. Incidentally noted are slight osteoarthritic changes involving both hips.

CONCLUSION:

1. Slight lumbar spondylosis with hypertrophic lipping and slight narrowing of the L4-L5 and L5-S1 disc spaces, 'rule out discogenic disease. If clinically indicated, CT of the lumbosacral spine may prove helpful in further evaluation.

2. Grade I spondylolisthesis of L5 on S1 with evidence of spondylolysis at L5 on the left.

3. Slight dextroscoliosis in the lumbar region and slight increased lordosis in the lumbosacral region.

M. Volz, M.D.

MV:ti

D: 10/19/20xx
T: 10/20/20xx

X-RAY REPORT	PT. NAME: DORN, JAY F. ID NO: RL-483091 ATT. PHYS: T. LIGHT, M.D.

FIGURE 9-7. Sample radiology report. (Reprinted with permission from Willis MC. Medical Terminology: The Language of Health Care, 1st ed. Baltimore: Williams & Wilkins, 1996.)

ments, procedures performed, improvements, setbacks, and, finally, the condition of the patient at the time of discharge.

The discharge summary is an excellent tool for members of the health care team involved in the patient's posthospital care. A patient who is recovering from a stroke may receive services from a home health nurse, a physical therapist, and a speech therapist. The discharge summary provides a snapshot of the patient's situation in one document.

Figure 9-8 is a sample discharge summary. Be sure it is in the office chart for the patient's first visit after hospitalization.

CENTRAL MEDICAL CENTER

211 Medical Center Drive • Central City, US 90000-1234 • PHONE: (012) 125-6784 • FAX: (012) 125-9999

DISCHARGE SUMMARY

DATE OF ADMISSION: 10/25/20xx   DATE OF DISCHARGE: 10/29/20xx

ADMITTING DIAGNOSIS:
Left ureteropelvic junction obstruction.

DISCHARGE DIAGNOSIS:
Left ureteropelvic junction obstruction.

PROCEDURE PERFORMED:
Left dismembered pyeloplasty and placement of stent.

BRIEF SUMMARY:
The patient is a 19-year-old male who was admitted to the hospital a month ago with left pyelonephritis. He was found to have a left ureteropelvic junction obstruction. The patient was brought to the hospital at this time for repair of the moderately to severely obstructed left kidney. A preoperative urine culture was sterile. The patient underwent the procedure without complication. A double-J stent was placed. The Jackson-Pratt drain was removed on the second postoperative day because of minimal drainage. The patient initially had urinary retention, but this resolved by the third postoperative day. He was doing fine at the time of discharge. His condition on discharge is good.

INSTRUCTIONS TO THE PATIENT:
1) Regular diet. 2) No heavy lifting, straining, or driving an automobile for six weeks from the day of surgery. He should also keep the incision relatively dry this week. 3) Follow up in my office in three weeks. 4) It is anticipated the stent will remain indwelling for six weeks and then will be removed cystoscopically at that time. 5) Discharge medication is Tylenol #3, 1-2 q 4 h p.r.n. pain.

_____
L. Zlatkin, M.D.

LZ:mr

D: 10/29/20xx
T: 10/30/20xx

DISCHARGE SUMMARY	PT. NAME:	MERCIER, CHARLES F.
	ID NO:	IP-392689
	ROOM NO:	444
	ATT. PHYS:	L.ZLATKIN, M.D.

FIGURE 9–8.   Sample discharge summary. (Reprinted with permission from Willis MC. Medical Terminology: A Programmed Learning Approach to the Language of Health Care, 1st ed. Baltimore: Lippincott Williams & Wilkins, 2002.)

Checkpoint Question

4. List the information found in a discharge or transfer summary.

TRANSCRIPTION RULES

The following section is not intended to be a complete list of rules, but it includes most of the general rules necessary in medical transcription. Different texts give different rules for punctuation, so it is recommended that you follow the guidelines of the American Association of Medical Transcription (AAMT), the source of these rules.

Abbreviations

When you use abbreviations in medical documents, your reader must be able to recognize or translate the abbreviation. Every licensed medical facility is required to keep a list of approved abbreviations, and this list should be updated regularly. Some facilities have local abbreviations that are specific to the facility. Like words in English, many abbreviations have two meanings. The use of capital letters can change the meaning entirely. For example, CC means chief complaint, but cc means cubic centimeters. For this reason, be very cautious in using abbreviations. Some abbreviations have become accepted because they are used more than the long form. BP has come to be easily recognized as blood pressure when used in the vital sign section of the report. In a hospital setting, the use of abbreviations in typed reports is forbidden. For example, you are not allowed to abbreviate the diagnosis on an operative report.

Most doctors' offices use standard abbreviations in the patients' charts, but when you are typing a formal report, it is risky to use abbreviations. If it is the policy of your facility to use abbreviations in letters and formal reports, spell out the words the first time the abbreviation is used, with the abbreviation following in parentheses. In general, "when in doubt, spell it out."

Capitalization

Knowing when to capitalize and when to use lowercase letters is a mark of an excellent transcriptionist. The rules about using capital letters you learned in grammar school still apply, but when you are transcribing medical records, capitals are used in additional situations.

Use capital letters:

1. For headings.
   CHIEF COMPLAINT or Chief Complaint
2. For eponyms (terms formed using the name of a person, usually the name of the researcher or physician who identified a disorder or the inventor of equipment, instruments, supplies, and so on), the second word in the phrase is not capitalized. *Note*: Recent revisions in punctuation guidelines eliminate the possessive apostrophe.
   Down syndrome   Foley catheter   Healy clamp
3. For trade or brand names of drugs and products. Do not capitalize generic names of drugs and products.
   diazepam   Valium
   tissue   Kleenex
4. For the genus of an organism. An example of this classification system of living organisms is *Staphylococcus aureus*. *Staphylococcus* is the genus and *aureus* is the species. A singular genus is capitalized and italicized. If the genus is plural or used as an adjective, it is lower case and not italicized. Use lowercase letters and italics for the species.
   as noun: *Staphylococcus aureus*
   as adjective: staphylococcal infection
5. For a department name when the name is the proper title of a place, but not for department names within a facility.
   The patient was taken to the emergency room.
   The patient was taken to the Forsyth Medical Center Emergency Room.
6. For proper names of languages, races, and religions.
   She is a 23-year-old Hispanic woman.
   Do not capitalize informal designations such as white or black.
7. For acronyms (words formed from initials of words in a phrase).
   NKDA (no known drug allergies)
   CABG (coronary artery bypass graft)
8. To draw attention to vital information, such as allergies.
   ALLERGIES: The patient is allergic to PENICILLIN.

Numbers

Traditional office technology courses teach the rules for using numbers, but many of those rules do not apply to medical documents. When those guidelines have the potential to cause confusion or harm a patient, you must be flexible enough to bend them. The safety of the patient is a goal of the transcriptionist.

Follow these guidelines for using numbers in medical reports:

1. Spell out the numbers one through nine in a narrative report (see guidelines 3 and 6 below). Ten and above are keyed as numerals (e.g., 10, 11) unless they begin a sentence, as in this sentence.
2. If you are using two numbers in one sentence, be consistent. It does not matter whether you choose numerals or words, but they should be consistent.
   Dr. Smith saw 14 patients today; one of them was only 2 days old.
   If using more than one number could cause confusion, spell out the one that is easiest and shortest.
   The patient states that she drinks 12 two-liter sodas per week.

3. Always use numerals with symbols. Do not key a space between the number and the symbol.

    100% oxygen

    $14.27 balance due

    #2 specimen

4. For balance and clarity, add a zero before and after a decimal point. The provider will say, "The specimen measures eight by five and a half by point six."

    Clear: The specimen measures 8.0 × 5.5 × 0.6.

    Unclear: The specimen measures 8 × 5.5 × .6.

5. Key a space between numerals and a unit of measurement, abbreviation, or symbol.

    10 mg%   40 mL   20 mm Hg

6. Use numerals for measurements of vital signs, laboratory values, age, height, weight, and so on.

    BP 110/70   Respirations 20

    Temperature 98.7°F   Wt. 140 lb.

    Pulse 80   Ht. 60 inch.

    FBS (fasting blood sugar) 98

7. Spell out ordinal numbers except in dates.

    She began feeling better the third day after surgery.

    The patient was seen on May 3.

8. Roman numerals are used with cranial nerves, obstetric history, electrocardiographic leads, types and factors, and cancer stages.

    Cranial nerves II through XII are intact.

    Limb leads II through V on the electrocardiogram were not making contact.

    The carcinoma is stage II.

Punctuation

One of the most important skills necessary to be an efficient and productive transcriptionist is the ability to punctuate without direction. Some physicians dictate punctuation, but you should not automatically type these directions unless they follow the AAMT's *Guidelines for Transcription.*

Apostrophes

Use an apostrophe:

1. To show possession

    The patient's appointment is Wednesday.

2. To form contractions

    She's having flu symptoms. (The apostrophe contracts *she* and *is*.)

    Note: "It is" can be shortened to "it's," but there is no apostrophe in the possessive:

    Its length is 4 cm.

3. With units of time and money when they are possessive

    We will give him a week's worth of medication.

    Nine months' gestation is standard.

    He bought 10 dollars' worth of gas.

4. For clarity when using one letter as a word

    The I's were not dotted.

    But not to form plurals

    DRGs

    WBCs

    I've had this dress since the 1970s.

    Unless it is possessive

    The CMA's uniform is neat and clean.

Commas

Use a comma:

1. Between items in a series (the last comma is optional).

    The patient is alert, oriented and talkative.

    Or

    The pain is bilateral, severe, and stabbing.

    Note: Do not use commas between items that modify each other. Even though this seems like a series of adjectives, it is really one unit.

    There is severe, stabbing, bilateral pain in the lower abdominal region.

    The first three adjectives modify *pain* and are separated by commas. "Lower" refers to the abdomen, not the region, so no comma is used.

2. To link two complete sentences that are separated by a conjunction.

    She is a very sick patient, and I will admit her immediately.

    But not when both clauses lack a subject and a predicate

    She is a very sick patient and needs to be admitted.

    "Needs to be admitted" does not contain its own subject. Therefore, no comma is needed.

3. After the conjunctive adverb.

    The medical assistant is in great demand; therefore, most schools have a waiting list.

4. After an introductory phrase or clause with a subject and a verb.

    After she has her chest radiograph, she will come back to the office.

    NO comma is needed when the sentence is reversed.

    She will come back to the office after she has her chest x-ray.

    Lightheaded, she sat down on the floor.

5. To set off clauses within a sentence that provide additional information.

    Electroencephalography, a test that assesses the electrical activity in the brain, is a diagnostic tool used by neurologists.

6. To set off parenthetical expressions.

    The pain, according to the patient, measures 10 on the pain scale.

7. With dates when using the year, place names, and long numbers.
    The patient was seen last on May 2, 2003.
    But: The patient was seen last on May 2 at 2:00 p.m.
    Duke University Medical Center is in Durham, North Carolina.
    Numbers over five figures:
    4500
    567,158,230
8. With quotations.
    The patient said, "I will quit smoking tomorrow."
9. To prevent confusion.
    "The physician came in, in order to see the patient."

Semicolons

Use a semicolon:

1. To separate main clauses that do not have a conjunction such as *and* or *but*
    The patient arrived 10 minutes late; she had car trouble.
2. To separate two main clauses if they are long or you need other commas within the sentence
    She had chest pain, nausea, and headache; and her daughter took her to the emergency room.

Colons

Use a colon:

1. After headings
    FAMILY HISTORY: The patient reports no family history of cancer.
2. To introduce a series after a complete clause but not after a verb
    The physician prescribed the following medications: Keflex, Darvocet-N 100, K Tabs and Prinivil.
    The physician prescribed Keflex, Darvocet-N 100, K-Tabs, and Prinivil.
3. To separate hours from minutes
    Your appointment is scheduled for 10:30 a.m.
4. After a salutation in a business letter
    Dear Dr. Johnsen:

Periods

In addition to ending sentences, periods are used:

1. With lowercase abbreviations
    a.m., p.m.   *But:* AM, PM   PhD
    Metric measurements do not use periods.
    They had to remove 3 ft. of her colon.
    We removed 15 mL of pleural fluid.

2. After an abbreviation that is a shortened part of a word
    American Association of Medical Assistants, Inc.
3. After a person's initials
    J. T. Weaver, MD

Quotation Marks

Quotation marks enclose:

1. A direct quotation
    The patient stated, "My friend recommended your office to me."
2. Words that are slang or thought to be a quotation.
    The patient stated he was "blown away" by his improved cholesterol reading.
    Jessica thinks her new boyfriend is "Prince Charming."
3. Titles of articles, short stories, subdivisions, and so on
    Please read "Making the Patient Comfortable" in the most recent issue of our professional journal.
    Table 9-1 presents rules for using other punctuation with quotation marks.

Slash Marks

In medical transcription, the slash mark is used:

1. In place of the word *per*. The provider says, "Give the patient one hundred percent oxygen at two liters per minute." You type:
    Give the patient 100% oxygen at 2 liters/minute.
    In some cases, the provider may not say "per," but you insert a slash.
    The student took the class on a pass/fail basis.
2. To separate options and alternatives.
    This is a pass/fail course.

Hyphens

Hyphens are used:

1. In compound words. The general rule is that when two words are used together to form a word, they are joined by a hyphen. Many compound nouns have been used long enough to be consolidated and are now accepted words in their own right. For example, spread-sheet has become spreadsheet.
    mother-in-law   figure-of-eight sutures
2. A hyphen can clear up confusion or ambiguity. For example, re-creation is quite different from recreation. Without the hyphen, the reader would misinterpret the meaning.
    We will *re-treat* with a different antibiotic.
    As opposed to
    We went on a weekend *retreat*.

T a b l e 9 – 1	**THE USE OF OTHER PUNCTUATION WITH QUOTATION MARKS**
Rule	**Example**
Place commas and periods inside quotation marks.	"Your bill, explained the patient, "has not come in the mail."
Place colons and semicolons outside quotation marks.	She said, "The doctor told me to come back on Friday"; however, he has no openings.
Place other punctuation inside quotation marks only if they belong in the quotation.	The student asked, "Is that going to be on the test?" *But* Did the patient say, "Yes, I'll come"?
Place commas and periods outside quotation marks when used with single letters or single words.	Even though she made an "A," she felt it was not her best work.

3. When joining the two words would result in two or more identical letters.

    post-traumatic   pre-enteric   pre-existing

Note: Otherwise, the hyphen is not used with these prefixes.

    postoperative infection   prehistoric

4. When spelling out the compound numbers twenty-one to ninety-nine.

    Fifty-eight percent of our patients are over sixty-five years old.

5. When using compound adjectives before a noun.

    high-frequency hearing loss

    well-developed frame

    22-gauge needle

    6-month-old infant

Remember, the hyphen is not used when the compound adjective follows the noun it modifies:

    The patient is 6 months old.

6. The hyphen is not used when adverbs modify adjectives.

    very high fever   quickly spreading cancer

7. When a compound adjective contains the suffix -free.

    symptom-free

8. When the compound includes an acronym.

    post-CABG care   pre-ICU lab results

9. When keying suture sizes.

    2-0 Prolene

Grammar

When a physician dictates a report using incorrect grammar, it is your job to correct the mistake. The physician expects you to produce an error-free report, even though he or she may overlook basic parts of speech and rules of sentence grammar. Although a thorough discussion of the grammar rules in the English language is outside the scope of this text, some basic rules should be mentioned. The most common errors made in medical transcription are those dealing with verb tense.

Always be sure that subjects and verbs agree in number.

One patient: The patient *is* alert.

More than one vital sign: His vital signs *are* normal

Always make sentences within a paragraph agree in tense and subject. Suppose the provider dictates, "The patient was seen in clinic today for pain in the left knee. The examination *is* negative." You will key, "The patient was seen in clinic today for pain in the left knee. The examination *was* negative."

Spelling

When in doubt about the spelling of a word or drug, always use a reference book, dictionary, or spell check to confirm the spelling. Keep in mind that computer spell check will check for spelling only, and a misused word will not be caught if it is spelled correctly. For example, "the patient was late four his appointment" will pass the spell check because "four" is spelled correctly, even though the transcriptionist meant to key "for."

Here are some basic spelling tips:

1. I comes before e except after c or when sounded like a as in neighbor and weigh.

    Examples: achieve, receive (the exceptions are either, neither, weird, leisure, and conscience)

2. For words ending in ie, drop the e and change the i to y before adding ing.

    Examples: die, dying; lie, lying

3. Words ending in o that are preceded by a vowel are made plural by adding s.

    Examples: studio, studios; trio, trios

Words ending in o that are preceded by a consonant form the plural by adding es.

    Examples: hero, heroes; potato, potatoes

4. Words ending in y preceded by a vowel form the plural by adding s.

    Examples: attorney, attorneys; day, days

Words ending in y that are preceded by a consonant change the y to i and add es.

    Examples: berry, berries; lady, ladies

5. The final consonant of a one-syllable word is doubled before adding a suffix beginning with a vowel.

    Examples: pin, pinning; run, running

If the final consonant is preceded by another consonant or by two vowels, do not double the consonant.

    Examples: act, acting; look, looked

6. Words ending in a silent e generally drop the e before adding a suffix beginning with a vowel.
     Examples: ice, icing; judge, judging
   The exceptions are dye, eye, shoe, and toe. The e is not dropped in suffixes beginning with a consonant, however, unless another vowel precedes the final e.
     Examples: argue, argument; pale, paleness
7. For all words ending in c, insert a k before adding a suffix beginning with e, i, or y.
     Examples: picnic, picnicking; traffic, trafficker

You must pay close attention to spelling when transcribing medical documents. Remember, in the medical world a misspelled drug or word can be dangerous.

TRANSCRIPTION SYSTEMS

Vast improvements have been made in dictating and transcribing capabilities and equipment over the past decade. Traditionally, the physician or health care provider uses a dictation machine with a handheld microphone to tape a report of a patient encounter or other correspondence. With the **analogue** or tape system, after the message is taped, the cassette tape will be removed and marked with some form of identification. Cassette tapes range in size from micro to standard.

Traditional Tape Dictation Systems

Each model of transcription machine is slightly different; however, most have the basic parts described next (Fig. 9-9).

- The foot pedal is used to start, stop, fast-forward, and rewind the tape.
- The speed control regulates the speed at which the tape plays. As a beginner, you want to keep the speed slow. As your listening and typing coordination improve, you will be able to increase the speed of the tape. When you become experienced with a particular

provider's voice speed, you will be able to set the speed control to match his or her voice speed and your typing speed.
- The tone dial can be adjusted to change the bass or treble of a provider's voice.
- The volume control is used to adjust the sound level.
- The headset is used to eliminate distracting external noises. It is not a good habit to share headset earplugs with fellow colleagues because an ear infection may be transmitted. Ear cushions that attach to the headsets should be used and washed or replaced often.
- The speaker allows the sound to be heard from a speaker in the transcriber instead of the headset. This feature is handy when the transcriptionist needs assistance or clarification in interpreting the dictation.
- Counters are available on most machines for ease in locating certain reports and to judge the length of a document.

Because every transcription machine is slightly different, you should read the instruction manual before you begin working on a unfamiliar machine. All instruction manuals should be kept in one central location in the office for easy access.

Tapes are usually transcribed in or near the medical records department. Tapes should be erased after the material has been transcribed, reviewed, and signed by the provider. Before discarding a worn-out tape, erase it completely to maintain confidentiality.

Digital Systems

The industry is moving toward a **digital** system, which converts the voice into digits, decodes it, and sends the voice directly to a transcriber through the telephone lines. The system integrates with a computer at the transcriptionist's desk, where a certain code is entered. This code will automatically produce the information and report format on the screen of the computer. In hospitals, most patient care units have dictation phones or ports for digital systems.

Voice Recognition Systems

Voice recognition software and digital voice recording systems have expanded and improved medical transcription. Some people predicted that the invention of voice recognition software would eliminate the need for medical transcriptionists, but the medical community has been slow to respond to the technology. Some limitations are difficult to overcome. For example, if the provider says "there," how does the computer know whether to type "there," "their," or "they're"? Accents, dialects, proper names, and garbled speech are challenges for transcriptionists no matter which system is being used. These same challenges face the inventors of voice recognition software. Even with sophisticated voice recognition systems, there will always be a need for

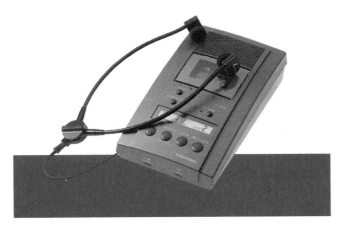

F I G U R E 9 – 9 . Transcription machines vary. Speed control is an important function of the machine.

WHAT IF

You are having trouble understanding a particular physician's dictation tapes because of a dialect or foreign accent. How should you handle this situation?

First, rewind the tape and listen again to the phrase. You can try to adjust the speed control to slow the pronunciation of the word. Consider what a word would sound like with the accent on a different syllable or using a short sound instead of a long sound of a vowel. Being familiar with the type of report being dictated will help you anticipate what the provider might be saying. If you are still uncertain about the word or phrase, leave a blank space for that word and continue transcribing. Edit the report to fill in the blank. Never guess! If you have difficulty understanding a provider, discuss the problem with him or her. Open communication will help you both make adjustments. Neither of you wants to take the chance of producing an erroneous report.

transcriptionists or medical language specialists to proofread, punctuate, and edit medical documents.

Transcription With Word Processing Software

When using word processing programs, you may use macros, templates, and other functions that record keystrokes or provide a blank format to speed the process of transcribing reports that contain the same text over and over again. For example, the format for a certain type of report or letterhead and normal dictation for ordinary examinations can be recorded for playback with a quick keystroke. Legal experts warn providers not just to report examination results as "normal." Instead, they should describe the negative findings. For example, when a patient's throat appears normal to the examiner, he or she should report, "The throat appears normal, with no redness or exudate" (pus).

Checkpoint Question

5. Describe the main difference between analogue and digital transcription equipment.

CHAPTER SUMMARY

Medical transcription is a growing industry. The person who possesses the necessary skills transforms vital information about a patient's care and treatment and is an important member of the health care team. Many medical assistants perform this important function in the medical office. The training you receive in your medical assisting education will enable you to perform at entry-level competency, but experience in transcribing will enhance your skills and make you a more desirable employee for medical offices. Medical information is crucial to patient care and must be prepared with proper grammar, punctuation, and spelling. Physicians depend on timely and accurate preparation of their reports to make decisions. This information is confidential and must be handled with great caution and integrity.

Answers to the Checkpoint Questions

1. A professional document should be well balanced and attractive with single spacing, double spacing between headings, and one-inch margins.
2. JCAHO requires that results of the H&P be placed on a patient's chart within 24 hours of admission to a hospital facility. The physician must sign the H&P report within a prescribed amount of time as well.

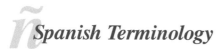

Spanish Terminology

Esto es una máquina de transcripción.	This is a transcription machine.
Yo no lo podría oír con los auriculares.	I couldn't hear you with the headphones on.
¿Qué escucha usted?	What are you listening to?
Escucho y escribo a máquina cartas para el doctor.	I am listening and typing letters for the doctor.

3. Subjective information is provided by the patient and is information that cannot be seen or measured. Examples are pain and nausea. Objective findings are reported by the examiner and can be observed or detected. Examples are rash and blood pressure.

4. The discharge, transfer, or death summary is a concise report of the reason for the patient's admission, tests performed, treatments given, results of those tests and treatments, procedures performed, improvements, setbacks, and, finally, the condition of the patient at the time of discharge.

5. The analogue system uses cassette tapes to record the voice, and the digital system uses digits that are converted and sent across the telephone lines.

 Websites

American Association of Medical Transcription
    www.aamt.org
Medical Transcription Jobs
    www.mtjobs.com
Medical Transcription Daily
    www.mtdaily.com

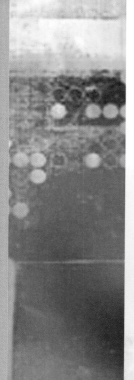

10

Computer Applications in the Medical Office

ROLE DELINEATION COMPONENTS

GENERAL: Communication Skills
- Recognize and respond effectively to verbal, nonverbal, and written communication
- Use electronic technology to receive, organize, prioritize, and transmit information

GENERAL: Operational Functions
- Perform routine maintenance of administrative and clinical equipment
- Apply computer techniques to support office operations

GENERAL: Instruction
- Locate community resources and disseminate information

GENERAL: Legal Concepts
- Perform within legal and ethical boundaries

ADMINISTRATIVE: Administrative Procedures
- Perform basic administrative medical assisting functions

CHAPTER COMPETENCIES

LEARNING OBJECTIVES
Upon successfully completing this chapter, you will be able to:
1. Spell and define the key words
2. Identify the basic computer components
3. Explain the basics of connecting to the Internet
4. Discuss the safety concerns for online searching
5. Describe how to use a search engine
6. List sites that can be used by professionals and sites geared for patients
7. Describe the benefits of an intranet and explain how it differs from the Internet
8. Describe the various types of clinical software that might be used in a physician's office
9. Describe the various types of administrative software that might be used in a physician's office
10. Describe the benefits of a handheld computer
11. Describe the considerations for purchasing a computer
12. Describe various training options
13. Discuss the ethics related to computer access

PERFORMANCE OBJECTIVES
Upon successfully completing this chapter, you will be able to:
1. Search a given topic on the Internet
2. Conduct a basic literary search

KEY TERMS

cookies	Ethernet	literary search	virus
downloading	Internet	search engine	virtual
encryption	intranet	surfing	

COMPUTERS PLAY A MAJOR ROLE in the physician's office. Computers are used for both clinical and administrative applications. A few examples of administrative applications are appointment scheduling, billing, staff scheduling, and insurance fillings. Clinical software programs are used for many areas, such as reading laboratory and radiology reports and helping the physician to prescribe medications. Computers promote communication among health care professionals and provide access to new treatment options. You will need excellent computer skills to work as a medical assistant. This chapter will help you to improve your existing skills. It provides a basic review of computer components. You will learn how the Internet is used in health care settings and some precautions. Various medical software applications will also be discussed. You will learn about training options and how to purchase a computer.

THE COMPUTER

A computer system is roughly divided into two areas, hardware and peripherals.

Hardware

Computer hardware consists of seven key elements (Fig. 10-1). Here is a review of their parts:

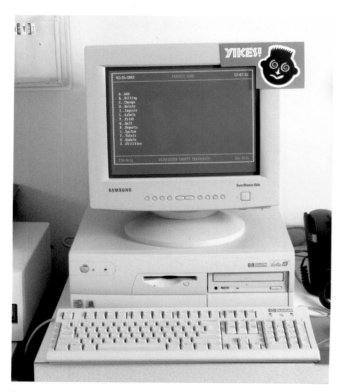

FIGURE 10–1. The computer consists of the CPU, keyboard, monitor, hard drive, printer, and secondary storage systems. Additional peripherals include the mouse, battery backup and modems.

- *Central processing unit.* The central processing unit (CPU), or microprocessor, is the circuitry imprinted on a silicon chip that processes information. The CPU consists of a variety of electronic and magnetic cells. These cells read, analyze, and process data and instruct the computer how to operate a given program. All CPUs function basically the same way, but chips differ dramatically in capabilities and speeds. Your CPU has many ports to connect the printer, mouse, and speakers. At minimum, it has two serial ports, one parallel port, and two universal serial bus (USB) ports. Serial ports are used for items like modems; parallel ports are used for connecting printers and backup drives to the CPU; and USB ports allow the computer to connect with various instruments.
- *Keyboard.* The keyboard is the primary means by which information is entered into the computer. Besides the typical letter and number keys, you will find special function keys that provide increased capabilities. Examples of special function keys are Alt, Ctrl, Insert, and Esc. Each of these keys has a specific function that is determined by the software program. These functions may include searching for and replacing words, moving blocks of text, indenting or centering text, and spell checking.
- *Monitor.* Monitors, also called the visual display terminals, come in various sizes and qualities. The quality of the image is based on the DPIs (dots per inch). The more DPIs, the clearer the picture. There are adjustment dials for brightness and contrast.
- *Hard drive.* The hard drive provides storage for programs, data, and files. The capacity of a hard drive (i.e., the quantity of program and data it can hold) is measured in megabytes or gigabytes. Originally, hard drives could hold 5 MB (equivalent to about 2,000 typed pages), but today they have much more capacity.
- *Printer.* The printer transfers information to paper (hard copy). Printers use various technologies, operate at various speeds, and print in either black or color. The printer allows you to generate bills, print letters, and produce a daily schedule. The two types of printers used in physicians' offices are dot matrix and laser. Dot matrix printers are used primarily for printing insurance forms. They should not be used to print patient discharge instructions unless the instructions can be clearly read. You should print all business letters on a laser printer.
- *Scanner.* A scanner allows you to take a picture or report and read it into the computer. You may scan laboratory reports, radiology reports, and discharge summaries into a patient's file. This is very helpful when a new patient arrives with reports from a previous physician. Patient education materials can also be scanned into the computer and then adjusted to meet the needs of your office. Keep in mind that you need to adhere to copyright laws.

• *Secondary storage systems.* All computers have multiple methods for saving data. Examples include floppy diskettes, compact disks, digital video disks, and zip drives. Cartridges are used by hospital for large storage systems. When saving any type of data, remember that good organization skills are essential. Name your files appropriately and place files in properly identified folders. Most computers have preset timing systems that automatically save data. Check your default setting and readjust as needed.

 Checkpoint Question

1. What do the CPU cells do?

Peripherals

Computers can have many peripheral connections. Three key computer peripherals that you need to know are:

• *Mouse.* The mouse can be used to control the cursor on the display screen. Although you cannot type in characters using the mouse, you can move or delete individual characters, words, or entire blocks of text with it. The track ball is an alternative to a mouse. Your finger rotates the ball to move the pointer. It takes less space than a mouse and is used based on personal preference.
• *Battery backup.* A battery backup allows the computer system to function in the event of a power failure. Batteries come in various sizes depending on the size of your computer and the amount of work to be done during a power failure.
• *Modem.* A modem is a communication device that connects your computer with other computers, including the Internet, online services such as bulletin boards, and electronic mail systems. The faster the modem, the faster the transmission. Modems may be connected through cable systems or through the telephone. Digital subscriber line (DSL) is the preferred method. To use a cable or DSL connection, your computer must have an **Ethernet** port or an Ethernet interface card.

 Checkpoint Question

2. Why should your computer have an Ethernet port or Ethernet interface card?

Care and Maintenance of the System and Equipment

As with any piece of equipment in the medical office, it is necessary to maintain your computer on a regular basis. Some general care guidelines follow:

• Place the monitor, keyboard, and printer in a cool dry area out of direct sunlight.

Box 10-1

BASIC CARE OF DISKS

Whether you are using a floppy diskette, CD or DVD disk, follow these guidelines:
• Always handle the disk by the label or jacket.
• Do not touch the inside of the disk.
• Store in a safe, cool dry place. Avoid high-moisture areas.
• Keep all food and liquids away.
• Never store near a magnetic field, such as a television screen or cellular telephone.
• Store in a vertical container designed for that purpose.
• Always label before storing. Write on the label sticker before sticking the label to the disk.

• Static electricity can cause memory loss, inaccurate data collection, and other adverse reactions. To control this problem, place the computer desk on an antistatic floor mat or carpet, or purchase a specific antistatic device.
• Use available accessories to care for your system. For example, use dust covers for the keyboard and the monitor when they are not in use. Antistatic wipes are available to use on the screen, and they should be used as an alternative to glass cleaners.
• When moving the computer, lock the hard drive to protect the CPU and disk drives.
• Keep keyboards free of debris and liquids, which can be hazardous to the keyboard, as it is directly plugged into the computer. Vacuum the keyboard periodically to eliminate dust particles under the key pads. Do not eat or drink while working on the computer.
• Be aware of any maintenance and warranty contracts for the computer system and do not hesitate to contact the service representative when needed. Some maintenance agreements require that a service representative clean and inspect the system on a regular basis.
• Handle data storage disks with special care. Box 10-1 provides some general guidelines.

INTERNET BASICS

Most physicians' offices can connect to the **Internet**. The Internet is used for both clinical and administrative reasons. The first thing you need to know is how to get your computer connected.

Getting Started and Connected

The Internet is used for access to the World Wide Web (www) and for electronic mail. To get connected, you will need an Internet connection company and appropriate Internet software.

There are three ways that your computer can connect to the Internet. One is an Internet service provider (ISP). The ISP is a company that connects your computer's modem to the Internet through the phone line. It is often called a dial-up service. This method provides the slowest service but is the cheapest. The second option is your cable television company. This system provides a faster connection. The third option is a digital subscriber line (DSL). This is the fastest connection but is not available in all areas. DSL is the most expensive connection system. If you need to download large files through the Internet, you should use either a DSL or cable connection. If you are having trouble accessing the Internet because of either slow service or connection troubles, speak to the physician or office manager to determine whether a different connection or ISP is needed.

Second, your computer will need a Web browser. A Web browser is software that communicates with your computer and the Internet. Two common examples are Internet Explorer and Netscape Navigator. Most computers are pre-loaded with a Web browser.

Clicking on the Web browser icon makes the actual connection to the Internet. Depending on how your system is set up, you may have to use a password. Box 10-2 gives you some guidelines on password use.

Checkpoint Question

3. Which two types of Internet connection are recommended for downloading large files?

Security

If you choose correct sites and follow some general safety tips, the Internet is a safe way to obtain and transfer patient information. Here are a few key points:

Box 10-2

PASSWORD USE

Here are some guidelines for passwords:
- Make unique passwords (combine letters and numbers)
- Do not use your initials, birth date, or phone number.
- Systemwide passwords that allow access to the computer should be changed after an employee has been fired.
- Do not share your password with your colleagues.
- Do not tape your password on the computer monitor or leave it on your desk.
- It is a good idea to have additional password verifications for certain secure sites (laboratory reports).

- Never send **any** patient information over the Internet to a site that does not have a secure sockets layer (SSL). This scrambles your information as it leaves your computer and unscrambles it when it arrives at its designated address.
- Look for a lock icon on the status bar.
- Set limits on your Web browser for **cookies**. A cookie is a tiny file left on your computer's hard drive from a website without your permission. By examining your cookies, a website can learn what sites you have visited, products that you have been searching, and files that you have downloaded. You may control your computer's cookies by setting limits on your Web browser software. Limit setters can generally be found on your toolbar under Internet options, then under either privacy or security.

Viruses

Virus protection is an important security issue. A virus is dangerous invader that enters your computer through some source and can destroy your files, software programs, and possibly even the hard drive. A worm is a specific type of virus that affects e-mail. Most computers come with virus protection software. This software will identify and stop harmful transmission. No virus protection is, however, 100% guaranteed. Some ways that you can protect your computer are:

- Do not open any attachments that are from unknown or suspicious sites.
- Update your virus protection software regularly. Most virus protection programs offer an updating service. Virus protection updates address new worms, as well.
- Remember, new viruses are detected daily.

Downloading Information

The Internet is filled with great patient teaching resources and other information. You may decide to copy some of this material into your computer. This is **downloading**. Downloading transfers information from an outside location to your computer's hard drive. Download only files that pertain to work. Do not download screen savers, news releases, recipes, or other personal information. Do not assume that you can photocopy any material that you have downloaded and distribute it. Always ask for permission from the author. Some government and professional medical websites state that their material can be freely copied and used. A good example of this is the United States Department of Agriculture (USDA) website that allows the food pyramids to be copied and used for teaching.

Working Offline

It is possible to access Web pages without connecting your computer to the Internet. To do this, save your commonly accessed sites on your Web browser. (If you are unsure how to do this, search your help topics for working offline). Then, to view the pages off line, click on the connection icon, select work off line, and locate your file. Remember, Web pages are regularly updated, and a page that you have saved to view off line may not be the latest version. Periodically view the online site and resave the site.

ELECTRONIC MAIL

Electronic mail (e-mail) provides many benefits to the health care system. It is estimated that about 6.6 trillion e-mail messages are sent every year. E-mail promotes good patient care, enhances communication, promotes teamwork, eliminates phone tag, and provides written documentation of messages. E-mail messages can't be guaranteed to provide confidentiality. Some general tips for using e-mail follow:

- Use the office e-mail address only to send work-related messages. Do not send personal messages.
- Do not participate in chain letters.
- Download your e-mail and read it off line unless you are using a DSL or cable connection.
- All e-mail messages should be professional.
- Read your e-mail's **encryption** feature and activate it. Encryption is a process of scrambling messages so that they cannot be read until they reach the recipient.
- Always leave a message on your e-mail system when you will be out of the office for a vacation or other reason. This message is automatically sent to the incoming e-mail senders. This alerts the sender that you will not be reading their message. Include the date when you will be returning to the office and instructions on whom they should contact in case of emergencies. This feature is often called "out-of-office assistant." An example of a good message: "I will be out of the office from 1/20 through 1/28. If this e-mail requires immediate attention, please forward it to Barbara Smith. I will respond to your e-mail when I return."

Checkpoint Question

4. What does the encryption feature do?

Access

Access to your e-mail account is through either Internet or intranet. The intranet is discussed later in the chapter. To access your e-mail, locate the mail icon, double-click it, and enter appropriate information. A password is generally required.

Composing Messages

When composing a message, follow the guidelines in Chapter 7 for writing business letters . Here are a few additional tips:

- Check your spelling, grammar, and punctuation before sending any messages.

- Keep messages short, concise, and to the point.
- Flag messages of high importance. This will alert the recipient that the message is important and should be read first. Do not overuse this feature. Flag only messages that warrant immediate response or attention. Never send an e-mail about a patient who is having an emergency. Always call or page the physician instead. An example of inappropriate e-mail is, "Ms. Smith's water broke. Do you want her to go the hospital or come into the office?"
- Use appropriate fonts and an appropriate font size.
- Generic or plain stationery should be used. Do not use stationery that has cute figures or looks busy.
- Always complete the subject line. Keep the subject line short and use only a few key words, for example, Staff meeting tomorrow.
- It is a good idea to restrict e-mail messages to only one topic.
- Paragraphs are not indented on e-mail messages. Skip a line between paragraphs.
- You can add a permanent signature to all outgoing e-mails. Your signature should include your name and phone number.

Address Books

Your e-mail software will allow you to create address books. An address book is a collection of e-mail addresses. Additional information, such as phone numbers, fax numbers, and street addresses, can be added. A few tips regarding address books are:

- Keep your addresses up to date.
- Organize your addresses in folders or categories. For example, one folder may contain all the cardiologists in the area, and another may contain just insurance-related addresses.

Attachments

An attachment is a file that is sent along with an e-mail. You attach a single file (letter) or several documents at one time. Remember these guidelines:

- When you receive an e-mail with an attachment, open the attached file or letter. File it in an appropriate place on your computer. If appropriate, print the attachment and distribute it as needed.
- If you are sending an e-mail and need to attach a file, compose your message first. Then attach the file by going into the tool bar and locating the menu for file attachments. Find the file on your computer and click to attach it. It is a good idea before sending the attachment to open it to be sure that you have selected the correct file or version of the document.

Opening Electronic Mail

Some general guidelines regarding opening an e-mail message follow:

- Open only your own e-mail messages unless otherwise instructed.
- After reading the e-mail, either delete it or place it in a folder. Do not allow multiple e-mails to clog your inbox.
- Always open flagged messages first and respond to them immediately.
- If you receive a message that you cannot address or resolve, forward the message to your supervisor and alert the sender that the message has been forwarded.
- If you start receiving bulk mail, either block the sender or ask to be deleted from that mailing list. This can be accomplished by clicking on "unsubscribe," usually at the end of the message.

 Checkpoint Question

5. Can you be 100% guaranteed that your e-mail transmissions are safe?

MEDICAL APPLICATIONS OF THE INTERNET

Besides e-mail, the Internet offers the World Wide Web, which provides health care professionals with great resources and information. Navigating through the Web quickly and efficiently takes skill and practice. The process of searching the Internet is called **surfing**. Surfing that is unorganized and not focused can be time consuming and unproductive.

Before surfing for information, you need to remember one important rule: Not all of the information on the Web is accurate or truthful. Anyone can post anything or make any claim. Since the information that you obtain from the Web will affect patient care, all steps must be taken to ensure that only accurate information is found and used. First, look for the HON (Health on the Net) seal. The HON seal (*www.hon.ch*) is a voluntary seal that indicates that the site has met certain standards for reliability and credibility. It does not certify that the information is correct or truthful, but it is a good starting point. Keep in mind that many good sites, for example governmental sites, do not have this seal. Box 10-3 provides you with some guidelines for selecting safe sites.

Search Engines

A **search engine** allows you to find sites that have the information that you need. There are numerous search engines (Google, Yahoo, Lycos, Excite, Dogpile). These sites are best used for searching out general information. Once you arrive at the search engine page, you must enter some

---

Box 10-3

SAFE SITE SELECTION GUIDELINES

Remember these key points when reading information on a website:

- Beware of phrases like breakthrough, medical miracle, secret formula.
- Avoid sites that advertise that they have cured a disease.
- Use caution when you see the phrase "ancient remedy."
- Use caution when you find a site that will treat a whole list of diseases with the same treatment.
- Do not believe every testimonial that you read.
- If the sites claims that the government is hiding information to cure a disease, use extreme caution.
- Use caution when the treatment can "only be bought here."
- If the site suggests that you not tell your doctor about it, stay away.
- See *www.quackwatch.com*.
- You can send complaints to the Federal Trade Commission at *www.ftc.gov* about sites that provide information that is misleading and wrong.
- Do not try to learn lifesaving skills, such as cardiopulmonary resuscitation, on the Internet. No matter how good the information or site is, you need to take a professional class.

---

key words. Your key words should be focused to limit the number of responses that you will get. For example, if you type in the key word "heart," you will get thousands of sites that pertain to the heart. Some of these sites will be referring to the heart as an organ and other sites will address how to mend a broken heart. If you had selected your key words to be "heart attack," however, you would narrow your search tremendously. To further narrow your search use the advanced search feature. Click on advance search and use the key words "heart and attack and prevention." By doing this, you will obtain the information you want faster and more efficiently. Unless you are using a medical search engine, avoid using medical terms. For example, use the word lung instead of pulmonary. When you need to find medical information, use a medical search or a megamedical site with links. Procedure 10-1 lists the steps necessary to search the Internet. See the listing of websites at the end of this chapter for some good places to start searching for medical information.

 Checkpoint Question

6. What is a search engine?

Procedure 10-1

Searching on the Internet

Equipment/Supplies

- Computer with Web browser software
- Modem
- Active Internet connection account

Steps	Purpose
1. Connect your computer to the Internet.	An Internet connection is necessary to search the Internet.
2. Locate a search engine.	A search engine is necessary to find information on the Internet.
3. Select two or three key words and type them at the appropriate place on the Web page.	Key words tell the search engine what to look for.
4. View the number of search results. If no sites were found, check spelling and retype or choose new key words.	The search engine was unable to find sites that can provide the information you requested.
5. If the search produced a long list, do an advanced search and refine your key words.	Reading through numerous sites is not time efficient.
6. Select an appropriate site and open its home page.	This allows you to view the information on the website.
7. If you are satisfied with the site's information, either download the material or bookmark the page. If you are unsatisfied with its information, either visit a site listed on the results page or return to the search engine.	Downloading or bookmarking the information gives you access to it in the future.
8. Complete this task within 10 minutes.	Quickly and effectively searching the Internet is necessary for good time management.

Professional Medical Sites

At the end of the chapters in this book you see various Web addresses listed that provide you with more information on that chapter's content. These are good starting points for professional topics. But keep in mind that Web addresses change frequently. If you are unable to access a site, try eliminating the letters and symbols after a slash (/). Use the primary site address. For example, suppose you want to enter this site: *www.fda.gov/cder/drug/consumer/buyonline/guide.htm*. If you cannot access that site, try *www.fda.gov* and advance from there. Most sites will link you automatically to a new home page. Also, depending on your Web browser, you may not have to type in **www**. In this case, you would just type in fda.gov.

The Internet can help you communicate with patients who speak a foreign language. Some websites translate phrases

and words. Box 10-4 lists sites that physicians are most likely to use. All medical specialties have their own special site. Hospitals have their own sites also. When you start working as a medical assistant, learn the Web addresses of the specialty of your physician and of local hospitals *(www.hospitalselect.com)*. For example, if you work for a neurologist, you will frequently use *www.aan.com* (American Academy of Neurology).

These sites will help you translate between English and Spanish:

- AltaVista
  www.altavista.com (click on translate)
- Free English to Spanish translations
  www.freetranslation.com

The CDC site is also available in Spanish. You can give this address to patients: *www.cdc.gov/ncidod/EID/spanish.htm*.

Box 10-4

SITES PHYSICIANS USE

Physicians and other health care professionals are likely to use these sites:

Journal of the American Medical Association	www.jama.com
New England Journal of Medicine	www.nejm.org
Lancet	www.lancet.org
Annals of Internal Medicine	www.annals.org
AMA	www.ama-assn.org
JCAHO	www.jcaho.org
CDC	www.cdc.org
Clinical trials	www.clinicaltrials.gov

Literary Searches

According to the American Medical Association, approximately 80% of practicing physicians regularly surf the Internet for medical research information. Most research information is found through a **literary search**. A literary search involves finding journal articles that present new facts or data about a given topic. Physicians who specialize in a given area and have conducted a controlled research study write these articles. Various databases can be used to do a literary search:

- OVID will search for articles as far back as 1966. It contains access to more than 4,000 professional journals. Its address is *www.gateway.ovid.com.*
- PubMed will search for journal articles back to 1966 from the National Library of Medicine.
- CINAHL contains journal articles published since 1982. It has primarily journals for nurses and other allied health care professionals.

Most literary search databases require an annual subscription fee. Once you arrive at the site, you can start to search for the information. First, enter your key words. To narrow the search, you can request journal articles from all countries or limit it to the United States. You can also limit the search by selecting a time line, such as the past 6 months. Once you have done your search, a list of articles will be displayed, and you can highlight the ones you wish to see. You will be asked whether you want to see the whole article or only the abstract. An abstract is a summary of the article. It is always a good idea to print only the abstracts and allow the physician to decide which full articles he or she will want to see. Fees for downloading the complete journal article vary. Abstracts can generally be downloaded free. Your local hospital librarian is often available to assist you with literary searches and may be able to get the article for free. Some libraries will

do searches for physicians on staff at no charge. Use this service if it is available.

Checkpoint Question

7. How is a literary search different from a search on an internet website?

Health-Related Calculators

The Web has numerous calculators that can be used for various health care topics:

- Basal metabolic rate calculator *www.global-fitness.com/BMR_calc.html*
- Due date calculator *www.babycenter.com/calculators/duedate*
- Ovulation calculator *www.babycenter.com/calculators/ovulation*
- Target heart rate *www.webmd.com/heartrate*

Insurance-Related Sites

The insurance world can seem like an endless maze of papers and regulations. The Internet can help you sort through and clarify some information. Your first stop should be the patient's insurance company. Its Web address is usually listed on the back of the patient's insurance card. Bookmark these sites. Chapter 16 will get into more details on this issue. A few sites that can also help you and your patients follow:

- For information on buying health insurance online: *www.ehealthinsurance.com.*
- The Medicare site (*www.medicare.gov*) discusses the basics of Medicare programs, eligibility, enrollment, drug assistance programs, and many frequently asked questions. This site will link you to various other options. You will also find links to report Medicare fraud and abuse.
- Patients who express concern about their health records being red-flagged because of an illness (HIV, cancer) can check a database that alerts insurance companies to "red-flagged" patients. This site is *www.mib.com*. There is a fee for using this site.

Patient Teaching Issues Regarding the Internet

Some of your patients will be very skilled at using the Internet. They can find enormous amounts of information regarding their disease, treatment options, medications. The guidelines discussed in Box 10-3 pertain to patients who surf the Internet. You cannot stop or limit the information that patients will search and find. Keep in mind that patients often turn to the Internet when they feel confused or hopeless about their disease or anger about the medical profession. If a patient communicates any such feelings, alert the physician.

Teach patients to acquire reliable medical information and advise them of the dangers on the Web. Some physician offices print brochures with recommended Web addresses. This is a very good education tool for patients. Box 10-5 gives you some good patient education sites. Some areas you should be aware of are discussed below.

Buying Medications Online

As the cost of prescription medications soar, patients look for options. It is possible to buy prescription medications over the Internet. A good Internet pharmacy will provide information on what the medication is used for, possible side effects, dosage recommendation, and safety concerns. If patients want to purchase prescriptions online, advise them to use only sites that are certified by the Verified Internet Pharmacy Practice Site (VIPPS). This certification comes from the National Association of Boards of Pharmacy and indicates that the site has been checked and is monitored for safety and quality care. Advise patients to purchase only medications that have been prescribed by the physician. Warn patients never to purchase medications from sites outside of the United States. These sites may not meet safety standards of the Food and

---

Box 10-6

MEDICATIONS THAT SHOULD NEVER BE BOUGHT ON THE INTERNET

According to the Federal Drug Administration, certain drugs should never be purchased on the Internet. These medications can cause serious harm if they are not prescribed correctly and the patient is not closely monitored.

- Accutane (isotretinoin)
- Actiq (fentanyl citrate)
- Clozaril (clozapine)
- Lotronex (alosetron hydrochloride)
- Mifeprex (mifepristone or RU-486)
- Thalomid (thalidomide)
- Tikosyn (dofetilide)
- Tracleer (bosentan)

Drug Administration (FDA). In addition, the FDA warns patients never to buy certain medications online because of their inherent dangers. Advise patients to use *www.fda.gov/cder/drug/consumer/buyonline/guide.htm* for consumer safety tips. Box 10-6 lists medications that the FDA warns people never to purchase online.

Some sites offer virtual prescribing. This means that the Internet user provides some information and asks for a prescription. For example, the patient may type in, "My cholesterol is too high. What medication will get it down?" The site will then ask the patient a few questions and select a medication. In other cases, the patient may simply request a medication: "I want some amoxicillin." In either case, the prescription is filled and mailed to the patient. Warn patients about the dangers of self-prescribing medications and alert the physician to any communication you have with the patient regarding this practice. Serious health risks can arise.

 Checkpoint Question

8. Name three safety tips to teach patients about buying medications on the Internet.

Financial Assistance for Medications

Patients who are having trouble paying for their prescription medications can find many financial resources on the Web. First, you should advise patients to search the drug company's home page, for example, *www.Pfizer.com*. Patients on Medicare will find assistance on *www.medicare.gov/prescription/home.asp*. Another good site is *www.needymeds.com/Mainpage.htlm*. Physicians can access *www.Rxhope.com* to find local financial resources for patients.

Box 10-5

GOOD PATIENT EDUCATION SITES

These sites provide good patient information:

American Dental Association
   www.ada.org/public/index.asp

American Sleep Apnea Association
   www.sleepapnea.org

Consumer Health Publications
   www.health.nih.gov

Merck Manual Home Edition
   www.merckhomeedition.com

National Attention Deficit Disorder Association
   www.add.org

Hotlines of National Library of Science
   www.nlm.nih.gov/hotlines

American Association of Poison Control Centers
   www.aapcc.org

Smoking cessation
   www.QuitNet.org

Sources for children with cancer
   www.cancersourcekids.com

Travel health
   www.cdc.gov/travel

Medical Records

Patients may choose to create their own "medical records" and store personal health information on sites. Patients who travel frequently may opt for this. Two sites that offer this are *www.personalmd.com* and *www.mywebmd.com*. Patients can store information about their medications, immunizations, laboratory tests, surgeries, and so on. For their own protection, patients should be discouraged from doing this. Instead, advise patients to download medical record forms, complete the printed copy, and store them safely.

Medical Record Forms

The American Health Information and Management Association provides forms online for patients to record their health histories. This is available at *www.ahima.org/consumer/index.html*. The American College of Emergency Physicians has an emergency consent form (*www.acep.org*) that parents can sign giving permission for another person to consent to their child to be treated in case of an emergency. This is valuable for parents who travel on business and have their child stay with a relative or friend.

Advance directives and legal forms for medical power of attorney are also available online. Patients should be advised to seek legal counsel and speak to the physician before completing these forms. The federal government does have cards available online for patients to complete and carry with them regarding their wishes to be an organ and tissue donor at *www.organdonor.gov/signup1.html*.

WHAT IF

Parents ask you how to keep their child safe on the Internet. What should you say?

First and foremost, explain to the parent that direct parental observation is the best method. Encourage parents to have an open and honest discussion with their child regarding the dangers on the Internet. Computers should be kept in living rooms or family rooms. Advise parents not to let children have a computer with Internet access in their bedroom. Parents can require a password to be entered for Internet access. This prevents access when the parent is not present. Most Web browser programs let the parent allow access only to "safe" sites. A few sites can add filters or safety nets to a child's computer. These sites are *www.netnanny.com,* Internet Guard Dog (*www.mcafee.com*), and CyberPatrol (*www.cyberpatrol.com*)

Injury Prevention

Injuries are a leading cause of death for children. The American Academy of Pediatrics (*www.aap.org*) has reference materials that can help parents with safety tips. The federal government sites (*www.cdc.gov and www.nih.gov*) also have good information that you can direct parents to search. The National Safe Kids foundation is another excellent resource (*www.safekids.org*). Questions regarding product recalls can be found at *www.cpsc.org*.

INTRANET

An **intranet** is a private network of computers that share data. Intranets, sometimes called internal webs, are used in large multiphysician practices. The only people with access to an intranet home page are people with an affiliation to the practice. Access may be limited to those within the offices or may allow for access from home computer systems. The benefits of an intranet are enhanced communication, quick access to needed information, and increased productivity. Common examples of data found on an intranet are:

- Policy and procedure manuals
- Marketing information
- Minutes from meetings and upcoming agendas
- Staff schedules
- Local hospital announcements or information
- Commonly used forms
- Internal newsletters
- Internal job postings
- Phone lists
- Video conference support
- Links to specialty sites

 Checkpoint Question

9. How does an intranet differ from the Internet?

MEDICAL SOFTWARE APPLICATIONS

The types of medical applications and their possibilities are endless. Every day, thousands of new software packages are released into the market. Upgrades and new versions of existing packages are also released daily. Each type of software program will have good benefits and will lack some features. The type of software that you will use will vary among different physician offices. The selection of software is based on the size of the practice, number of physicians, specialty, and the affiliated hospital's software. If the hospital software is compatible, interchanging information is relatively easy. Physician and office manager preferences play a role in the software selection. Other factors include how many users can use software at one time, can the software be used with multiple windows open, and how often does the company plan to update it.

MEDICAL SOFTWARE COMPANIES

Numerous companies sell medical office software programs. Here are a few sites that you can visit:

Advanced Medical Management
www.amdsoftware.com

AltaPoint Practice Management
www.altapoint.com

American Medical software
www.americanmedical.com

EZ Claim medical billing
www.ezclaim.org

Find Medical Billing Software
www.findaccountingsoftware.com

Medical Manager
www.medicalmanager.com

Medical Software products
www.medsoftware.com

NextGen
www.nextgen.com

Plexis Health Care
www.plexisweb.com

SoftAid
www.soft-aid.com

Web-based appointment scheduling
www.compassscheduling.com

Never buy or install a new software program or update an existing version without permission from either the office manager or the physician.

Learning to use a particular software program and navigate quickly and efficiently through its features takes time. Most programs come with a tutorial program. On-site training is often included in the purchase price of major software applications. Training options will be discussed later in the chapter.

Medical software applications can be divided into two main groups: clinical and administrative. Clinical software packages help the physician or health care professional provide the best possible medical care to patients. Administrative software packages focus on tasks to keep the office flowing efficiently and financially strong. The next sections introduce you to what types of software capabilities are available and most commonly used. Keep in mind that new technologies are emerging every day. Box 10-7 lists some companies that sell medical software.

Clinical Applications

Clinical software is designed to help the physician, nurse, medical assistant, or other health care professional provide the most efficient, safest, and most reliable health care available. Here are some examples of the benefits that clinical software programs can bring into the physician's office:

1. Create a **virtual** patient chart. A virtual chart is a paperless chart in which all documentation is stored on computer. Some offices create dual charts (virtual and paper), and other offices will keep one or the other. The advantages to a virtual charting system are that it saves filing space, increases access to patients' charts for all staff members, eliminates hunting for misplaced charts, and keeps the charts better organized and neater. Since the charting is done through keyboarding, the notes are always readable.

2. Clinical software can maintain an up-to-date list of clinical tasks organized by employee's name. For example, suppose you just discharged a patient and made a note on his chart that you need to check his laboratory tests tomorrow. The task manager would automatically assign this task to your list of duties for tomorrow. Or a physician may discharge a patient and want you to call that patient in the morning for a follow-up. The physician could assign this task to your list. This promotes organization and decreases the potential for tasks to get overlooked or forgotten.

3. The software available for prescription management and drug information is tremendous. A good program that focuses on pharmaceutical information will decrease medication errors, increase patient satisfaction, and provide better patient care, and it can be financially beneficial to the patient and to the practice. At minimum, the software should enable the physician to find the patient's name in a database, virtually write the prescription, and download it directly to the patient's pharmacy. This allows the pharmacist to fill the prescription before the patient arrives. Thus the patient gets the medication much faster. More important, since most prescription filling errors are due to physicians' poor handwriting, this potentially lethal error is prevented. Most medication software packages red-flag the physician if the prescription is contraindicated for the patient. Medications can be contraindicated because of a particular disease (e.g., asthma or diabetes), interaction with other medications the patient is taking, or an allergy. For example, assume the physician has written a prescription for Bactrim, which contains a sulfonamide. The software would find in the patient's medical record that the patient is allergic to sulfonamides. The computer would alert the physician, and the physician would select a different medication. Software also allows the physician to save the patient money. Each insurance company and hospital has a formulary of medications that it reimburses. If the physician orders a medication that is on the patient's insurance formulary, the patient saves money. If the physician selects a medication

outside the formulary, the insurance company may refuse to pay some or all of the cost of the medication.

4. Computer programs can insert laboratory reports directly into the patient's records. This is more time efficient than faxing or manually recording the results. It also eliminates transcription errors. Most software will alert the physician when a new laboratory report has been received. Laboratory reports of serious or life-threatening findings will still be telephoned to the office.

5. Perhaps one of the greatest technologies is the importing of the actual imaging study into a patient's chart. Some software allows the physician to see the radiograph or computed tomograph from the office. Without this program, the physician gets a typed written report, such as "chest radiograph shows left lower lobe infiltrate." With this technology the physician can see the radiograph itself and thus make better clinical decisions.

6. Plastic surgeons use a wide variety of image reconstruction programs in their office. This software allows the physician to insert a picture of the patient and contrast it with the expected outcomes of the surgery. This helps patients both to decide whether the surgery is warranted and to develop realistic expectations of the surgery.

7. Many physicians' offices have a special defibrillator called an automated external defibrillator (AED). Once the AED is used on a patient, the information from the machine must be downloaded to the patient's chart for legal documentation. After use, the AED is attached to a desktop computer, and the AED sends the report into the computer and then into the patient's record. If the patient's chart is not on computer, the data can be printed on paper and placed in a conventional chart.

8. Some programs can help you with telephone triage. Triage is sorting patients. The software allows you to select a caller's topic and displays a list of relevant questions. The software also provides you some instructions for the patient. For example, assume you have a caller with abdominal pain. You type the key words abdominal pain, and a list of questions appears. These programs log the calls with the date, time, and instructions. This provides legal protection for you.

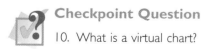

Checkpoint Question

10. What is a virtual chart?

Administrative Applications

There are hundreds of administrative software packages available for physician offices. Most systems have a combination of features. At present, the Medical Manager system is the most commonly used software in physician offices.

Some examples of benefits administrative software can bring to the physician's office follow:

1. Appointment making and tracking are more efficient with a computer program than with a book format. Good appointment software will allow you to enter appointments quickly and make changes more easily. It should allow for an unlimited comment area near the patient's name. The comment area allows you to add special notes, such as "patient is requesting a pregnancy test." Appointment software can keep a waiting list of patients who are looking for appointments or wanting to move their appointment date and time to the first available. Appointment software can also automatically print notices to remind patients of the need to make appointments. For example, the program can be set to alert patients who have an annual Pap smear to be sent a letter each year reminding them when it is time for the next one. Appointment software can be integrated with other physicians' offices to allow you to have access to their appointment books. This allows you to see when the next available appointment is. For example, assume your physician makes a referral for Mr. Mannual to see a dermatologist. You would be able to view the schedule of the dermatologist and see when he could get an appointment and then later see if he went for his appointment. Software programs allow appointments to be made only when certain equipment is available. For example, the patient needs a biopsy that is done with a particular laser machine. The machine is available only on Tuesdays, so the program would automatically set the appointment for the patient on a Tuesday.

2. Software can allow you or the office manager to track patient flows. This can be helpful to adjust staff scheduling needs, with more help at the busiest hours or days and less staff on slower days. It can alert managers to productivity of staff members. For example, one physician may average 45 minutes per patient, while another may average 30 minutes. This allows you to schedule appointments at various intervals and thus promotes patient flow. It can track the time patients wait in the waiting room or examination room. Examining such information allows the staff to change the office flow to decrease waiting times or to indicate the need for additional staff. It can also highlight the days when patients are most likely to cancel their appointments. Patient demographics can be obtained, used for marketing, and allow the office to apply for special funding based on patient demographics.

3. Software programs are needed to send insurance claims electronically. You will be able to send claims and track their progress. This allows for faster reimbursement to the practice and can identify problems of reimbursement earlier. The programs

that you will use should have access to numerous plans and can be updated frequently and easily.

4. Software programs can allow integration with insurance companies and other businesses to allow for automatic quick payment and posting. This saves time and is less complicated to use them traditional accounting books.

5. Physicians' offices should have software that allows for credit card authorization. A variety of card types should be available (Visa, MasterCard, American Express).

6. Insurance software can allow you to check for patient eligibility. Most programs have enough room for the addresses and phone numbers of the primary, secondary, and tertiary providers. Case manager names should be added when available. Software can also allow for preadmission certifications to completed and electronically submitted. Preadmission or preauthorization allows you and the patient to verify that the insurance company will cover the procedure or admission. Some software programs come with codes (ICD-9, CPT, HCPCS) and anesthesia codes preinstalled.

7. Some programs aim to comply with the Health Insurance Portability and Accountability Act (HIPAA). HIPAA is a federal act that requires all health care professionals to follow a variety of privacy and confidentiality rules; these programs allow you to document your adherence to these rules and regulations. For more information on HIPAA, visit *www.hipaa.org*.

8. Other programs alert you to send collection letters. These programs have a variety of template collection letters. Always double-check the information before sending a collection letter. More information on how to collect past due accounts is discussed in Chapter 13.

9. A variety of financial software programs track accounts receivable and accounts payable. You may need to adjust the billing cycles to meet the needs of the office in which you are working. Software programs can also automate the tickler system.

10. Automated payroll software can automatically calculate tax deductions and other deductions. You will be able to arrange for direct deposit of employee checks through these software programs.

11. You will find transcription systems in most physicians' offices. These programs help you transcribe various medical reports quickly and effectively. Transcription is covered in Chapter 9.

12. A medical office can't effectively run without a word processing system. These systems help you write letters and other types of documentation.

13. An important part of any administrative software is the section that handles the personnel records. Contracts, disciplinary reports, performance evaluations, and so on can all be stored in a virtual personnel record.

Paging System Software

Most physicians carry a pager. In some offices, other staff members may also be assigned pagers. Always double-check to make sure that the physician you are paging is the one on call. Most paging systems allow you to type alphabetic (alpha) messages versus a numerical code. A numerical message is simply a telephone number. An alpha message is a written message that is displayed on the pager; for example, "Call the office regarding Ms. Home's blood gas results." Here are some guidelines regarding paging:

- Always provide a return phone number unless you are asking the physician to call the office.
- Watch your spelling on alpha pages.
- Keep the message short and concise.
- Keep track of what time the message was sent and repage if there is no response.
- If it is an emergency page and there is no response, repage or page another physician as per office policy.
- Never give out pager numbers to patients or sales representatives.
- If you are given a pager, do not give the pager number to anyone. Insert fresh batteries when the battery icon is first showing; treat the pager with care and respect. Notify the office manager immediately if is lost or stolen.

 Checkpoint Question

11. What is an alpha page message?

PowerPoint

Physicians are often asked to do formal presentations. These presentations may be made to other physicians, support group meetings, hospital staff meetings, and professional inservices. The most popular program used to write presentations is PowerPoint. Using this software, the physician will create slides. The slides can then be shown on a projection screen by connecting a computer to a projector. Most often a laptop computer is used. You may be asked to print slides or handouts for the program or to transfer files. Use the tutorial software for tips on making presentations.

Meeting Maker

Meeting Maker is a common package that promotes internal coordination of meetings and calendars. This system is primarily used in large practices with multiple offices and multiple administrative personnel. This is how the system works: Everyone is listed as user. Each user enters his or her schedule into a personal calendar. Calendars can be seen daily, weekly, or monthly. For example, you may type in, "Monday, Middletown office, 8 A.M.–4 P.M.; Tuesday, Southside office, 10A.M.–5 P.M.." The system allows you to view other people's calendars. It is possible to allow other people to enter data to your calendar. You can also maintain a list of tasks and print your schedule. If you are asked to arrange a staff meeting, you enter the names of the people who should come, and the computer will select a date and time that is convenient for everyone.

HANDHELD COMPUTERS

According to the American Medical Association, approximately 23% of physicians use a handheld computer, or personal digital assistant (PDA). A handheld device can do almost anything that your desktop computer can do. Companies that make PDA software can be found at these three Web addresses: *www.pdacortex.com, www.skyscape.com,* and *www.handheldmed.com.* At minimum, handheld computers come with software that can do these functions:

- Address book
- Calendar
- Memo pad
- E-mail
- Word processing

Information can be entered into the handheld device either with a stylus (pen) or on a small keyboard. It is possible to attach a regular-size keyboard to a PDA. Information can be sent back and forth between a PDA and a desktop computer in either of two ways. The PDA can be placed in a cradle that is connected via a cable to the desktop ("hot sync"), or information can be sent via e-mail. PDAs can beam information among themselves (business cards, memos) and can attach their modem through a cellular phone for Internet access.

Physicians often add software that allows them to:

- Access patients' charts
- Set up a virtual office
- View financial data
- Use pharmacy and formulary dosing tools
- Access Micromedx (drug information, toxicology, databases)
- View procedures that they may not routinely do, enhancing lifesaving skills

PURCHASING A COMPUTER

Purchasing a new office computer system or updating an existing one is a very important business decision. All key members of the staff should be consulted prior to such a purchase and should be actively involved in selecting the hardware and software. Here are some general guidelines to follow when shopping for a computer and software:

- Determine your specific needs. For example, do you need both clinical and administrative applications?
- Visit physicians' offices and clinics to see what other medical office staff are using. Ask questions: How user friendly are the programs? How long did it take to educate the staff? What does the staff like and dislike about the programs?

- Try out many software packages. Most have demonstrator disks that can be used to evaluate the system.
- Interview and compare different computer vendors. Find out:
  1. How long they have been in service
  2. How many service representatives they have and whether they are available 24 hours a day
  3. Specifics of the system
  4. Specifics of any service and warranty contracts they provide
  5. What training they provide and at what additional cost
  6. How to transfer data into the new system
  7. How much the system costs
  8. Whether the software can be customized and at what cost
  9. What is their response time for service or technical support calls

Independent computer consultants can be hired to evaluate your particular office and make specific recommendations. This option is often more expensive initially but can save money in the long run.

TRAINING OPTIONS

To achieve the optimal benefit from any computer or software package, you must be trained in its use. There are a number of ways that this can be accomplished:

- The company from which the computer was purchased may provide personnel to train you and other staff members.
- A user manual will come with your system. You can refer to it when you have problems.
- Help screens installed with every software package allow the user to self-teach. The disadvantage of this method is that it is often time consuming.
- Most software packages come with a tutorial. This is an on-screen short course on the use of the software.
- Most computer manufacturers and software programs will have a service called a help desk, which provides technical support. It is usually accessed by calling a toll-free number and is manned by computer professionals who can answer your questions concerning the system.

A combination of these methods is the best approach to learning about your computer and software.

COMPUTER ETHICS

The computer is a must in all physicians' offices. Its capabilities are endless. It can, however, lead to invasion of patients' privacy and unethical behavior. Some key points to keep in mind are:

- Never give out your login password. New employees must be issued their own password.

- Never leave a screen open with patient information and walk away from the computer. Exit the file.
- Only key people need access to sensitive patient information. Some programs, such as those with laboratory results, should have individual passwords.
- Physicians can often access patient data (e.g., radiology and laboratory reports) from the hospital computers. The hospital gives the physician a special code. It is not appropriate for the physician to share this with staff members. If you are using another person's password to get patient information, you should contact the administrator of the program and get your own code.
- Do not use the office Internet access for your own pleasure. It is inappropriate to surf the Internet for personal reasons while at work.
- E-mails should be read only by the person to whom they were sent. To avoid conflicts, the physician should have his or her own e-mail account, and the practice should have a generic e-mail address. It is never appropriate for you to receive personal e-mail messages on the office's e-mail address. It is also inappropriate to access your personal e-mail while at work.
- Sensitive patient data should not be sent via e-mail from one office to the other unless it is clearly known that the recipient of the e-mail is the only one with access to it. It is a common practice to send patient information to the consulting physician. This information may include cancer diagnosis, HIV testing, and drug abuse reports. Extreme caution must be used.
- If you are allowed access to local laboratories to obtain laboratory results, it is to be used only on patients in your practice. It is unethical and illegal to obtain other people's reports. For example, if your son had a throat culture done at the pediatrician's office and sent to the laboratory you have access to, you should not look up his results.
- Do not take advantage of your position in the medical field. Remember, you have a legal and ethical responsibility to protect patient information.

CHAPTER SUMMARY

Computers are an essential piece of technology in the medical office. As a medical assistant, you will use the computer for both clinical and administrative tasks. Computers will help you perform your job more efficiently, timely, and professionally. Computers also promote good patient care. You will be able to communicate with various health care professionals by using electronic mail. The Internet plays a key role in medicine. Patients, physicians, and medical assistants use the Internet to find new medical cures and for seeking current information about various health topics. You will need to be able to navigate the Web quickly and safely. It is essential that you stay abreast of computer technology, as it changes and improves daily.

Critical Thinking Challenges

1. Log on to the Internet and locate a search engine. Search for a medical topic. It can be administrative or clinical. What are your key words? How many sites are listed? Now, using the same key words, use the advanced search engine. How many sites are listed? What are the benefits of using the advanced search method?
2. Select any five Web addresses listed in this chapter. View their home page. What benefits did the sites offer? What information or topics were missing or appeared inaccurate?
3. Review Box 10-3 about how to select a site safely. Find three websites that use these types of phrases or words. Do you think these sites are misleading? Do you think they pose a danger to patients?
4. Formulate a list of questions that you can ask a vendor before buying a computer system. Include questions regarding software applications.
5. Create a patient education pamphlet about the Internet. The pamphlet may focus on a particular disease process or contain broad information. Make sure you provide at least six Web addresses.

Answers to Checkpoint Questions

1. The CPU cells read, analyze, and process data and instruct the computer how to operate a given program.
2. Your computer should have an Ethernet port or Ethernet interface card so that it can be connected to a cable or DSL provider.
3. The two types of Internet connections that are recommended for downloading large files are DSL and cable.
4. The encryption feature scrambles messages as they leave your site and unscrambles them when they arrive at the receiver's site.
5. You cannot be 100% guaranteed that your e-mail messages are secure, but you can take many steps to safeguard them.
6. A search engine allows you to find the sites that will have the information that you need quickly and efficiently.
7. A literary search is different because it is searching for a professional journal article that addresses a topic versus searching for general information.
8. Three safety tips that you need to teach patients about buying medications online are: (1) buy medications only from a site with a VIPPS certification; (2) buy only medications for which they have prescriptions; and (3) buy medications only from sites within the United States.
9. The intranet is a private network of computers; the Internet is a global network of computers.

10. A virtual chart is a paperless chart that holds all necessary documents on the computer.
11. An alpha paging message is a written message that is displayed on the pager.

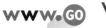 **Websites**

OSHA ergonomics
www.osha-slc.gov/SLTC/ergonomics/index.html

Websites that offer additional information
www.tifaq.com
www.healthfinder.gov
www.medlineplus.gov
www.healthcentral.com
www.mywebmd.com
www.Mayoclinic.com
www.familydoctor.org
www.raredisease.org (this site has a database of over 1,000 rare diseases and over 900 drugs that can be used to treat rare diseases)

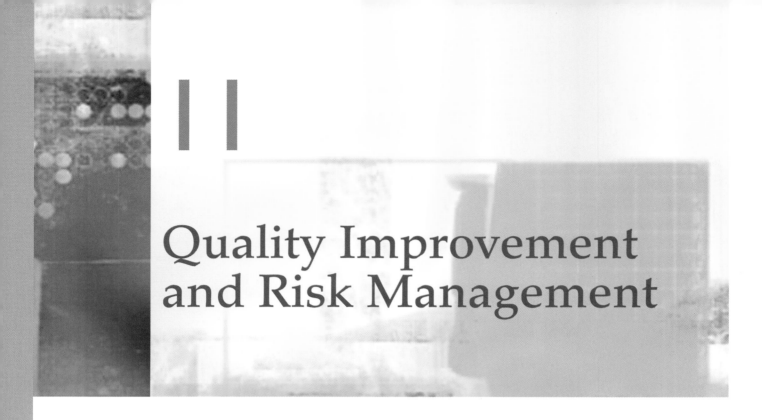

Quality Improvement and Risk Management

CHAPTER OUTLINE

ROLE DELINEATION COMPONENTS

GENERAL: Professionalism
- Display a professional manner and image
- Demonstrate initiative and responsibility
- Work as a member of the health care team
- Adapt to change
- Enhance skills through continuing education

GENERAL: Legal Concepts
- Perform within legal and ethical boundaries
- Document accurately
- Implement and maintain federal and state health care legislation and regulations
- Comply with established risk management and safety procedures

CHAPTER COMPETENCIES

LEARNING OBJECTIVES
Upon successfully completing this chapter, you will be able to:

1. Spell and define the key terms
2. List four regulatory agencies that require medical offices to have quality improvement programs
3. Describe the accreditation process of the Joint Commission on Accreditation of Healthcare Organizations
4. Describe the intent of the Clinical Laboratory Improvement Amendments Act
5. Describe the intent of the Health Insurance Portability and Accountability Act
6. Describe the steps to developing a quality improvement program
7. List five guidelines for completing incident reports
8. Explain how quality improvement programs and risk management work together in a medical office to improve overall patient care and employee needs

PERFORMANCE OBJECTIVE
Upon successfully completing this chapter, you will be able to:

1. Complete an incident report

KEY TERMS

Centers for Medicare & Medicaid

Clinical Laboratory Improvement Amendments Act

expected threshold

incident reports

Health Insurance Portability and Accountability Act

Joint Commission on Accreditation of Healthcare Organizations

Occupational Safety and Health Administration

outcomes

quality improvement

sentinel event

task force

QUALITY IMPROVEMENT (QI) is the commitment and plan to improve every part of an organization. Its goal is both to meet and to exceed customers' (patients') expectations and employees' needs. QI plans examine the way care is delivered, analyze problems in the delivery system, and investigate methods to correct the problems. Although quality medical care has been a concern of health care providers for many years, formal QI plans were not always required. In the mid 1980s, health care settings were required to develop quality assurance (QA) plans. The purpose of a QA plan was to "assure" patients that they received good medical care. QA plans often created mounds of statistical data to prove that the physicians and staff were doing a good job. QA plans did not focus on improving care, only on acquiring statistical data. Therefore, physician offices now focus on QI plans. These plans require that you collect the data and then use the information to improve and provide quality health care.

In this chapter, we discuss why health care organizations have QI programs, the process for developing and maintaining QI plans in a medical office setting, and risk management. We also discuss the agencies that mandate physician offices to have QI programs.

QUALITY IMPROVEMENT PROGRAMS IN THE MEDICAL OFFICE SETTING

Quality improvement programs let an organization scientifically measure the quality of its products and services. A health care organization's success depends on patient satisfaction and patient **outcomes**. The patient's outcome is the final result of the care that he or she received. For example, Mrs. Brown arrives in the office with a laceration on her leg. The cut is sutured, and in 6 days she returns for suture removal. The wound healed without complications. The patient's outcome was acceptable. Patient outcomes are reported to various regulatory agencies. At present, only hospitals are required to post report cards about patient outcomes. Legislative bills now in Congress would require all health care settings to report patient outcomes. Patients can review report cards and other regulatory agencies' reports on various websites. Then, patients can select the health care organization that best meets their needs in terms of professional services and personal care.

Quality improvement programs have many other benefits for all health care organizations. These benefits include the following:

- Identifying system failures or delays in patient care
- Improving patient and family customer service
- Improving patient outcomes and satisfaction
- Improving employee efficiency and productivity
- Improving company morale
- Encouraging teamwork within the institution or organization

Regulatory Agencies

Quality improvement programs exist in medical office settings because of these benefits and because regulatory agencies require such programs. The primary regulatory agencies that mandate QI programs are the **Joint Commission on Accreditation of Healthcare Organizations** (JCAHO), **Occupational Safety and Health Administration** (OSHA), **Centers for Medicare & Medicaid** (CMS), and state public health departments. Some other organizations and associations have requirements for QI programs. These associations require QI data along with applications for research or grant money and for specific accreditation of services. For example, the American Diabetes Association may require an endocrinologist to receive a certification in diabetes care to provide QI data on diabetic patient outcomes. The three major agencies are discussed next.

Joint Commission on Accreditation of Healthcare Organizations (JCAHO)

The JCAHO is a private agency that sets health care standards and evaluates an organization's implementation of these standards for health care settings. Prior to the mid 1990s, the primary focus of the JCAHO was on evaluating hospitals and in-patient care institutions such as nursing homes. In 1996, the JCAHO expanded its jurisdiction to outpatient and ambulatory care settings. This change was, in part, due to the shift of patient care from inpatient to outpatient services. The JCAHO sets standards and evaluates the care in the various health care settings. Box 11-1 lists various types of freestanding facilities for which the JCAHO sets standards and provides accreditation.

The JCAHO surveys these centers and then assigns them an accreditation title. A survey is on-site evaluation of the organizations facility and policies. Participation in the JCAHO is voluntary for health care organizations; without accreditation, however, the health care organization may not be eligible to participate in particular federal and state funding programs, such as Medicare and Medicaid. In addition, accreditation indicates to the community that an organization has met basic practice standards, which is important for marketing its services.

 Checkpoint Question

1. What are the benefits to a health care organization that has obtained an accreditation from the JCAHO?

JCAHO Accreditation Process. The process of obtaining and maintaining accreditation by the JCAHO occurs in various stages:

1. The health care organization files a survey application and a business associate agreement with the JCAHO. The business associate agreement is a new require-

Box 11-1

TYPES OF FACILITIES

The Joint Commission on Accreditation of Healthcare Organizations accredits a variety of health care settings. These are some types of centers that can be accredited:

- Ambulatory care centers
- Birthing centers
- Chiropractic clinics
- Community health organizations
- Corporate health services
- County jail infirmaries
- Dental clinics
- Dialysis centers
- Endoscopy centers
- Group practices
- Imaging centers
- Independent practitioner practices
- Lithotripsy centers
- Magnetic resonance imaging centers
- Oncology centers
- Ophthalmology surgery centers
- Pain management centers
- Podiatry centers
- Physician offices
- Rehabilitative centers
- Research centers
- Sleep centers
- Student health centers
- Women's health centers

ment that is part of the Health Insurance Portability and Accountability Act regulations. These regulations are discussed later in the chapter. The application, which is sent from the JCAHO headquarters, consists of inquiries regarding the following:

- Ownership of the organization
- Demographics (e.g., address and phone number)
- Types of services provided
- Volume of patients served per year

2. The health care organization prepares for the survey by reviewing each JCAHO standard and assessing its own compliance. JCAHO standards can be found in its publications or on its website. In addition, the organization to be inspected reviews and updates all policy and procedure manuals. Personnel records are checked for accuracy and completion. Staff members are taught about the survey process and provided with sample questions that they may be asked during the survey.

3. The JCAHO informs the health care organization of the date, time, and duration of the survey. The length of the survey depends on the size and complexity of the setting. A first-time survey visit usually lasts 2 to 4 days. The JCAHO surveyors who specialize in health care standards conduct the survey.

4. The JCAHO conducts the survey, which consists of reviewing patient records, interviewing patients and family members, and touring the facility. Employees are interviewed to determine whether they know

where the policy and procedure manuals are kept, what is in the manuals, and safety rules. An exit conference in which preliminary findings are discussed is held between the surveyors and the administration (leadership) of the health care organization.

5. The JCAHO mails the accreditation decision to the health care organization within 60 days after the survey. An organization can appeal to the JCAHO for reevaluation of its assigned title. The organization receives a certificate indicating the level of accreditation that it has achieved. The certificate is posted at the facility.

6. If the initial site review identified some unsatisfactory areas, a second survey, called a focus survey, may be required to prove that corrections have been made. This type of survey generally lasts 1 to 2 days. After 3 years (the period for which accreditation by the JCAHO is valid), the health care organization submits a renewal application, resuming the cycle. Approximately 50% of the JCAHO standards are directly related to patient safety issues. As of January 2003, all site surveys are based on a new set of national goals aimed at improving the overall safety of patient care in hospitals and in other health care settings. All settings must show that they have reached these six goals:

- Improved accuracy of patient identification. (Always use two methods to identify patients.)
- Improved effectiveness of communication among caregivers. (Physician offices and hospitals must standardize abbreviations, acronyms, and symbols used in documentation. All sites must also have a policy stating what abbreviations and symbols cannot be used.)
- Improved safety of using high-alert medications. (These medications are given only in hospitals by registered nurses. Examples of high-alert medications are chemotherapy agents and potassium injections.)
- Eliminate wrong-site, wrong-patient, and wrong-procedure surgeries. (All steps must be taken to prevent procedures on a wrong patient. Wrong procedures can be simple errors, such as drawing blood from a wrong patient, to serious life-changing mistakes.)
- Improved safety of infusion pumps. (Examples of infusion pumps are pain management devices and insulin administration devices.)
- Improved effectiveness of clinical alarm systems. (All alarms must be checked on a regular basis and must be audible to everyone.)

In addition, the JCAHO requires accredited health care organizations to have a **sentinel event** policy and alert forms. A sentinel event is an unexpected death or serious physical or psychological injury to a patient. Box 11-2 lists some examples of sentinel events. Anytime a sentinel event occurs, the organization must determine the cause, implement

EXAMPLES OF SENTINEL EVENTS

These are examples of sentinel events that are reportable to the JCAHO:

- Any patient's death, paralysis, coma, or other major loss of function associated with a medication error
- Any suicide of a patient in a setting where the patient is housed around the clock, including suicides following elopement from such a setting
- Any procedure on the wrong patient, wrong side of the body, or wrong organ
- Any intrapartum maternal death and any death of a newborn weighing more than 2500 g that is not due to a congenital condition
- Any fall by a patient that directly results in death or major permanent loss of function
- Hemolytic transfusion reactions involving major blood group incompatibilities

improvements to prevent a repeat occurrence, and monitor the effectiveness of its plan. The JCAHO publishes a newsletter, *The Sentinel Event Alert*, discussing reported events to alert other facilities to potential problems, and copies can be viewed on its website. The sentinel event alert has raised awareness in the health care community and in the federal government about the occurrences of adverse events and ways these events can be prevented.

Physicians who perform office-based surgery need to follow the standards set forth by the JCAHO in the *Standards Manual for Office-Based Surgery*. The manual addresses certain standards, such as customer service, quality of care, qualified and competent staff levels, patient safety, leadership, and improving care and health. The manual provides the standards, the intent or purpose of the standards, and some tips for compliance. Box 11-3 displays a sample standard. If office-based surgeries are performed where you work, you should be familiar with these standards. Questions on how to implement these standards can be answered via the JCAHO website or through its hotline.

Checkpoint Question

2. What is a sentinel event?

Occupational Safety and Health Administration

OSHA is a federal agency that regulates health and safety concerns in the workplace. OSHA requires that QI programs be in place to protect the health and welfare of patients and employees. OSHA's mission is to save lives, prevent injuries, and protect the health of America's workers. Many rules under OSHA affect your job. Examples are rules for bloodborne pathogen protection, use of personal protective equipment (PPE), tuberculosis prevention, management of bio-

SAMPLE STANDARD

The practice demonstrates respect for the following needs of patients:

Standard	Intent	Tips for Compliance
RI.1.5 Privacy	Confidentiality of information gathered during treatment Privacy during care Security of self and property	Private examination rooms and treatment areas Staff members who demonstrate concern for patients' privacy Gowns provided when clothing must be changed
RI.1.6 Communication	Effective communication that considers hearing, speech, and visual impairments	Interpreters available when needed Staff age-specific training Patient information packets, educational materials, and consent forms available in the patients' languages
RI 1.7 Resolution of complaints	The right to complain about care and to have complaints reviewed and resolved	Documentation on investigation of patients' complaints or issues regarding care

hazardous waste, ergonomics, and laser protection. Laser protection is needed if you are working with a physician who is operating a laser in the office. These rules and other guidelines can be found on the OSHA website. Unlike the JCAHO, compliance with OSHA regulations is not voluntary. Noncompliance with OSHA regulations can result in fines and closure of the health care organization.

 Checkpoint Question

3. What is the mission of OSHA?

Centers for Medicare & Medicaid Services

The Centers for Medicare & Medicaid Services (CMS) [formerly the Health Care Financing Administration (HCFA)], a division of the United States Department of Health and Human Services, regulates and runs various departments and programs, including Medicare and Medicaid. This group is assigned to monitor and follow two key regulations that will affect your job as a medical assistant. These two laws are the **Clinical Laboratory Improvement Amendments Act** (CLIA) and the **Health Insurance Portability and Accountability Act** (HIPAA).

Clinical Laboratory Improvement Amendments Act. CLIA (Public Law 100-578) was originally written in 1988 and was aimed a streamlining the standards and quality of all laboratory settings. There are three levels of testing complexity. Laboratory sites and physician offices may perform tests only to the level of their certification. The three levels are low complexity, moderate complexity, and high complexity. Most physician offices perform only low- to moderate-complexity tests. Examples of low-complexity tests are urine dipsticks, fecal occult blood packets, urine pregnancy tests, ovulation kits, centrifuged microhematocrits, and certain blood glucose determinations. Examples of moderate-complexity tests are white blood cell counts, Gram staining, packaged rapid strep test, and automated cholesterol testing.

As the CMS has expanded, many amendments have occurred, with the latest one (CMS-2226F) occurring on January 24, 2003. The amendments aim at further reducing the potential for errors. Most laboratory errors occur in specimen collection and handling. Laboratory settings must have a complete and comprehensive QI program that studies and corrects problems associated with specimen collection and handling. Box 11-4 lists examples of errors in collecting and handling specimens.

Health Insurance Portability and Accountability Act. The HIPAA has four main objectives. They are to ensure health insurance portability for all people, reduce health care fraud and abuse, enforce standards of health information, and guarantee security and privacy of health information. Health insurance portability ensures that all working Americans

---

Box 11-4

ERRORS IN SPECIMEN COLLECTION

Errors in handling specimens or collecting them can occur in many ways. These errors can lead to errors in patient care. In most of these cases, the laboratory will not do the test and will dispose of the specimen. Another specimen will have to be collected from the patient. Here are some common errors:
- Wrong container used for specimen
- Container's expiration date passed
- Wrong patient's name on the label
- Wrong physician's name on the label
- No date or time on the label
- Patient's identification number not matched to laboratory slip
- Messy or illegible label
- Specimen label not matched to laboratory slip
- Specimen not stored at right temperature
- Laboratory slip not completely filled out

---

have access to health insurance and can take that insurance along if they leave the job. Some key requirements of the HIPAA are:

- Each physician practice must designate a privacy officer. This person is responsible for maintaining the privacy and security of all patients and ensuring compliance with the HIPAA.
- Physician offices must post a note in all waiting room areas that explains the practice's privacy policies.
- Policies and procedures must ensure that patients' safety and confidentiality are protected.

You will need to focus and guarantee security and privacy of all patient health information. There are specific guidelines on how you can transmit electronic transactions. Information must be encrypted before it is sent electronically. Many software programs can help physician offices to comply with these new regulations. The government is planning on implementing new laws that will require digital signatures to be sent with electronic data to decrease the potential for fraudulent Medicare claims. You can stay abreast of these new changes and regulations through the CMS website.

Physician offices must take appropriate steps to ensure that any company they are associated with also follows HIPAA regulations. Physician offices often have a variety of business partnerships that help keep the office flowing professionally and effectively. Some examples of business partnerships are cleaning services, document-shredding companies, laboratory and specimen transport personnel, and temporary staffing agencies. Contracts among physicians and their business partners should reflect that the business adheres to HIPAA regulations. For the JCAHO to meet HIPAA regulations and ensure security and privacy of patient information during the site visit, health care settings being surveyed must sign a business associate agreement prior to inspection.

Checkpoint Question

4. What governmental agency would you look to for additional information on HIPAA and CLIA regulations?

State Health Departments

Each state has a specific agency to license and monitor health care organizations. Each state has specific guidelines for required QI programs. As in participation with OSHA regulations, participation with state regulations is not optional. The rules and regulations vary among states. It is important that you be aware of the regulations in your state. For example, in some states medical assistants cannot administer medications, while in other states they can. Using your Internet search engine, type in key words "public health department" and look for your state's health department website.

DEVELOPING A QUALITY IMPROVEMENT PROGRAM

The size and complexity of an organization's QI program depends on the organization's particular needs. In large hospitals, numerous committees may be assigned to monitor and implement QI plans. Examples of QI plans are fall prevention, needlestick surveillance, and laboratory contamination rates. The committees will consist of staff members, including physicians. Most hospitals have a specific person assigned to oversee all of these committees.

In the medical office and ambulatory care settings, QI programs tend to be more informal. Usually the office manager or senior physician is responsible for monitoring and implementing QI plans. As more outpatient centers become accredited by the JCAHO, however, QI programs have become more structured. A few examples of quality issues that can be monitored in the physician offices are:

- Patient waiting times
- Unplanned returned patient visits for the same ailment or illness
- Misdiagnosed illnesses that are detected by another partner in the practice
- Patient or family complaints
- Timely follow-up telephone calls to patients
- Patient falls in physician's office or office building
- Mislabeled specimens sent to the laboratory
- Blood specimens that are coagulated or contaminated

Seven Steps for a Successful Program

The following seven steps are essential for creating an effective QI program:

1. *Identify the problem or potential problem.* All organizations can improve their delivery of patient care. Suggestions for improving care can come from many resources, including the following:
   - Office managers
   - Physicians (recommendations and complaints)
   - Other employees (e.g., nurses and medical assistants)
   - Patients (interviews)
   - Incident report trending (discussed later)

   The person responsible for QI in the medical office reviews all QI problems or potential problems and selects the one to be addressed first. Problems given top priority are those that are high risk (most likely to occur) and those that are most likely to cause injury to patients, family members, or employees.
2. *Form a task force.* A **task force** is a group of employees with different roles within the organization brought together to solve a given problem. In a medical office, the task force usually consists of a physician, nurse, medical assistant, and office manager. In large hospitals, various department managers are generally involved.
3. *Assign an expected threshold.* The task force establishes an **expected threshold** (numerical goal) for a given problem. Thresholds must be realistic and achievable. For example, if the problem is needlestick injuries, the expected threshold is a realistic number of employee needlestick injuries that the task force considers acceptable in a given period. For instance, the threshold may be one employee stick per month. It is not realistic to set the goal at zero; this may be optimal but is not achievable.
4. *Explore the problem and propose solutions.* The task force investigates the problem thoroughly to determine all potential causes and possible solutions. After various solutions are discussed, the task force decides what solution or solutions are to be implemented.
5. *Implement the solution.* The key to successful implementation of the solution is staff education. All staff members must be taught about the problem and the plan to decrease the problem. The type of implementation will be based on the problem. For example, if the problem is patients falling at the entrance to the building, fixing the problem is likely to be complex and expensive. It may involve reengineering and construction of new walkways. If the problem is mislabeling or misspelling patient's names on laboratory specimens, the implementation will be simpler, possibly printing labels from the computer database.
6. *Establish a QI monitoring plan.* After implementation, the solution must be evaluated to determine

whether it worked and if so, how well. QI monitoring plans have three elements:
- Source of monitoring, that is, where the numerical data will be obtained (e.g., medical record review, incident reports, laboratory reports, office logs)
- Frequency of monitoring, that is, how often the data will be monitored and tallied (e.g., once a week, once a month)
- Person responsible for monitoring, that is, who collects the data and presents the results in graphic form, allowing for easy comparison of data from before and after implementation of the solution

7. *Obtain feedback.* The members of the task force must review the graphs in relation to their expected threshold. Did they meet the threshold? If yes, the problem has been resolved. If the threshold was not met, the task force must determine whether the expected threshold was unrealistic or the solutions were inadequate. In either case, the problem has not been resolved; therefore, the task force must review each of the steps and make appropriate changes.

Checkpoint Question

5. How does an organization select problems for a QI program?

RISK MANAGEMENT

Risk management is an internal process geared to identifying potential problems before they cause injury to patients or employees. Potential problems are related to risk factors. A risk factor is any situation or condition that poses a safety or liability concern for a given practice. Examples of risk factors are poor lighting, unlocked medication cabinets, failure to dispose of needles properly, and faulty patient identification procedures. Such factors may lead to patient falls, medication errors, employee needlesticks, and mistakes in therapeutic intervention. Risk factors for a particular health care organization are identified through the trending of incident reports.

One of the most challenging problems for risk managers is to prevent noncompliance with regulatory agencies. As discussed earlier, numerous agencies regulate health care settings, and these rules and regulations change frequently. You can stay up-to-date with new changes by reading newsletters from these organizations, attending your state and local professional meetings, and frequently visiting various professional websites.

Incident Reports

Incident reports, sometimes referred to as occurrence reports, are written accounts of untoward (negative) patient, visitor, or staff events. Such events may be minor or life or limb threatening. The insurance company that provides the institution's liability insurance often requires incident reports.

An incident report is written or completed by the staff member involved in or at the scene of the incident. The report is reviewed by a supervisor for completion and accuracy and is then sent to a central location. In a hospital, incident reports are sent to the risk manager. In a medical office, incident reports are usually given to the office manager or the physician. Depending on the type of event and organizational policy, a physician may or may not document the event on the incident report. If an unusual event happens to a patient, however, the physician should assess the patient and document the findings on the incident report.

Checkpoint Question

6. What is an incident report?

When to Complete an Incident Report

Even in the safest settings, undesirable things can happen to patients. These events sometimes result from human error (e.g., giving the wrong medication), or they may be idiopathic. Idiopathic means that something occurred for unknown reasons and was unavoidable (e.g., an allergic reaction). Incident reports must be completed even if no injury resulted from an event. A few examples of situations requiring an incident report are:

- All medication errors
- All patient, visitor, and employee falls
- Drawing blood from a wrong patient
- Mislabeling of blood tubes or specimens
- Incorrect surgical instrument counts following surgery
- Employee needlesticks
- Workers' compensation injuries

The rule of thumb is, when in doubt, always complete an incident report. Many health care professionals are reluctant to complete incident reports, owing to various myths, which are discussed in Box 11-5.

Information Included on an Incident Report

Although every agency has its own form, the following data are always included on an incident report (Fig. 11-1):

- Name, address, and phone number of the injured party
- Date of birth and sex of the injured party
- Date, time, and location of the incident
- Brief description of the incident and what was done to correct it
- Any diagnostic procedures or treatments that were needed
- Patient examination findings, if applicable
- Names and addresses of witnesses, if applicable
- Signature and title of person completing form
- Physician's and supervisor's signatures as per policy

Box 11-5

MYTHS ABOUT COMPLETING AN INCIDENT REPORT

Myth	Fact
If I complete an incident report, I will get fired.	Employers want incident reports to be completed for documentation of events. You are more likely to get fired for *not* completing one.
Incident reports go into my personnel file.	They are not placed in your file. They are stored separately. Supervisors may document discussions or education that you were given about the incident.
If I complete the incident report, I am admitting that I am at fault.	Incident reports do not imply fault. They document the evidence.
I need to photocopy the incident report and save it at home for my own legal protection.	You may find yourself in more trouble if you copy the document and store it at home. Most incident reports contain confidential patient information, and it is illegal to copy private patient information and store it at home.

Guidelines for Completing an Incident Report

When completing an incident report, follow these guidelines:

1. State only the facts. Do not draw conclusions or summarize the event. For example, if you walk into the reception room and find a patient on the floor, do not write, "Patient tripped and fell in reception area," because that draws a conclusion. Instead, document the incident as follows: "Patient found on the floor in the reception area. Patient states that he fell" (Fig. 11-2).
2. Write legibly and sign your name legibly. Be sure to include your title.
3. Complete the form in a timely fashion. In general, incident reports should be completed within 24 hours of the event.
4. Do not leave any blank spaces on the form. If a particular section of the report does not apply, write n/a (not applicable).
5. Never photocopy an incident report for your own personal record.
6. Never place the incident report in the patient's chart. Never document in the patient's chart that an incident report was completed. Only document the event in the patient's chart. (By writing in the medical record that an incident report was completed, it opens the potential for lawyers to subpoena the incident report, should there be a lawsuit.)

Trending Incident Reports

After incident reports are completed, they are reviewed and tracked to highlight specific patterns. The resulting statistical data can be used to identify problem areas, which can be corrected through QI programs. Examples of statistical data that can be found in incident reports follow:

• Particular days of the week when most negative events happen (if most events occur on Friday afternoons,

perhaps staffing on Friday afternoon should be reevaluated)
• Most common area for patient falls (if most falls happen in the lobby, a QI program may need to be established to assess why falls occur there)
• Medications that are routinely given incorrectly (educating staff and using colored labels to highlight similar drug names may correct this)
• The age group most likely to have problems (if most of your incident reports reflect problems in the geriatric population, a QI program focusing on geriatric care may be needed)
• Incident reports should be kept in a special file in the manager's office (some managers file these reports

WHAT IF

You give the wrong medication, and the patient has a bad reaction to it. Would you be better off not documenting the medication error?

NO! By not documenting the incident, you place yourself at risk. These risks can include allegations of falsifying medical records, tampering with medical records, and failing to follow reporting policies and procedures. On the incident report, do not say, "I gave the wrong medication"; just state the facts: "X medication was ordered. I gave Y medication." Then document whom you told and when, what you were advised to do, and any other pertinent information. Your supervisor or the risk manager may call the medical office's insurance company to alert them to the incident. If the incident results in a malpractice lawsuit, an accurately completed incident report can prove helpful to your organization's attorney.

INCIDENT REPORT FORM
PRIVILEGED & CONFIDENTIAL

Patient Stamp

☐ Inpatient ☐ Outpatient ☐ Visitor ☐ Volunteer ☐ Other   *NOT A PART OF THE MEDICAL RECORD–FORWARD TO RISK MANAGER WITHIN 72 HOURS*

Name	Age	Sex	Admit Date	Location of Incident	Room #

Diagnosis	Date of Incident	Time AM/PM	Date of Report	Person Reporting & Title (print)

CONDITION BEFORE INCIDENT
☐ Alert ☐ Disoriented ☐ Unconscious ☐ Agitated
☐ Confused ☐ Sedated ☐ Uncooperative ☐ Other

Activity Orders
☐ Adib ☐ BRP ☐ BRP c help
☐ With assist ☐ CBR
☐ Up in chair ☐ BSC

Signature

INCIDENT (please check all items that apply)   FALLS

FALLS	PREFALL FACTORS	RESTRAINTS	RISK CONDITIONS	CURRENT MEDICATIONS
☐ Fall from Bed ☐ Fall from Chair ☐ Fall from Bedside Commode ☐ Fall from Stretcher ☐ Fall from Wheelchair ☐ Fall from Toilet ☐ Fall while Ambulatory ☐ Other_____	☐ Bed Up ☐ Bed Down ☐ Brake On ☐ Y ☐ N ☐ Not working ☐ Siderails Down ____ 2 Up ____ 3 Up ____ 4 Up ____ Climbed Out	Restraints Ordered ☐ Y ☐ N Restraints in Use ☐ Y ☐ N Type: ☐ Vest ☐ Wrist ☐ Ankle 　　　☐ Secured Mittens ☐ Tied ☐ Untied by: 　____ Staff 　____ Patient 　____ Family/S.O. Call light in reach ☐ Y ☐ N Fall follow-up program initiated prior to fall ☐ Y ☐ N	☐ Weakness ☐ Decreased Mobility ☐ Confusion ☐ Neuro/ortho diagnosis ☐ Cardiovascular diagnosis ☐ Inpaired Vision ☐ History of Syncope ☐ Poor Nutritional Status ☐ Incontinence ☐ History of fall last 6 months Safety Education given prior to fall: ☐ None ☐ Patient ☐ Family/S.O.	☐ None ☐ NTG ☐ Diuretics ☐ Cathartic preps/enemas ☐ Antihypertensives ☐ Antiseizure ☐ Antidepressants ☐ Antiemetics ☐ Antipsychotics ☐ Analgesics/Hypnotics ☐ Narcotics ☐ Cardiovascular

Environment: ☐ Floor wet ☐ Y ☐ N　　　　☐ Free from obstacles ☐ Y ☐ N Describe: _____
　　　　☐ Night light on ☐ Y ☐ N ☐ N/A　☐ Objects not in reach-searching for _____

MEDICATION VARIANCE, Including IV & Blood Product(s)	PROCEDURE VARIANCE	MISCELLANEOUS
☐ Incorrect Pt. Identification ☐ Incorrect IV Solution ☐ Incorrect Dosage ☐ Incorrect IV Rate ☐ Incorrect Route ☐ Incorrect Count/Missing Med ☐ Incorrect Time ☐ Topical Substance Reaction, ☐ Incorrect Med Given 　 including Tape ☐ Incorrect Med Dispensed ☐ Allergy Not Documented ☐ Med Omitted ☐ Contrast Reaction/Complication ☐ Med Transcription Error ☐ Medication Past Due 1 hour ☐ Incorrect Blood Given 　 or more ☐ Pharmacy Notified ☐ Other_____ ☐ Infiltration ☐ Blood Reaction ☐ Med Reaction	☐ Record Error ☐ Transcription ☐ Incorrect Pt. Identification ☐ Omitted Treatment ☐ Delayed Treatment ☐ Omitted Diagnostic/Lab ☐ Delayed Diagnostic/Lab ☐ Traumatic Venipuncture ☐ Break in Sterile Technique ☐ Incorrect Surgical Count–Sponge ☐ Incorrect Surgical Count–Needle ☐ Incorrect Surgical Count–Instrument ☐ Retained Foreign Body ☐ Other: ☐ Documentation Error ☐ Consent Variance ☐ Improper Prep of Pt. ☐ NPO Violated ☐ Radiation/Toxic Chemical Exposure ☐ X-ray Interpretation Discrepancy ☐ Airway/Intubation Problem ☐ Incorrect Level of Heat/Cold Applied ☐ Incorrect Procedure/Treatment ☐ Unordered Procedure/Treatment ☐ Equip./Product Malfunction ☐ User Error ☐ Equipment Unavailable	☐ AMA/Elopement ☐ Admitted c Pressure Sore ☐ Damaged/Lost Teeth/ 　 Denture ☐ Injury During Transport ☐ Self Inflicted Injury/Suicide ☐ Malpositioning/Incorrect 　 Body Alignment ☐ Pt. Self Extubation ☐ Tube/IV Catheter Out ☐ Accidental Strking Against 　 an Object ☐ Fainted ☐ Pt. Dissatisfied/Pt. 　 Threatened Law Suit ☐ Transfer to Critical Care 　 p incident ☐ Behavior Out of Norm. ☐ Other:_____

INJURY (please check all items that apply) All serious/significant injuries must be described on reverse side　　　**PROCEDURE/LABOR & DELIVERY/NURSERY**

SERIOUS	SIGNIFICANT	SUPERFICIAL
☐ None ☐ Spinal Cord Injury ☐ Injury to Nerves ☐ Brain Injury ☐ Surgery to Wrong Pt. ☐ Incorrect Surgical Procedure ☐ Shock ☐ Trauma Causing Internal Injury ☐ Hemorrhage ☐ Death ☐ Unscheduled Return to OR ☐ Other:	☐ None ☐ Major Infiltration ☐ Hospital Acquired Decubiti ☐ Burn ☐ Fracture ☐ Sprain/Strain Joint/Muscle ☐ Injury to Blood Vessel ☐ Dislocation of Joint ☐ Open Wound Needing Medical Care ☐ Adverse Effect Due to Med/Anesthesia/Transfusion ☐ Adverse Effect Due to Exposure to Toxic Chemical ☐ Complication Due to Mechanical Device ☐ Prolongation of Hospital Stay ☐ Anoxia/Respiratory Distress ☐ Cancellation of or after induction of anesthesia	☐ None ☐ Unknown ☐ Abrasion ☐ Bruising ☐ Blister/Skin Tear ☐ Skin Prick ☐ Laceration ☐ Rash/Hives ☐ Other:

☐ Newborn with apparent Cerebral dysfunction
☐ Newborn with APGAR of four (4) or less at five (5) minutes
☐ Newborn with serious birth trauma
☐ Precipitous Delivery
☐ Unattended Delivery

MEDICAL DEVICE/EQUIPMENT RELATED

Equipment involved: _____
Manufacturer: _____
Serial #: _____
Asset #: _____
Biomedical Dept. Notified: _____ Date
Tagged & Removed from Service: _____ Date/Time

Maintain all components of device such as connectors, adaptors, tubings, etc. Document all readings/settings.

DO NOT ADJUST OR CLEAR ANY READINGS.

AMA FOLLOW-UP

Reason for leaving: _____
Patient admitted <24 hours ☐ Yes ☐ No
Patient/S.O. Teaching: ☐ Completed ☐ Partial ☐ None ☐ Patient Uncooperative

FIGURE 11–1. Sample incident report.

(continued)

Description of event: _____

_____

_____

_____

_____

_____

_____

_____

_____

_____

_____

_____

_____

_____

_____

_____

Physician notified: ☐ Yes ☐ No   Name of Physician (print): _____
Physician Remarks: _____

_____

_____

_____

_____

_____

_____

_____

| Physician Signature | Date |

Supervisor/Manager Investigation/Follow-up Action: _____

_____

_____

_____

_____

_____

_____

| Supervisor/Manager Signature | Date |

Witness: Name (print)	Department/Shift	Address	Phone

| Risk Manager Signature | Date |

F IGURE 11–1. *(Continued)*

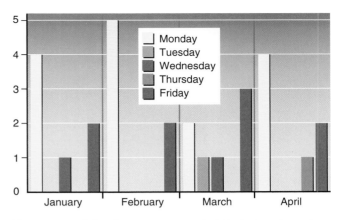

FIGURE 11–3. Frequency of mislabeled specimens by day of the week and by month.

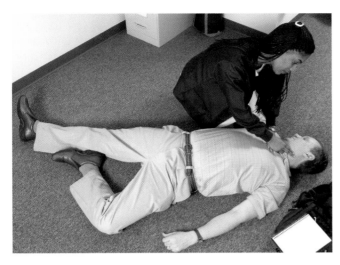

FIGURE 11–2. When writing an incident report, document only the facts. Do not draw conclusions. Always be honest, and never falsify the information.

according to dates, whereas others file them according to the problem)

PUTTING IT ALL TOGETHER: A CASE REVIEW

Following is a case study in which the elements of successful QI and risk management programs are put into action.

You are working in a busy family practice. The average number of patients seen daily is 92. The physicians, nurses, and medical assistants are responsible for labeling specimen containers before they go to the laboratory. On the average, 15 specimens are collected daily. The hospital laboratory that analyzes the specimens reports that an average of seven specimens are mislabeled monthly.

The office manager brings to a staff meeting a graph (Fig. 11-3) depicting the number of mislabeled specimens that occurred over a 4-month period. She notes that most mislabelings occurred on Monday and Friday afternoons. It is decided that this is a significant patient care issue and that a QI program to address and resolve the problem is needed.

A task force is formed. It includes a physician, a nurse, and a medical assistant. The task force identifies the problem as a high-risk issue and assigns the expected threshold to be fewer than two mislabeled specimens per month. The task force identifies the factors related to the problem, which includes lack of sufficient labels in patient rooms, high patient volumes on Monday and Friday afternoons, and overall need for educating all staff members about the importance of labeling specimens correctly.

Solutions to these three problems are created:

Problem: *insufficient labels in the rooms.*
Solution: *Additional specimen labels are placed in every room. Also, specimen labels will be already printed and waiting for patients who arrive for an anticipated specimen collection (stool, urine, skin biopsy).*
Problem: *large volume on Monday and Friday afternoons.*
Solution: *The medical assistant's hours will change to 10:00 A.M. to 6:30 P.M. on Monday and Fridays instead of 8 A.M. to 4:30 P.M. This creates more staff coverage during peak hours.*
Problem: *lack of knowledge.*
Solution: *A representative for the hospital laboratory will conduct an in-service for all staff members. He or she will explain the implication of mislabeled specimens and how they can impair patient care. Lets say*

Spanish Terminology

¿Vio usted lo que pasó?	Did you see what happened?
¿Cayo usted?	Did you fall?
¿Está lastimado usted?	Are you hurt?
¿Quiere usted ver un doctor?	Do you want to see a doctor?
Usted necesita obtener una radiografía.	You need an x-ray.

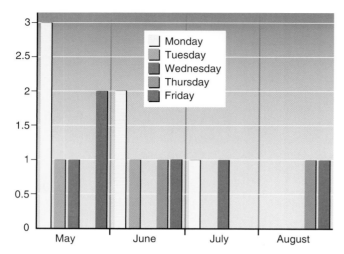

F I G U R E   1 1 – 4 .   Frequency of mislabeled specimens by day of the week and by month after a QI plan was carried out. Note the change in the numerical system on the graph.

that both Mrs. Brown and Mrs. Lisien came into the office for skin biopsies. The specimens were taken and placed in bottles. The bottles were put next to each other on the shelf. The name labels were reversed on the specimens. One specimen showed a malignancy. Which patient would get treated? The wrong patient would be treated, causing unnecessary expense and distress, while the patient with the malignancy would not be treated and might get sicker.

After these steps were taken, a new graph was developed showing the improvement (Fig. 11-4). Because the threshold has been met, the task force does not think any more changes are needed, and the QI mislabeling program is ended.

CHAPTER SUMMARY

Quality improvement programs have many benefits to heath care organizations. They can identify potential problems for patients and employees. After identifying the problem, the task force can create solutions to resolve them. QI programs are also required by various agencies. Four important agencies are the JCAHO, OSHA, CMS, and your state health department. You must stay alert to new regulations from these agencies. More information about various health care regulations can be found through their websites, newsletters, and professional organizations. Patients place trust in all health care workers and health care settings. We must all work hard to provide good quality care to all patients every time they are treated.

Critical Thinking Challenges

1. Create a list of potential patient or employee problems that could be solved with a QI program. Be sure to include some administrative, clinical, and laboratory examples. Then select three problems and develop a list of solutions for each problem.
2. List 10 reasons to complete an incident report. Select one of these reasons and complete the incident report. (Photocopy the incident report from the chapter.) Be sure to review the guidelines for completing an incident report. Make sure your description of events on page 2 follows these guidelines.
3. Search the JCAHO website. What information can you find regarding sentinel events? What steps can be taken to prevent them?
4. Privacy of patient information is essential. Write a policy that aims at protecting patients' privacy. What steps can you take to ensure patients' privacy? Would you make a good privacy officer? Why or why not?

Answers to Checkpoint Questions

1. The benefits of being accredited by the JCAHO are that the health care organization is eligible for state and federal funding programs and that accreditation proves to the community that the facility has met basic standards of care.
2. A sentinel event is an unexpected occurrence involving a death or serious physical or physiological injury to a patient.
3. OSHA's mission is to save lives, prevent injuries, and protect the health of America's workers.
4. Centers for Medicare & Medicaid (CMS) are responsible for HIPAA and CLIA regulations.
5. QI programs should be selected to address problems that are high risk and those most likely to cause injury to patients, family members, or employees.
6. An incident report is a written account of untoward or negative events involving patients, visitors, or employees.

   Websites

Centers for Medicare & Medicaid Services
    www.cms.gov
Clinical Laboratory Improvement Amendments Act
    www.cms.hhs.gov/clia/
Health Care Report Cards
    www.healthgrades.com
Health Insurance Portability and Accountability Act
    www.cms.hhs.gov/hipaa
Joint Commission on Accreditation of Healthcare Organizations
    www.jcaho.org
Occupational Health and Safety Administration
    www.osha.gov

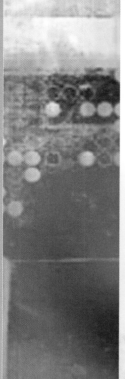

12

Management of the Medical Office Team

CHAPTER OUTLINE

ROLE DELINEATION COMPONENTS

GENERAL: Professionalism
- Demonstrate initiative and responsibility
- Work as a member of the health care team
- Adapt to change
- Enhance skills through continuing education
- Promote the practice through positive public relations

GENERAL: Legal Concepts
- Perform within legal and ethical boundaries
- Follow employer's established policies dealing with the health care contract
- Implement and maintain federal and state health care legislation and regulations
- Comply with established risk management and safety procedures
- Recognize professional credentialing criteria
- Develop and maintain personnel, policy, and procedures manuals

GENERAL: Communication Skills
- Recognize and respond effectively to verbal, nonverbal, and written communications
- Serve as a liaison

GENERAL: Operational Functions
- Perform inventory of supplies and equipment
- Perform routine maintenance of administrative and clinical equipment
- Apply computer techniques to support office operations
- Perform personnel management functions
- Negotiate leases and prices for equipment and supply contracts

ADMINISTRATIVE: Administrative Procedures
- Perform basic administrative medical assisting functions
- Understand and adhere to manage care policies and procedures
- Negotiate managed care contracts

ADMINISTRATIVE: Practice Finances
- Manage accounts receivable
- Develop and maintain fee schedules
- Manage renewals of business and professional insurance policies
- Manage personnel benefits and maintain records
- Perform marketing, financial and strategic planning

CHAPTER COMPETENCIES

LEARNING OBJECTIVES
Upon successfully completing this chapter, you will be able to:
1. Spell and define the key terms
2. Describe what is meant by organizational structure
3. List seven responsibilities of the medical office manager
4. Explain the five staffing issues that a medical office manager will be responsible for handling
5. List the types of policies and procedures that should be included in a medical office's policy and procedures manual
6. List five types of promotional materials that a medical office may distribute
7. Discuss three financial concerns that the medical office manager must be capable of addressing
8. Discuss four legal issues that affect medical office management

PERFORMANCE OBJECTIVES
Upon successfully completing this chapter, you will be able to:
1. Write a job description
2. Create policy and procedures manuals

KEY TERMS

Americans with Disabilities Act	compliance officer	job description	policy
budget	Family and Medical Leave Act	mission statement	procedure
		organizational chart	

A SUCCESSFUL MEDICAL practice needs an effective medical office management process. This process must be a team effort among the physicians, nurse managers, and the office manager. This chapter provides an overview of medical office management as well as a discussion of a medical office manager's specific responsibilities.

OVERVIEW OF MEDICAL OFFICE MANAGEMENT

Each medical office is organized in a slightly different manner, depending on the size and complexity of the setting.

Organizational Structure

The medical office's organizational structure, or chain of command, is depicted in an **organizational chart**, a flow sheet that allows the manager and employees to identify their team members and to see where they fit into the team. Figure 12-1 displays a sample organizational chart for a physician's office in which there is a partnership between two physicians. In this example, it is assumed that the physicians have an equal partnership in the practice.

Checkpoint Question

1. What is the purpose of an organizational chart?

The Medical Office Manager

The medical office manager must be multiskilled, multitalented, and able to prioritize a variety of issues, juggle responsibilities, and communicate effectively with patients, staff, and physicians. In some settings, the medical office manager may be referred to as the business manager. Managers may be nurses, medical assistants, or administrative support personnel. Although the qualifications and educational requirements for the position vary greatly among health care organizations, a successful medical office manager must be:

- Flexible
- A positive role model for employees
- Honest and fair
- A good communicator
- A resource person for employees
- Supportive of all management decisions
- Well organized
- Able to focus on a given task
- Able to resolve conflicts
- Able to see the big picture

A medical office manager's responsibilities include varied tasks:

- Communicating with patients, physicians, and staff
- Handling staffing issues

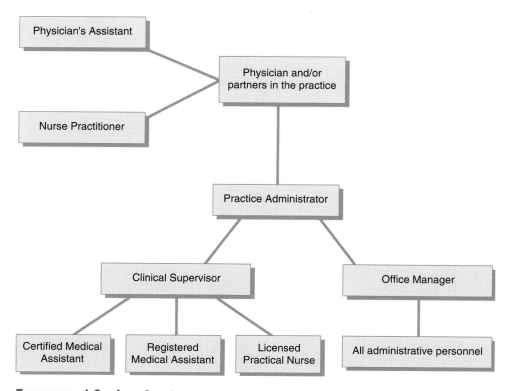

FIGURE 12-1. Sample organizational chart.

- Writing and revising policy and procedures manuals
- Developing promotional materials
- Handling financial concerns
- Handling maintenance and inventory
- Ensuring that the staff receives appropriate education

RESPONSIBILITIES OF THE MEDICAL OFFICE MANAGER

Communication

Perhaps one of the hardest and yet most important aspects of being an effective manager is being able to communicate with fellow employees, colleagues, physicians, and patients. (The techniques for effective communication are discussed in Chapter 3.) You must be a good listener, have good interpersonal skills, and be aware of your own nonverbal language.

Communicating With Patients

Communication with patients on a management level can often be challenging. Patients come to you with a variety of complaints, such as incorrect billing, poor care, or long waits to see physicians. Of course, you must always be diplomatic. Your goal should be to correct the problem in a timely and professional manner and to alleviate any negative feelings the patient may have.

Communicating With Staff

Communication with staff members can be difficult, depending on the number of employees, number and locations of satellite centers, and the variety of shifts that are in place. There are three ways to promote communication with staff members: staff meetings, bulletin boards, and communication notebooks.

Staff Meetings. Staff meetings should be scheduled at a predictable frequency and time to allow the staff to plan (e.g., they might be held the first Monday of every month at 8 A.M.) Meetings should never be canceled except in a true emergency.

Staff meetings must be well organized and should begin and end on time. Agendas should be created prior to the meeting and posted for staff review. (See Chapter 7 for information on agendas.) The agenda should be followed as closely as possible. Individual staff concerns or complaints should not be handled during a general staff meeting; the meeting should remain focused and constructive and not turn into a battleground for staff disagreements. Minutes should be taken and kept in a notebook for staff to review as needed. (See Chapter 7 for information on minutes.)

Staff meetings should be conducted in a private area out of patients' sight and hearing (Fig. 12-2). All interruptions except for emergencies should be avoided.

Have the telephone covered by an answering service or a prerecorded message informing callers of the time the staff will be unavailable. Lock the door and place a sign with the time the office will reopen. Of course, you will give clear instructions to callers or visitors who have an emergency. The personnel manual should clearly state the attendance policy for staff meetings. In addition, some offices include attendance as a duty in each employee's job description (statement of work-related responsibilities). To improve attendance at staff meetings, consider serving food or including an educational presentation.

Bulletin Boards. Bulletin board postings allow employees to get a quick and easy look at new polices or procedures. To encourage staff members to read the postings, make sure the bulletin boards are attractive, well organized, and updated regularly. It is a good idea to have employees initial all messages on the bulletin board after reading them.

Communication Notebooks. A simple notebook can serve as a two-way communication tool: You can write messages to employees, and they can write back to you. Such a notebook is usually kept in the staff lounge. Again, staff members should initial any important messages after reading them. If the message is directed to you, be sure to respond as soon as possible.

Communicating Electronically

E-mail has become popular and is an easy and time-saving way to communicate with staff. Messages can be printed and kept in a binder for easy reference. E-mail messages eliminate the need for memos that must be posted or circulated. Your e-mail system will provide you with an address book that can be customized to include groups such as all employees, all clinical employees, employees and physicians, and so on.

Sometimes, the stress of daily duties prevents managers from communicating with staff members on a personal level. To be an effective manager, you should communicate not

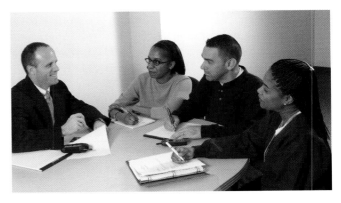

FIGURE 12-2. Staff meeting being conducted in a private area.

only bad news but also positive messages to your employees. You can communicate positive messages through birthday and holiday cards and employee recognition awards.

Checkpoint Question

2. What are three ways to promote communication with staff members?

Staffing Issues

Staffing issues will occupy most of your time as an office manager. These concerns include writing job descriptions, hiring new employees, evaluating present employees, taking disciplinary actions, handling terminations, and scheduling.

Writing Job Descriptions

Each job must have a description. The purpose of a **job description** is to inform the employee about the duties and expectations for a given position. Job descriptions also help you in interviewing applicants and evaluating existing employees.

Each employee should receive a copy of his or her job description at the time of hiring and after any revisions to the description are made. Some medical offices have a policy requiring the employee to read and sign the job description at the time of hiring.

Formats for writing job descriptions vary among offices. In general, the following elements are included: job title, supervisor, position summary, hours, location, employment requirements, physical requirements, duties, and the evaluation process (Fig. 12-3). The description should also include the date it was written and date of any revisions.

If possible, involve staff members in writing and revising their job descriptions. Employee participation leads to greater cooperation.

Hiring and Interviewing Employees

Only after creating or reviewing an existing job description can you begin the process of interviewing and hiring a new employee. Finding applicants for most medical office positions is usually not a problem. You can seek applicants through advertising in local newspaper classified sections,

LEGAL TIP

Verify the credentials of an applicant by calling the appropriate state licensing board or certification registry. Is the applicant's license or certification current? Unfortunately, some people are dishonest and unethical. A person who is not misrepresenting himself or herself will not mind you checking. A CMA's status can be obtained by calling 1-800-ACT-AAMA. Many state medical assisting societies also have certification registries. Try going to the particular profession's website.

placement personnel at local schools that offer medical assisting programs, networking, and employment agencies.

All applicants should complete an application. State laws vary regarding the types of questions that can be asked on applications. In general, you must avoid any questions pertaining to an applicant's age, sex, race, religion, and physical or mental disabilities. If your medical facility requires a criminal background check and drug testing, the form should include this information with a place for the applicant to give necessary permission with a signature. Any employee application form should be reviewed by legal counsel prior to its use. It is always a good idea to request that the applicant bring a résumé to the interview.

Before interviewing an applicant, prepare a list of questions. Again, use caution; under law you are not permitted to ask about some topics. During the interview, assess the applicant's ability to do the following:

- Perform technical skills
- Treat patients in a caring manner
- Fit into your organization
- Communicate in a professional yet friendly manner
- Remain flexible

Evaluating Employees

All employees must be evaluated annually. The evaluation should be a positive experience for the employee. Employee evaluations must be fair, accurate, and objective. Some type

ñ Spanish Terminology

Busco un trabajo.	*I am looking for a job.*
¿Tiene usted cualquier abîerto?	*Do you have any openings?*
¿Dónde estan las aplicaciones?	*Where are the applications?*
Soy el director.	*I am the manager.*

Job Description

Title: Medical Assistant

Supervisor(s): Clinical Supervisor

Office Manager for Administrative Duties

Position summary: This is a 40-hour position that will require the employee to perform various duties including administrative, clinical, and laboratory procedures. Scheduling will be variable to meet the needs of the office.

Hours: Hours will vary to meet the needs of the office. Hours will rotate from 8:00 AM–4:30 PM and 10:00 AM–6:30 PM. You will be expected to work one Saturday per month.

Location: Our main office is located at 129 South Main Street. The satellite office is located at 56 West Road, Suite 102. This position will primarily require you to work at our main office. However, occasional days may be assigned at the satellite office.

Employment Requirements: The employee must have graduated from a medical assisting program. CMA or RMA is preferred. The employee must have a current CPR and First Aid card. One year of experience or completion of an externship is preferred.

• *Language skills:* The employee must be able to read and interpret documents and respond appropriately (verbally and/or in writing). Must be able to document in a professional manner.

• *Mathematical skills:* The employee must be able to add, subtract, multiply, and divide whole numbers and fractions.

Physical requirements: The following are physical requirements for this job: Standing: 6–8 hours/day; Sitting: 6–8 hours/day; Lifting: 50 pounds; Twisting and rotating: 45 degrees; Squatting: As needed to assist patients or to perform office tasks.

Duties: You will be expected to perform the following duties after completing the orientation process. This is a partial list; and other duties can be added as necessary.

Administrative:

Scheduling appointments	Processing mail
Transcribing documents	Operating the telephone
Filing	Providing patient education
Completing insurance forms	

Clinical/Laboratory:

Operating centrifuge	Obtaining vital signs
Performing phlebotomy	Administering vaccines and other medications
Performing HCT/HGB/CBC	as ordered
Performing pregnancy and monospot tests	Providing patient education
Obtaining visual acuities	Assisting the physician as directed

Evaluation process: Three evaluations will be conducted in the first year. Thirty days from start date, ninety days from start date, and then at the one-year anniversary date. Following the first year of employment, annual evaluations will be done.

I have read my job description, and I understand what is expected of me. I am able to physically perform all the required duties.

Signature of employee: _____   Date: _____

Signature of supervisor: _____   Date: _____

Signature of supervisor: _____   Date: _____

Dates: original JD - 1977, revised March 1998.

FIGURE 12–3. Sample job description.

of written evaluation should be given to the employee to read, sign, and comment on. Most forms ask employees to list their objectives and goals for the coming year. Figure 12-4 displays a sample evaluation form. Some organizations call evaluations performance appraisals.

New employees should be evaluated 1 month after their start date, again in 90 days, and then at their 1-year anniversary date. This process helps new employees gain confidence and improve weaknesses.

Taking Disciplinary Action

Most offices have policies regarding documentation of disciplinary action. Disciplinary actions can be verbal or

Employee Evaluation Form

Employee: _____

Evaluation Date: _____

Job Title: _____

Ratings:

Traits	Score
Appearance	
Communication Skills	
Attendance	
Quality of work	
Reliability	
Initiative	
Other:	
Total Score:	

Rating scale:

5—excellent

4—above average

3—meets job expectations

2—below job expectations

1—does not meet job expectations

Supervisor comments:

_____

_____

Employee goals for the next year (to be completed by employee):

_____

_____

_____

Employee Comments:

_____

_____

_____

Supervisor signature: _____   Date: _____

Employee signature: _____   Date: _____

FIGURE 12–4.   Sample employee evaluation form.

written. Verbal warnings are generally done for a first-time minor occurrence (e.g., not showing up for work and not calling in). A note should go into the employee's file stating that a verbal warning was given, the date, any actions that were taken, and any comments that the employee made.

Written notices are used for more serious problems (e.g., breaching patient confidentiality, substance abuse) or recurrent minor ones. Employees should sign any written warning notices. These documents can be used as evidence in the event that the person is fired and brings a lawsuit for wrongful discharge. Figure 12-5 shows a sample written disciplinary action form. Determine whether the employee's credentialing agency should be notified of serious infractions.

Terminating Employees

Having to terminate (fire) an employee is never an easy or pleasant task. It is essential that policies regarding termination be followed precisely. All disciplinary actions must be clearly and objectively stated. Terminating employees for unlawful reasons or failing to follow the organization's termination policy can result in lawsuits against you and the office. Some reasons for termination:

- Excessive tardiness or absenteeism
- Inappropriate dress or behavior
- Alcohol or drug use
- Endangering patients

WHAT IF

You receive a call requesting a reference for an employee who was fired. What should you say?

Be careful! This situation can turn into a legal nightmare if not handled appropriately. If you give a wonderful report to the potential employer and say, "She was great; never had any problems," you and the office may be sued by the former employee for wrongful discharge. In court, you would be asked: "If she was so wonderful, why did you fire her?" On the other hand, if you say, "She was a terrible employee, and we fired her," you can be sued for defamation of character. Because of the legal concerns in providing employment references, most organizations have a policy stating that the only information to be released is verification of employment dates and job titles. When in doubt, give no information. Ask for the caller's name and phone number; discuss the issue with the physician in charge, and then return the phone call.

- Lying or stealing
- Falsifying medical records or time sheets
- Breaching patient confidentiality

Scheduling

The primary goal of scheduling is to meet the needs of the office. The secondary goal is to meet the requests of your employees. You must be fair in scheduling and always follow your organization's policies for weekend and holiday or personal day requests. If possible, employees should be given time off with pay when attending seminars and meetings of their professional organization. This practice will keep morale high and encourage employees to stay current with their skills. Depending on the number of employees that you have to schedule and the complexity of the hours or shifts, you can either schedule by hand or use a computer program. If your organization is small and cohesive, you may want to assign a senior staff member to do the scheduling, or you might allow the employees to self-schedule. No matter what scheduling format is used, you are ultimately responsible for ensuring that the appropriate number and type of employees needed are scheduled.

Discipline Record

Employee Name: _____ #: _____ Date of Warning: _____

Warning

Date of Violation: _____ Time: _____ Place: _____
Description of Violation:

_____

_____

_____

_____

_____

_____

_____ Verbal Warning   Action To Be Taken:
_____ Written Warning   _____
_____ Probation _____ Days   _____
_____ Suspension _____ Days   _____
_____ Termination   _____

_____   _____
Supervisor's Signature   Date

Employee's Remarks

Do you agree with the details above: Yes: _____   No: _____

Comments: _____

_____

_____

Employee's Signature: _____   Date: _____

FIGURE 12-5. Sample disciplinary action form.

Requests for time off should be put in writing. Depending on the size of the organization, such requests may have to be received by a given date or time. For example, the policy may read, "A request for a day off in May may have to be submitted by April 15. Any requests for time off filed after the cutoff date will be approved whenever possible." This eliminates repeated adjustment of the staffing schedule.

Checkpoint Question

3. What is the medical office manager's primary goal in scheduling?

Policy and Procedures Manuals

Every business needs written rules and regulations to ensure that its practices are within legal and ethical boundaries. Employees need written procedures to ensure consistency in the practices of the business. In the outpatient medical facility, these written policies and procedures are *required* by regulatory and accrediting agencies.

It is the office manager's responsibility to coordinate the orientation and training of any new employee. A personnel manual that includes the organization's policies and outlines step-by-step procedures for each task performed in the facility becomes the new employee's information source. Even veteran employees may have to refer to the proper procedure for a task. As new procedures become available or existing procedures are changed, this is added to the procedures manual.

Most organizations create *a policy and procedures manual* that is written, maintained, and regarded as one document. A **policy** is a statement regarding the organization's rules on a given topic. A **procedure** is a series of steps required to perform a given task. Policies and procedures must be written in a clear, concise, and understandable format. Each policy or procedure is signed by the employees, indicating they have read, understand, and will adhere to the policy or procedure. Policies regarding medical office management are signed by the physician and supervisory staff.

Tips for Writing Personnel Manuals

- Form a personnel committee. If staff members help develop the policies and procedures, they are more likely to follow them.
- Determine the rules and regulations of the office with the physician and managers.
- Contact local organizations, medical offices, or ambulatory care centers and ask for copies of their personnel manuals including policies and procedures.
- Research state and federal laws that regulate the medical office.
- Ensure compliance by appointing a **compliance officer**.

- Personnel manuals must be kept in a central location and be available to each employee for review.
- Review all policies and procedures annually to assess for currentness and accuracy.

Types of Policies and Procedures. There are many types of policies and procedures. In general, the following areas are included in a policy and procedures manual:

1. Mission statement
2. Organizational structure
3. Human resources, or personnel
4. Quality improvement and risk management
5. Clinical procedures
6. Administrative procedures
7. Infection control

Section 1: mission statement. A **mission statement** describes the goals of the practice and whom it serves. Often a mission statement provides a philosophical look at an organization. It is generally one to two paragraphs long (Fig. 12-6).

The mission statement should not only be included in the policy and procedures manual; it should also be available to patients. Often it is framed and placed in the waiting room or printed in the practice brochure.

Section 2: organizational structure. The organizational chart is included in this section along with policies regarding the following:

- Chain of command
- How and when to contact various members of the team
- Coverage for managers
- Physician on-call policies

Section 3: human resources, or personnel. This section consists of policies relating to staff responsibilities, benefits, and rules and regulations for employees. Box 12-1 lists the kinds of policies found in this section of the manual. A sample human resources policy is displayed in Figure 12-7.

Section 4: quality improvement and risk management. This section includes policies outlining who is in charge of quality improvement, the steps for developing a quality improvement plan, and explanations of incident reporting. (See Chapter 11.)

Section 5: clinical procedures. Any task that requires intervention with a patient should be listed in this section. (Some offices separate laboratory procedures into a different section for convenience.) In addition, clinical procedures should include specific infection control guidelines for the particular procedure, patient education guidelines, and instructions for documentation. Sample documentation forms should be included in this section. It is a good idea to complete the sample form correctly so that it can serve as a model. In the medical office, these procedures may vary slightly to meet the needs of the office, physicians' requests, or manufacturers' guidelines.

Section 6: administrative procedures. This section includes procedures on all tasks that the administrative office staff must

Procedure 12-1

Creating a Procedures Manual

Equipment/Supplies

- Word processor
- 3-ring binder
- Paper

Steps	Reason
1. Gather product information; consult government agencies, as needed. If the procedure is for using new equipment, ask the sales representative for educational pamphlets. Some companies offer printed sample procedures.	This ensures that you are using products and equipment according to the manufacturer's suggestions and that you are practicing within legal and ethical boundaries.
2. Title the procedure, e.g., Infection Control Procedure for Handwashing.	A logical, easily identifiable format will allow easy retrieval.
3. Number the procedure, e.g., "HR 14" means human resource section, policy 14.	All policies and procedures should be numbered to allow for easy access and identification.
4. Define the overall purpose of the policy. This should be a sentence or two at most explaining the intent of the procedure.	Provides the staff with a rationale for the policy.
5. List any necessary equipment or forms. Include everything needed to complete the task. Also indicate so if no special equipment or forms are necessary.	The employee will be prepared before beginning the procedure if he or she has everything needed at hand.
6. List each step with its rationale. The steps must be complete and in order. Never assume the reader knows how or when to perform a given step, such as handwashing. The employee will be able to follow specific steps, ensuring patient safety.	Listing the steps in order promotes compliance and accuracy for policy completion.
7. Provide spaces for signatures. Administrative procedures are signed by the physician and office manager. Clinical procedures usually are signed by the clinical manager and a physician. Employees must have a space to sign.	The employee's signature will verify that he or she has read and understands the policy.
8. Record the date the policy was written. If changes are needed, the procedure is rewritten, signed, and dated again. The previous dates also are generally listed.	By recording the date, you ensure that you are reading the most current revision. It will also help you know when a new revision should be considered.

perform. Sample forms should also be included and updated as necessary. Examples of administrative tasks follow:

- Accounting and bookkeeping
- Appointment scheduling
- Collections
- Computer care and operations

- Insurance filings
- Medical records management
- Mail and postal machines operations

Section 7: infection control. Depending on the length of this section, some offices opt for a separate manual dedicated to infection control and prevention. Examples of these policies are:

North Shore Family Practice is a group practice dedicated to providing quality care through compassion, innovation, performance and education. It is our goal to provide medical care to the community of Rochester, New York. The physicians, nurse practitioners, and all staff members are committed to working together as a team to provide the patient with the best care possible.

F I G U R E 1 2 – 6 . Sample mission statement.

- Types of personal protection equipment available
- Biohazardous waste disposal
- Handling of various disease identities
- Handling of employee exposures and needlesticks
- Documentation required by the Occupational Safety and Health Administration (OSHA)
- Employee education for infection control

Checkpoint Question

4. Which seven elements must be included when writing a policy or procedure?

Box 12-1

TYPES OF HUMAN RESOURCES POLICIES

Absentee policies	Jury duty
Cafeteria plans	Office hours
Confidentiality policy	Orientation
Continuing education requirements	Overtime reports
	Parking
Disciplinary action procedures	Payroll
	Personal phone calls
Emergency procedures	Resignations
Employee benefits (health and dental insurance)	Sexual harassment
	Sick leave and family leave
Evaluation and performance appraisals	Staff meetings
	Tardiness
Grievance procedures	Termination process
Grooming, uniforms, appearance	Time recording
	Vacation days
Holiday coverage and compensation for holidays	

Benjamin William, MD
2295 Matthews Drive
Boca Raton, Florida 33432
POLICY AND PROCEDURE MANUAL

Policy title: Human Resources, Call offs
Purpose: The purpose of this policy is to advise all employees of the policy for call offs and to prewarn employees regarding the disciplinary steps that will be taken as a result of not complying with this policy.
Equipment/Forms necessary: No equipment or forms are required.
Explanation:

- If you are going to call in sick, you must call in two hours prior to your assigned time. Messages should be left with the answering service if the office is not open.
- If you have personal days accrued, you can use them for compensation.
- If you are going to be out sick for more than three consecutive working days, you will need to obtain a physician's note to document the illness.
- Employees are allowed six (6) call offs per year without disciplinary action. Seven (7) call offs will result in a verbal warning regarding attendance. Eight (8) call offs will result in a written warning. Nine (9) call offs will result in termination. Exceptions to disciplinary action will be reviewed on an individual basis and are at the joint discretion of the office manager and physician.

Susan Rogers, RMA
Office Manager

Benjamin William, MD

date: original policy - 06/96, revised 07/98
HR: 14

F I G U R E 1 2 – 7 . Sample human resources policy.

Developing Promotional Materials

The medical office manager is often responsible for developing and distributing promotional literature for the practice. Depending on the budget, promotional materials can be created and produced at commercial printing shops or done in the office with desktop publishing programs. Examples of promotional materials follow:

- Education pamphlets and booklets for patients
- Practice brochure
- Newsletters
- Holiday cards
- Birthday cards (usually used by pediatricians)
- Newspaper articles
- Yellow pages
- Direct mail
- Business cards

Follow these guidelines when creating promotional materials:

- Double-check all spelling and grammar.
- Ensure accuracy.
- Use clear and specific language.
- Avoid abbreviations and complex medical terms.
- Use brightly colored materials.

If you are using a commercial printer, be sure to review the proofs carefully before the final printing.

Financial Concerns

Budgets

A **budget** is a financial planning tool that helps an organization estimate its anticipated expenditures and revenues. Budgeting has many purposes for an organization:

- Forcing the manager and physician to plan
- Causing managers and staff to become cost conscious
- Promoting communication among staff and managers
- Helping the organization achieve a financial goal

The medical office generally has both an operating and a capital budget. Operating budgets consist of all costs to run the office. These include but are not limited to payroll, office and medical supplies, education, promotional materials, and electricity and telephone services. Capital budgets consist of large outlays of money. These usually include large purchases (usually over $500), building maintenance, property management, and equipment.

Developing and writing a budget takes practice and instructions from the financial officer or physician. In general, the previous year's expense report is reviewed, revenues are projected for the following year, and figures are assigned to ensure that income balances with the outgoing expenses.

Checkpoint Question

5. What are the two basic types of budgets?

Payroll

Another financial concern for the manager is payroll. All employees expect to receive the correct amount of pay on time, and those expectations must be met. Payroll is a complex task that must satisfy state and federal laws regarding deductions for Social Security and other taxes. Because of this and because payroll is so time-consuming, some offices outsource this service (see Chapter 15).

Petty Cash

Most offices keep a small amount of cash in the office. Petty cash is used to purchase small items (e.g., postage, emergency office supplies) or to reimburse employees for small items. It is essential that the office manager keep close tallies on the petty cash fund. Most offices have some form of a petty cash receipt. Petty cash must be kept in a separate drawer from the change box (see Chapter 14).

Maintenance and Inventory of Supplies

One of the medical office manager's key responsibilities is to keep the office neat, clean, and well organized. Most offices have an outside cleaning agency to maintain the lobby, examination rooms, and offices. Special attention to waiting room toys is necessary because they can pose a safety threat to children (see Chapter 5). Staff should be encouraged to check the lobby periodically for neatness and to assist in routine cleaning and straightening.

Service Contracts

The medical office manager is responsible for keeping track of all service contracts. A **service contract** is an agreement between the medical organization and a service company in which the company agrees to perform regular inspections of and care for a specific piece of equipment. Service contracts are usually obtained for copiers, computers, fax machines, and other large and expensive pieces of equipment.

Inventory

Extensive amounts of supplies are needed to run a medical office. As a medical office manager, you must develop a logical system to keep track of them. There should be a policy outlining who is responsible for ordering supplies and the procedure for ordering. There also must be some process to check that deliveries of supplies are complete and accurate.

Education

Staff Education

The medical office manager must keep the staff up to date on medical procedures, drugs and vaccines, insurance coding and billing regulations, and any other topics that promote good patient care. In addition to these topics, annual education is usually conducted on cardiopulmonary resuscitation (CPR), infection control, and fire and electrical safety. Most allied health professionals are required to accumulate continuing education units (CEUs). CMAs must receive 60 CEUs every 5 years to retain the CMA credential. The office manager may choose to keep a file for each employee with the necessary documentation. This will assist the staff in the recertification process.

As the medical office manager, you should select an educational topic for each month. In some offices, the educational topic is covered during the monthly staff meetings, whereas other offices have separate educational programs. After choosing the monthly topic, select an appropriate presenter. Suggestions for presenters include colleagues, physicians, sales representatives, local hospital staff development coordinators, and specialists. Presenters for CPR classes must be CPR instructors who are approved by a national organization. To promote attendance, create informative flyers and distribute them to all staff members. Keep attendance records for all classes given.

In addition to formal educational programs, there are other ways to keep your staff up to date. For instance, educational videos can be rented or purchased for staff viewing; consider developing a posttest to assess for comprehension. Also, many professional magazines have continuing education articles on various topics, usually accompanied by a posttest. Finally, staff members should be sent to one or two seminars a year. Outside seminars help increase employee productivity, self-esteem, and retention.

Patient Education

All members of the health care team must constantly contribute to educating patients. As a manager, you may not provide patient education directly, but you are responsible for assisting the staff in performing this task. You can help the staff with patient education by creating booklets, developing posters, and by teaching your staff how, when, and what to teach patients and families.

Patient education brochures should be colorful and easy to read. Close attention to spelling, grammar, punctuation, and accuracy is essential. All brochures should be reviewed by a physician. Depending on your office's clientele, the brochures should be printed in various languages. Refer to Chapter 4 for more details on creating patient education brochures.

Manager Education

Managers should attend workshops and conferences and read appropriate printed materials to enhance their knowledge and skills in managing a medical office. All new managers can benefit from courses on time management, stress management, solving personnel conflicts, and budget preparation. Memberships in professional organizations can also assist the new office manager. Two such organizations are:

Medical Office Management Association
1355 South Colorado Boulevard, Suite 900
Denver, CO 80222-3331

Professional Association of Health Care—Office Managers
Suite 102
2929 Langley Avenue
Pensacola, FL 32504-7355

LEGAL ISSUES REGARDING OFFICE MANAGEMENT

Americans with Disabilities Act

Formerly called the Rehabilitation Act, the **Americans with Disabilities Act** (ADA) was expanded in 1994. All companies with more than 15 employees must comply with regulations designed to meet the needs of people with physical and mental disabilities. This act requires that all buildings be accessible to physically challenged people. Following is a partial list of ways the medical office can comply with this act:

- Entrance ramps
- Widened rest rooms and doors to be wheelchair accessible
- Elevated toilet bowls for easier transferring from wheelchairs
- Easy-to-reach elevator buttons
- Braille signs
- Access to special telephone services to communicate with hearing-impaired patients

Sexual Harassment

Sexual harassment of any employee or patient is illegal. Sexual harassment comes in many forms. As a medical office manager, it is your responsibility to be alert for signs of harassment and to have in place a policy for handling complaints regarding this.

Family and Medical Leave Act

The **Family and Medical Leave Act**, approved in 1993, allows an employee to leave his or her job for up to 12 weeks (unpaid) to meet family needs (e.g., the birth or adoption of a child; serious illness of a child, parent, spouse, or self). Employers must hold the employee's job position or offer the employee a position of similar nature on return.

LEGAL TIP

Many acts and regulations affect health care organizations and their operations. As a medical office manager, you must keep current on all legal updates. Most states publish a monthly bulletin that reports new legislation. Every state has a website that will link you to legislative action. Read these regularly. Each office should have legal counsel who can assist in interpreting legal issues. It is important for a new manager to meet with the medical office's attorney to discuss legal concerns for the practice.

Other Legal Considerations

The Clinical Laboratory Improvement Amendments (CLIA) of 1988 contain specific rules and regulations regarding laboratory safety.

OSHA is a federal agency that sets standards for employee safety. OSHA regulations are also discussed in Chapter 11.

The Joint Commission on Accreditation of Healthcare Organizations (JCAHO) is a private organization that sets standards for health care administration. The JCAHO is discussed in Chapter 11.

Each state also has specific laws regarding patient care, insurance billing, payroll management, and so forth that a medical office manager must understand.

Checkpoint Question

6. What are some legal issues of concern to the medical office manager?

CHAPTER SUMMARY

Effective management of the medical office is essential for a health care organization to succeed in the competitive marketplace. A good manager must be able to perform a variety of tasks in an organized and efficient manner. These tasks include communicating with patients and staff, handling staffing issues, developing policy and procedures manuals, creating promotional materials, preparing budgets, and overseeing educational programs. In addition, the medical office manager must keep current on legal requirements related to office operations.

Critical Thinking Challenges

1. Review the list of qualities that a manager should have. Which ones do you have? How would you acquire the others? Should any other qualities be listed?
2. Review the types of sections that are often included in policy and procedures manuals. Now assume that you are to help a physician set up a practice. How would you organize your policy and procedures manual? Create one sample sheet for each section of your manual. Be sure to include all necessary elements when you write your policies and procedures.
3. Write a description of your ideal job. How would you go about finding this position?

Answers to Checkpoint Questions

1. An organizational chart is a flow sheet that allows the manager and employees to identify their team members and to see where they fit into the team.
2. Three ways to communicate with staff members are through bulletin boards, staff meetings, and communication notebooks.
3. The primary goal of scheduling is to ensure that the needs of the office are met.
4. The elements that must be in a policy or procedure are document name, purpose, equipment or forms needed, steps or explanations, signatures, numbering system, and dates.
5. The two basic types of budgets are operating and capital.
6. Some of the legal issues are the Americans with Disabilities Act, sexual harassment laws, Family and Medical Leave Act, CLIA, and OSHA.

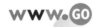 **Websites**

Medical Group Management Association
    www.mgma.org
Physician Practice Group
    www.physicianspractice.com
Family Leave Act/Department of Labor
    www.dol.gov
Americans with Disabilities Act/U. S. Department of Justice
    www.ada.gov
    www.usaoj.gov

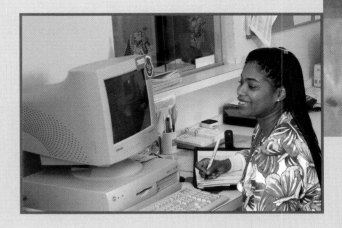

Managing the Finances in the Practice

Good management of finances is essential for a medical practice to succeed. This unit introduces you to various aspects of medical office finances, beginning with a chapter on credit and collections, in which you learn the process of collecting fees. Next, you will learn bookkeeping and banking skills to register the fees that you have collected. Medical offices must also pay various people, and this information is covered in the following chapter. Most of the income for the physician's practice is through insurance reimbursements. To be able to collect fees from insurance companies, you must understand coding. This information is covered in the last three chapters. A financially strong practice is good for the patients, the community, and you.

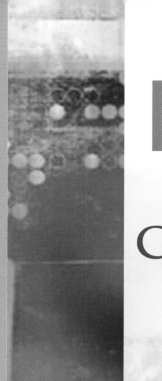

13

Credit and Collections

CHAPTER OUTLINE

FEES
    Fee Schedules
    Discussing Fees in Advance
    Forms of Payment
    Payment by Insurance Companies
    Adjusting Fees

CREDIT
    Extending Credit
    Legal Considerations

COLLECTIONS
    Legal Considerations
    Collecting a Debt
    Collection Alternatives

ROLE DELINEATION COMPONENTS

GENERAL: Legal Concepts
- Perform within legal and ethical boundaries

ADMINISTRATIVE: Administrative Procedures
- Perform basic administrative medical assisting functions

ADMINISTRATIVE: Practice Finances
- Apply bookkeeping principles
- Manage accounts receivable
- Manage accounts payable
- Document and maintain accounting and banking record

CHAPTER COMPETENCIES

LEARNING OBJECTIVES
Upon successfully completing this chapter, you will be able to:
1. Spell and define the key terms
2. Explain the physician fee schedule
3. Discuss forms of payment
4. Explain the legal considerations in extending credit
5. Discuss the legal implications of credit collection
6. Describe three methods of debt collection

PERFORMANCE OBJECTIVES
Upon successfully completing this chapter, you will be able to:
1. Use an aging schedule
2. Write a collection letter

KEY TERMS

adjustment	credit	participating providers	professional courtesy
aging schedule	installment	patient co-payment	write-off
collections			

THE MEDICAL PRACTICE MUST operate in a financially sound manner to continue to serve the patient's needs. The office depends on the fees generated by patient visits, laboratory work, and in-office procedures. Without these fees, the medical office would be unable to pay for staff, office space, and supplies. Therefore, collecting fees, whether paid by the patient, an insurer, or a third party, is essential for the medical practice to succeed. Box 13-1 shows how to determine whether your office is collecting fees satisfactorily.

FEES

Fee Schedules

Generally, the physician sets the fees for office visits, laboratory work, and in-office procedures based on the UCR concept: (1) U (usual) fair value of the service; (2) C (customary) competitive rates charged by other physicians; and (3) R (reasonable), that which meets the other two criteria. Fee setting also considers the resource-based relative value scale (RBRVS), by which fees are based on the relative value of a particular service and adjusted for geographical differences. (See Chapter 16 for more information about UCR fees and Chapter 18 for more information about RBRVS.) A physician's fee schedule also takes into consideration the costs of operating the office, such as rent, utilities, malpractice insurance, salaries, and so on. A list of the services and procedures

Code	Key	Mod	Par Fee	Non Par Fee	Limiting Charge
50010			$690.30	$655.79	$754.16
50010			$690.30	$655.79	$754.16
50020			$1,112.72	$1,057.08	$1,215.64
50021			$522.30	$496.19	$570.62
50040			$1,009.84	$959.35	$1,103.25
50045			$921.52	$875.44	$1,006.76
50060			$1,116.74	$1,060.90	$1,220.04
50065			$1,128.28	$1,071.87	$1,232.65
50070			$1,172.52	$1,113.89	$1,280.97
50075			$1,451.88	$1,379.29	$1,586.18
50080			$976.28	$927.47	$1,066.59
50081			$1,336.92	$1,270.07	$1,460.58
50100			$1,033.66	$981.98	$1,129.28
50120			$945.54	$898.26	$1,033.00
50125			$980.30	$931.29	$1,070.98
50130			$1,010.09	$959.59	$1,103.53
50135			$1,110.42	$1,054.90	$1,213.14
50200			$138.72	$131.78	$151.55
50205			$696.55	$661.72	$760.98
50220			$1,015.02	$964.27	$1,108.91
50225			$1,168.36	$1,109.94	$1,276.43

FIGURE 13-1. Sample Medicare fee schedule.

offered in an office along with descriptions, procedure codes, and prices must be available to patients. Federal regulations require that a sign to this effect be posted in the office.

There may be several fee schedules based on the reimbursement schedules of different insurance companies. **Participating providers** are those who agree to participate with managed care contracts and other third-party payers in exchange for building a solid patient base. Patients covered under participating plans will have a different fee schedule from patients who are private pay (paying with no money from insurance). Each managed care plan, workers' compensation company, Medicaid carrier, and Medicare has a different fee schedule. See Chapter 16 for further discussion of third-party payers.

A Medicare fee schedule has three columns. A participating fee is the amount paid to physicians who participate or agree to accept a certain fee. A nonparticipating fee is the amount paid to physicians who do not have agreements with Medicare. A limiting charge is the amount a physician can charge a Medicare patient. Figure 13-1 is a sample Medicare fee schedule.

Discussing Fees in Advance

It is always a good policy to discuss fees with patients in advance. This ensures that patients are aware of the charges. Patients will need to know in advance whether the medical office is a participating provider with their insurance carrier. Managed care companies usually require that the patient pay

---

Box 13-1

DETERMINING A PRACTICE'S COLLECTION PERCENTAGE

Medical practices should evaluate their method of collections periodically to determine the effectiveness of their practices. A collection analysis lets you identify the strengths and weaknesses of the system.

To do a collection analysis, determine the monthly production from the first day of each month to the last day. This will be the total charges posted to all patients' accounts. Next determine the revenues the practice received. Computer systems will automatically total payments received during a specified time. Divide revenue by production to determine the collection percentage. Analysis of the collection percentage should reveal the percentage of the collection of all outstanding debts to the practice.

Collection percentage =
monthly production ÷ monthly revenue received

Most medical practices average 8 to 20% loss yearly. Experts consider a collection percentage above 80% to be reasonable. Performing a 2-year collection percentage comparison analysis will help you evaluate past collection effectiveness.

a certain share of the bill, known as the **patient co-payment,** or co-pay. A good and easy way to initiate a discussion of fees is by providing an office brochure that lists not only the office's address, telephone number, and hours but also office policies regarding fees and collections, third-party payments, and how they are handled. Patients should understand that co-pays are to be paid at the time of service. Such information should be included in the office brochure. Many offices post a sign in the waiting area stating this.

Always collect the entire amount due from a new patient on the first visit. Most problems associated with collection (acquiring funds that are due) come from patients who go from one practice to another. Be sure you get a picture identification, such as a driver's license, on a patient's first visit.

Forms of Payment

Depending on the medical office's policies, the patient can usually pay for services in one of two ways: with cash or by personal check. If a new patient is paying by check, get two forms of identification. Many larger practices accept credit and debit cards (Visa, MasterCard, Discover) also. By agreeing to accept a credit card payment, the medical office also agrees to pay the credit card company a percentage (usually 1.8%) of the total charge. Although this may seem costly, it is sometimes more cost effective to receive payment by credit card than to receive it in installments—or not at all—from the patient.

Payment by Insurance Companies

By far the largest proportions of fees are paid by insurance companies. Therefore, it is imperative that patients' insurance information be kept current. Most medical practices require that a patient submit a medical insurance card for each visit; this way, changes in insurance can quickly and easily be noted. Always make a copy of both sides of the patient's insurance card and staple it to the appropriate section of the chart for billing reference.

Adjusting Fees

Sometimes, **adjustments** (changes in a posted account) must be made to a standard fee, as when the medical office accepts a set insurance rate for a service that is lower than the practice's rate. You must charge the patient the normal fee for the service; when the insurance carrier sends payment, however, the explanation of benefits (EOB) will show how much you may collect for the service. The difference between the physician's normal fee and the insurance carrier's allowed fee will be adjusted in the credit adjustment column on the patient's account.

Other fee adjustments include **professional courtesy** fees, in which other health care professionals are charged a reduced rate. The physician may choose not to charge a fee at all; this too is considered a professional courtesy and should not be confused with writing off a fee. (A **write-off** is cancellation of

an unpaid debt; these generally can be claimed on the practice's federal taxes.) Again, you charge the normal fee and then adjust the designated amount in the adjustment column with "professional courtesy" in the description column.

Checkpoint Question

1. To avoid collection problems, what should you get from a new patient on the first visit?

CREDIT

Extending Credit

It is not always possible for patients to pay the entire bill when such costs are incurred. Depending on the medical office's policy, **credit** may be extended to patients on an installment plan. Collection experts have estimated that billing one patient costs the practice about $8 per month. This total includes the time it takes to prepare the statements, the supplies needed, and so on. Extension of credit to a patient is a decision that is often made solely by the physician.

Legal Considerations

When a medical practice extends credit to a patient, it may charge interest on the patient's unpaid balance. If this is the case, the medical office is legally required to disclose this information to the patient, along with any other fees or charges incurred by the patient's acceptance of credit. This legal documentation, called a truth-in-lending statement, must be filed in the patient's medical chart.

Different states have different laws concerning the extension of credit. Generally, credit cannot be denied based on age, gender, race, marital status, religion, national origin, or source of income (e.g., if a patient receives public assistance). If your facility has given credit to one patient, you typically may not refuse the same arrangement to another patient. Some states have laws limiting the amount of interest that can be charged. The practice's accountant should be able to provide the information required by the state and municipality.

Checkpoint Question

2. On what grounds should credit *not* be denied?

COLLECTIONS

When a patient has an unpaid bill or has not paid an installment per a credit agreement, those funds must be collected. Collecting an unpaid debt is costly to any business. Collecting fees can also be time consuming, and collecting practices are regulated by a variety of consumer protection laws. Many medical practices outsource their billing to companies specializing in billing and debt collection.

Box 13-2

RULES FOR TELEPHONE DEBT COLLECTION

When attempting to collect a debt by telephone, a debt collector may not:

1. Contact the patient at his or her place of employment if the employer objects
2. Tell anyone other than the patient or responsible party about a debt without court authorization
3. Contact the patient before 8:00 A.M. or after 9:00 P.M.
4. Contact the patient at all if the patient has filed for bankruptcy
5. Harass or intimidate the patient; that is, use abusive language, provide false or misleading information, or pose as someone other than a debt collector

Box 13-3

COLLECTING DEBTS FROM A PATIENT'S ESTATE

When a patient dies, the family needs time to grieve and accept the death. Collecting debts from an estate requires professionalism and tact. Never contact the family regarding a debt immediately after a patient's death. Most offices have a policy stating that family members of deceased patients will not be contacted until a week after the funeral. At the appropriate time, call the next of kin listed in the patient's chart. Offer your sympathy and ask for the name of the patient's executor, the individual responsible for handling the patient's affairs after death. The executor may be an attorney, spouse, friend, or other relative. Call the executor and introduce yourself. Obtain the executor's address and send a final bill. It is important that all claims on a patient's estate be made promptly. In case the estate does not have enough funds to meet all of its debts, the probate court will decide the priority list for debt collection.

Legal Considerations

Certain procedures should be followed in attempts to collect a debt. A debt collector—in this case, the administrative medical assistant or billing clerk—must exercise reasonable restraint when contacting a patient about a bill. Box 13-2 displays guidelines for collection attempts by phone.

Attempting to collect a debt from a patient's estate requires particular diplomacy. Box 13-3 offers some guidelines to follow in such a situation.

Collecting a Debt

Monthly Billings

The easiest way to collect a debt or an installment is by monthly billing. Once a month, the medical office sends bills to its patients who have unpaid balances. Larger offices set up a billing cycle and divide the alphabet, sending statements once a week to each selected group. For example, patients with names beginning with the letters A to G might be billed

on the 1st of the month, H to N on the 8th, O to S on the 15th, and T to Z on the 22nd. If your facility changes a billing cycle, you are legally required to notify patients of the change 3 months before the change takes effect.

The uncomputerized office normally just copies the ledger cards of the patients who owe balances. It is important to make each entry on the ledger card with consistency and provide a key for office codes or abbreviations. The patient should be able to understand each entry. When a practice is computerized, the staff can easily send statements. Medical office software usually gives the option of printing a separate message at the bottom. For instance, you may add "Happy Holidays" to every patient's December statement or "Time for your flu shot" in the September statements.

If the account is on an **installment** plan, the patient receives a bill that lists the amount due for that month, any third-party payments or adjustments applied to the account, the total amount due, and the amount the patient owes. This

ñ Spanish Terminology

Necesito recoger el total en su cuenta.	I need to collect the balance on your account.
¿Puede pagar usted algunos de su deuda?	Can you pay some of your balance?
Esto es una carta de la colección.	This is a collection letter.
Usted debe este dinero a esta oficina.	You owe this office money.

way, the patient has the option of paying more than is due for that particular month (and thereby reducing the amount of any interest charged) and is aware of the current balance.

Aging Accounts

Unpaid accounts must be monitored to determine how far overdue or in arrears they are. Aging of an account is calculated from the first date of billing, not by the procedure date. For example, a patient has an office visit on January 5 and the first statement is sent on February 1. The account will not be past due until March 1.

For this purpose, the medical office keeps an **aging schedule** that lists the patient's name, balance, any payments, and comments, such as reminders or second notices sent. Such a schedule can be kept on a large sheet of paper or by a comprehensive computer billing program. Figure 13-2 is a sample of a manual report. Figure 13-3 shows a computer screen that automatically places the amounts charged under the proper heading based on the age of the account. This account shows that $132 of the charges are current, or less than 30 days old. The $95 represents charges that were incurred and posted at least 120 days ago.

Aging of accounts is a measure of the practice's ability to collect its fees. Nearly all fees (80%) should be collected within 30 days. If the aging shows a high percentage (50%) of fees being collected 30 days or more after billing, the practice's billing and collection procedures should be reviewed.

Collecting Overdue Accounts

The three most common ways of collecting an overdue account are sending an overdue notice to the patient, telephoning the patient to let him or her know the account is overdue, and informing the patient at the next office visit.

Overdue Notices. With a manual system, overdue notices are fairly simple to prepare. Often, they consist of a copy of the patient's monthly billing with the words "overdue" or "second notice" stamped in red. Alternatively, a form letter with spaces for the patient's particulars may be sent. Figure 13-4 is a sample collection letter. If a computer billing program is used, the computer often can automatically generate overdue notices.

Telephoning the Patient. If written notices bring no response, you may have to telephone the patient to inquire about an overdue account. Always ask when payment may be forthcoming and document the reply on the patient's account. If payment is not received as promised, contact the patient again.

Aging of Accounts Receivable Report: April 30, 2003			
Patient Name	**Account Number**	**Due Date**	**Amount**
Accounts 30 Days Past Due:			
Doe, John C.	000-00-0000	3/6/03	625.00
Graham, Paula R.	000-00-0000	3/29/03	450.00
O'Toole, William Q.	000-00-0000	3/13/03	25.00
Parker, Mary W.	000-00-0000	3/25/03	299.00
Reeves, Chris A.	000-00-0000	3/11/03	58.00
South, Cheryl C.	000-00-0000	3/8/03	385.00
Yarkony, Ralph M.	000-00-0000	3/11/03	108.00
Accounts 60 Days Past Due:			
Forest, Patricia L.	000-00-0000	2/19/03	476.00
Heany, Beverly O.	000-00-0000	2/13/03	57.00
Thomas, Walter T.	000-00-0000	2/27/03	185.00
Accounts 90 Days Past Due:			
Glick, Rhonda K	000-00-0000	1/4/03	28.00
Payne, Robert A.	000-00-0000	1/25/03	456.00
Accounts 120 Days or More Past Due:			
Baird, Jane C.	000-00-0000	10/3/02	45.00
Wallace, Michael S.	000-00-0000	12/15/02	349.00
Total Overdue Accounts Receivable			**$3,546.00**

FIGURE 13–2. Sample aging of accounts receivable report.

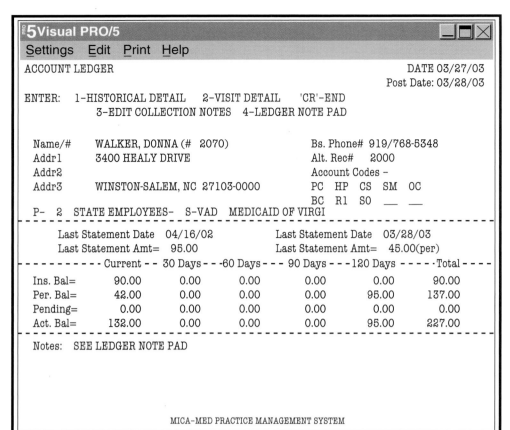

```
┌────────────────────────────────────────────────────────────────────┐
│ ⁵⁵Visual PRO/5                                          _ □ ✕        │
├────────────────────────────────────────────────────────────────────┤
│ Settings  Edit  Print  Help                                         │
│ ACCOUNT LEDGER                              DATE 03/27/03            │
│                                             Post Date: 03/28/03      │
│                                                                      │
│ ENTER:  1-HISTORICAL DETAIL    2-VISIT DETAIL    'CR'-END            │
│         3-EDIT COLLECTION NOTES   4-LEDGER NOTE PAD                  │
│                                                                      │
│   Name/#    WALKER, DONNA (#  2070)      Bs. Phone# 919/768-5348     │
│   Addr1     3400 HEALY DRIVE             Alt. Rec#   2000            │
│   Addr2                                  Account Codes –             │
│   Addr3     WINSTON-SALEM, NC 27103-0000  PC  HP  CS  SM  OC         │
│                                           BC  R1  SO  __  __         │
│   P-  2  STATE EMPLOYEES-  S-VAD  MEDICAID OF VIRGI                  │
│ - - - - - - - - - - - - - - - - - - - - - - - - - - - - - - - - - - │
│     Last Statement Date  04/16/02    Last Statement Date  03/28/03   │
│     Last Statement Amt=  95.00       Last Statement Amt=  45.00(per) │
│ - - - - - - - Current - - 30 Days - - 60 Days - - 90 Days - - 120 Days - - - Total - - - │
│   Ins. Bal=   90.00      0.00     0.00      0.00      0.00     90.00 │
│   Per. Bal=   42.00      0.00     0.00      0.00     95.00    137.00 │
│   Pending=     0.00      0.00     0.00      0.00      0.00      0.00 │
│   Act. Bal=  132.00      0.00     0.00      0.00     95.00    227.00 │
│ - - - - - - - - - - - - - - - - - - - - - - - - - - - - - - - - - - │
│ Notes:  SEE LEDGER NOTE PAD                                         │
│                                                                      │
│                                                                      │
│                                                                      │
│              MICA-MED PRACTICE MANAGEMENT SYSTEM                     │
└────────────────────────────────────────────────────────────────────┘
```

F I G U R E 1 3 – 3 .
Sample computer screen.

Family Practice Associates
2345 Oak Street
Forest, OR 77777
(234) 567-8900

June 23, 2003

Mary W. Parker
300 Red Bird Lane
Lake, OR 77771

Dear Ms. Parker:

It has recently come to our attention that your account with our office is slightly overdue. Your balance of $299.00 is over 30 days past due. Please pay this amount as soon as possible. If you are having trouble paying this amount, please call our office and make arrangements to pay your balance.

If you have recently paid this amount and your payment is on the way to us in the mail, please disregard this letter. If you have any questions or concerns, feel free to contact me at the phone number above.

Sincerely,

Kathy Porter
Accounting Manager

F I G U R E 1 3 – 4 .
Sample collection letter.

WHAT IF

A patient who has an overdue account wants to schedule an appointment. What should you do?

As a medical assistant, you are not responsible for deciding whether a patient who has an outstanding balance gets to be seen by the physician. Schedule the appointment, then discuss the issue privately with the physician. Ethically, the physician may opt to care for the patient until the disorder is resolved. Legally, the physician is obligated to care for this patient until the physician–patient relationship is terminated (see Chapter 2).

In-Office Reminders. A patient can be reminded of an overdue balance when he or she comes to the office to see the physician. To handle this situation discreetly, simply give the patient a copy of the most recent overdue notice. Once again, ask when payment may be forthcoming and follow through. Computer systems may offer the option of a flashing computer screen when the patient's overdue account is retrieved. This alerts anyone working with the patient either to discuss payment or to refer the patient to someone in the office who will explain that payment is expected.

Collection Alternatives

Sometimes, it is more cost effective for **collections** to be handled outside the medical office. Three common options include collection agencies, small claims court, and credit bureaus. Collection agencies specialize in collecting debts. For either a fee or a percentage of the debt, the collection agency attempts to collect the monies due by the methods listed earlier. In addition, the collection agency can represent the medical practice in small claims court and can have the bad debt listed with credit-reporting agencies.

LEGAL TIP

The Fair Debt Collection Act

The Fair Debt Collection Act is a federal law that states how and when a collector can attempt to collect a debt. It is a violation of the law to threaten to send a patient to a collection agency if you do not intend to do so. Unlawful threats can result in a lawsuit for harassment against the caller. Box 13-2 shows the guidelines for telephoning patients to attempt to collect a debt.

The medical practice can, of course, sue patients in small claims court or list patients with credit bureaus itself, but it is often more time and cost effective to hire an outside agency.

Checkpoint Question

3. What are three ways of collecting overdue accounts?

CHAPTER SUMMARY

The financial status of a medical office is based on the ability of the staff to collect the physician's fees. This must be done in a professional manner and in accordance with state and federal laws. Technology affords the medical office the ability to streamline procedures, and collection practices are more efficient with computer systems. Aging accounts and communicating with patients in a fair and professional manner ensures a constant cash flow and success in managing the finances of the outpatient medical practice.

Critical Thinking Challenges

1. Under what circumstances might a patient need credit? To what local resources could you refer this patient?
2. A patient has an overdue account balance. What steps would you take to collect the debt?
3. Create a collection letter for a patient account that is 60 days' overdue. Create a collection letter that you would send to a patient's executor or patient's estate.

Answers to Checkpoint Questions

1. On a new patient's first visit, collect the entire amount due and get a picture identification.
2. Credit cannot be denied based on age, gender, race, marital status, religion, national origin, or source of income.
3. Overdue accounts can be collected by sending overdue notices, telephoning patients, and informing patients at the next office visit.

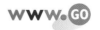 **Websites**

Credit and Collections World
www.collectionsworld.com

Fair Debt Collection Practice/Federal Trade Commission Statutes
www.ftc.gov

National Credit Systems
www.nationalcredit.com

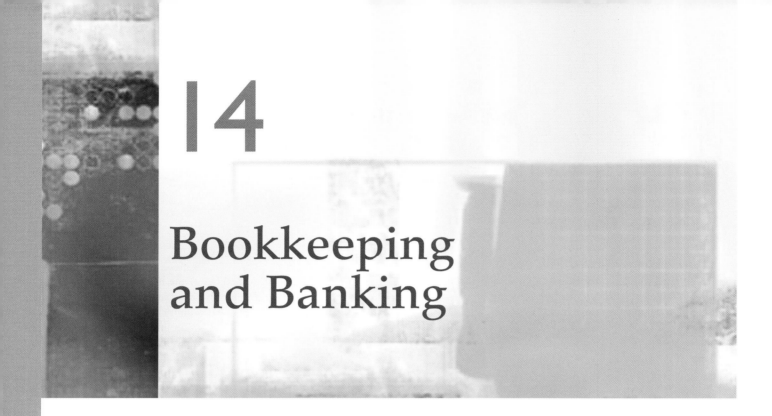

14

Bookkeeping and Banking

CHAPTER OUTLINE

DAILY BOOKKEEPING

MANUAL ACCOUNTING
Pegboard Bookkeeping System
Posting a Charge
Posting a Payment
Posting a Credit
Posting a Credit Adjustment
Posting a Debit Adjustment
Posting to Cash-Paid-Out Section
of Day Sheet

COMPUTER ACCOUNTING
Posting to Computer Accounts
Computer Accounting Reports

BANKING
Banks and Their Services
Bank Fees
Types of Checks
Writing Checks for Accounts
Payable

Receiving Checks and Making
Deposits
Reconciling Bank Statements

PETTY CASH

ROLE DELINEATION COMPONENTS

GENERAL: Legal Concepts
- Perform within legal and ethical boundaries

ADMINISTRATIVE: Administrative Procedures
- Perform basic administrative medical assisting functions

ADMINISTRATIVE: Practice Finances
- Apply bookkeeping principles
- Manage accounts receivable
- Manage accounts payable
- Document and maintain accounting and banking records

CHAPTER COMPETENCIES

LEARNING OBJECTIVES
Upon successfully completing this chapter, you will be able to:
1. Spell and define the key terms
2. Explain the concept of the pegboard bookkeeping system
3. Describe the components of the pegboard system
4. Identify and discuss the special features of the pegboard day sheet
5. Describe the functions of a computer accounting system
6. List the uses and components of computer accounting reports
7. Explain the services and procedures of the bank

PERFORMANCE OBJECTIVES
Upon successfully completing this chapter, you will be able to:
1. Record financial transactions, such as charges, payments, credits, and adjustments to patient ledger cards
2. Balance a day sheet
3. Complete a bank deposit slip and make a deposit
4. Reconcile a bank statement
5. Write a check
6. Maintain a petty cash account

KEY TERMS

accounts payable	bookkeeping	debit	posting
accounts receivable	charge slip	encounter form	returned check fee
adjustment	credit	ledger card	service charge
balance	day sheet		

BOOKKEEPING AND BANKING are important facets of medical office management. In most medical practices, bookkeeping and banking involve maintaining both patient and office account records, including petty cash, **accounts receivable** (money owed to the practice), and **accounts payable** (money owed by the practice). Most medical practices use computer accounting systems, although some smaller practices and satellite offices still use manual systems. In large outpatient medical conglomerates with many sites, a central billing office may handle bookkeeping and billing. Some practices outsource their billing and related accounting functions. Although daily bookkeeping practices are handled in the office, the office also employs an accountant who receives reports of the daily financial functions.

DAILY BOOKKEEPING

Bookkeeping is defined as an organized and accurate record-keeping system of financial transactions for a business. The daily financial transactions of a medical office include patient payments that arrive through the mail, patient payments from patients seen in the office, and patient charges that are added to the accounts receivable. Most medical practices use the single-entry bookkeeping system.

The foundation of accounting is this equation:

$$\text{Assets} = \text{liabilities} + \text{equity}$$

Assets are all things of value owned by or relating to the practice. Liabilities are monies owed. Equity refers to the amount of capital the physician has invested in the practice. Because the two sides of the accounting equation must always **balance** (be equal), each transaction requires a **debit** (charge) on one side of the equation and a **credit** (payment) on the other side of the equation; the amount of the debit and credit must be equal. Double-entry systems are usually used by accounting firms and corporations.

Most medical facilities use the *cash basis* type of accounting, which means that income is considered as income only when money is collected and that payables (money owed) are considered expenses only when money is paid.

The most popular formats for daily bookkeeping are the manual pegboard system and computer systems.

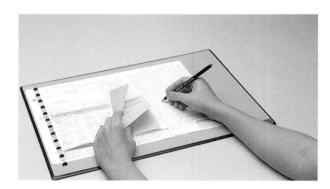

FIGURE 14–1. Sample day sheet with ledger card and charge slip. (Courtesy of Control-o-fax, Waterloo, IA.)

MANUAL ACCOUNTING
Pegboard Bookkeeping System

The pegboard, or write-it-once, bookkeeping system uses a board with pegs running down the left side. The pegs hold a **day sheet**, or daily journal, in place on the board. All transactions for the day are recorded on this day sheet. Each patient has a ledger card (record of the patient's financial activities). When a patient transaction occurs, the bookkeeper places the ledger card over the day sheet and the **charge slip** (preprinted patient bill) over the ledger card on the next available entry line and makes the appropriate entry on the ledger card. Figure 14-1 is a sample day sheet.

Day sheets come with a sheet of carbon paper; thus, the entry recorded on the ledger card, even when a charge slip is not used, is also recorded on the day sheet. When a payment received in the mail is posted, for example, no charge slip is needed. As the day progresses, each patient's ledger card is placed on the next available line on the day sheet, so that the day's entries appear consecutively. At the end of the day, all of the transactions are added.

The various components used in a pegboard system and the specific steps for recording patient transactions are discussed in greater detail next.

Day Sheet

The day sheet keeps track of daily patient transactions, such as charges for services to patients, payments received from pa-

ñ *Spanish Terminology*

Esto es su total.	This is your balance.
Esto es su crédito.	This is your credit.
No pague esta cuenta.	Do not pay this bill.
Su cheque se volvió para fondos de insuficiente.	Your check was returned for insufficient funds.
Su cuenta ha sido mandada a una agencia de la colección.	Your account has been sent to a collection agency.

tients and insurance carriers, and adjustments to patient accounts. A day sheet should be kept for each day that the physician sees patients; on busy days or for practices with more than one physician, more than one day sheet may be required.

The day sheet has several sections: a deposit slip, distribution columns, a section for payments, a section for adjustments, and a section for **posting** proofs (listing financial transactions in a ledger).

The deposit slip is a detachable portion of the day sheet. All payments received are noted on the deposit slip, and at the end of the day it is separated from the day sheet and deposited with that day's payments.

The distribution columns are used to assign charges for various services. How these columns are used depends on the needs of the individual practice. In a group practice, each practitioner has his or her own column. Some practices may assign columns to the various insurance plans they accept. Finally, these columns can be used to provide information on quality improvement issues. The distribution columns, re-

gardless of how they are assigned, provide the physician with important information about how the practice earns its income.

An **adjustment** is an entry to change an account. The adjustments section allows for reductions in office fees, as with professional courtesy discounts and insurance disallowances. The adjustments section also allows for crediting an account for uncollectible monies without using the payment column. It can also be used to return charges to an account if the patient's payment has been returned by the bank for insufficient funds.

The posting proofs section is where the day's totals are entered and the day sheet is balanced, much as one would balance a checkbook. Once the day sheet is complete, each column or section is totaled individually. It is best to total each column twice to make sure that no errors have been made. After all the columns have been totaled, the posting proofs section is filled out.

If the posting proofs do not balance, an error has been

Procedure 14-1

Balancing the Day Sheet

Equipment/Supplies

- Calculator
- Current day sheet with yesterday's previous balance total
- Carbon
- All ledger cards with transactions on the day sheet
- Pencil
- Pen

Steps	Reason
1. Determine if all entries are complete.	If all charge slips listed on the day sheet are not returned to you, the day sheet will not balance. Make sure you have finished the transaction on each account.
2. Add each column with a calculator and place the total in pencil in the appropriate column.	Day sheets include a portion for performing a daily proof (verifying the accuracy of the entries). Using pencil will enable changes if needed.
3. Add the totals from today to the totals from the previous day sheet.	A running total is kept by placing the ending figure for each day under the column for the beginning figure on the next day's sheet. This gives you a total accounts receivable amount at any time.
4. To verify the accuracy of the entries: • Add the total of the previous balance column to the total of the current balance column • From this total, subtract the totals of the payment and adjustment columns • This amount equals the current balance	This allows for double verification of current totals.
5. When the totals are verified, go back over them in pen.	Day sheets are legal documents that are retained. They must be written in ink.

Box 14-1

BASIC BOOKKEEPING TIPS

- Always use black ink; do not use pencil.
- Write legibly.
- *Never* erase or white-out errors. Draw a single line through the incorrect entry, record the correct information, and initial the change.
- Always double-check each entry.

made on the day sheet. To locate the error, go over each transaction one by one. Add the previous balance to the fee or subtract the payment from the previous balance to check whether the new balance listed is correct. If the posted charges are correct, total each column again. Do not erase or white-out errors, but draw a line through the erroneous entry and enter the transaction on a new line. When you reenter a transaction on the day sheet, use the ledger card again. Box 14-1 outlines some basic bookkeeping tips.

The day sheet is important because it keeps track of accounts receivable. The accounts receivable total changes every time a charge, payment, or adjustment is made to an account. You should perform a trial balance at the end of each month. Add the totals of each ledger card with an outstanding balance. The total should match the running total kept on the day sheet. This practice ensures the accuracy of your financial records.

Completed day sheets are filed chronologically in a ledger (a book of accounts) with the most recent day sheet on top. Completed day sheets are important legal documents and must be kept for at least 7 years for tax purposes. They should be stored in a safe, dark area to avoid loss or fading.

Checkpoint Question

1. What are five sections of a pegboard day sheet?

WHAT IF

You cannot balance the day sheet.
What do you do?

First, take a short break. Then return to the day sheet and double-check each entry and your arithmetic (a common error is transposing numbers, such as entering 69 instead of 96). If you are still unable to find the error, ask a colleague to check the day sheet. After all attempts to balance the sheet have been exhausted, notify the physician or office manager.

Ledger Cards

The **ledger card** is a financial record for each patient. Most ledger cards include areas for the responsible person's name, address, telephone number, and insurance information. Fig. 14-2 is a sample ledger card. Other information, such as employment information and primary and secondary insurance information, may appear on the ledger card. Patient information appears on the top of the ledger card; the bottom portion is used to record the patient's financial activities.

Many practices use photocopies of an individual's ledger card as a bill, mailing the photocopy to the patient each time payment is required. If you use a copy of the ledger card for billing, make sure that no information other than the billing name and address is visible through the window of the envelope. Allowing other information to be visible is a breach of privacy.

The ledger card is a legal document and should be kept for the same length of time as the patient's medical record. Ledger cards are filed alphabetically in a ledger tray. A medical practice may require more than one ledger tray. Ledger cards with outstanding balances are kept separate from paid ledger cards; this makes it easier to photocopy the monthly bills or find a ledger card when a patient calls about an outstanding bill. If the office uses only one ledger tray, the ledger cards with outstanding balances are filed alphabetically in the front of the ledger tray, with the paid ledger cards filed alphabetically in the back.

Encounter Forms and Charge Slips

The **encounter form** and the charge slip are preprinted patient statements that list codes for basic office charges and have sections for the patient's current balance and next ap-

DATE	REFERENCE	DESCRIPTION	CHARGES	CREDITS PYMNTS.	ADJ.	BALANCE
		BALANCE FORWARD →				

FORM MR 10   PLEASE PAY LAST AMOUNT IN BALANCE COLUMN ⬎

FIGURE 14-2. Sample ledger card.

pointment. Most encounter forms and charge slips have three-part copies:

1. The first copy is kept by the facility for auditing purposes (all are numbered).
2. The second copy is given to the patient for insurance filing (if the patient files the insurance claims).
3. The third copy, which has a carbon line at the top to match your ledgers and day sheets, is given to the patient as a receipt of services.

Charge slips are smaller versions of an encounter form and are designed to be used in conjunction with ledger cards. They often have different-colored no-carbon-required (NCR) copies. Figure 14-3 shows a computer-generated encounter form and a charge slip used in a manual system.

Checkpoint Question

2. How do ledger cards and encounter forms differ?

Posting a Charge

The charge column of the day sheet is for original charges incurred for services received by the patient from the physician or staff on a specific date. Examples include office visits, electrocardiogram, blood work, hospital visits, consultations, and fees for returned checks. Charges in a medical office are based on a fee schedule or list of charges determined by the usual, customary, and reasonable charges of similar providers in similar localities who practice under similar circumstances. Fee schedules are discussed further in Chapter 16. Procedure 14-2 outlines the steps for posting a charge.

Posting a Payment

Payments received by the practice may include insurance checks received in the mail, money orders, credit card payments, or cash received from patients. Procedure 14-3 outlines the steps for posting payments and adjustments.

Posting a Credit

Sometimes an account is overpaid, either by the patient or the insurance company. Such an overpayment is termed a credit (money owed to the patient or insurance carrier). This will show on the patient's ledger card as the last balance, with brackets (e.g., [25]) indicating a credit. Brackets are used to show the opposite of the column's normal meaning. For example, the balance column normally shows patients' debits, or amounts patients owe to the doctor. Brackets around an amount indicate the opposite, namely, that the doctor owes the patient money.

Credits are handled in one of two ways: (1) the credit stays on the account and is subtracted from the charges on

the patient's next visit, or (2) the patient is mailed a refund for the amount of the overpayment. How an overpayment is handled depends on office policy and the amount of the overpayment. Generally, overpayments under $5 are left on account as a credit, whereas overpayments over $5 are refunded.

Posting a Credit Adjustment

The adjustments section is used to indicate nonstandard office fees and to credit an account for uncollectible monies. Below are three specific situations that require a credit adjustment.

Example 1. The physician wishes to give a registered nurse a 25% professional discount on charges incurred for an office visit. You enter the fee from the fee schedule in the charge column, show in the description column an office visit with a professional discount of 25%, and put the 25% in the adjustment column. Assume an office visit is $40. You put $40 in the charge column and $10 (25% of $40) in the adjustment column. The patient owes your facility $30 for this visit.

Example 2. Most medical offices participate with certain insurance groups, which means the physician has signed an agreement with the insurance carrier to accept the fee for services set by that carrier instead of the physician's normal fee. Again, you must charge the same fee for the same procedure. When payment is received, however, the explanation of benefits from that carrier will show the agreed-on amount for that procedure. You will post the payment in the normal way, but you must write off the difference between the physician's standard fee for this procedure and the agreed-on amount. Assume the doctor charged $40 for an office visit and the insurance carrier's agreed-on amount was $35. You would post $40 in the payment column and $5 in the adjustment column to arrive at the agreed-on amount.

Example 3. Most facilities request that you write off the balance of an account when you turn it over to a collection agency to keep better control of the accounts receivable. Therefore, if the patient's balance is $1200, you would show "collection agency" in the description column of the ledger and put the $1200 in the adjustment column, which would bring the balance to 0. Procedure 14-4 lists the steps for posting an adjustment.

Checkpoint Question

3. What do brackets around an amount listed in a column indicate?

Posting a Debit Adjustment

Generally, a credit adjustment reduces the patient's account balance, whereas a debit adjustment adds to the patient's account balance. Below are three specific situations that require a debit adjustment.

Patient Name: _____

Patient ID #: _____ DOB: _____ Sex: _____

PCP: _____

SSN: _____ Financial Class: _____

Phone: _____ (home) _____ (work)

Medical Record #: _____ Date of Service: _____

Benefit Pkg: _____ Copay $ _____

Encounter #: _____

Service Provider: _____

Appt. Status: ☐ Scheduled   ☐ Same Day   ☐ Walk-in

Check-in Time: _____   Check-out Time: _____

Escorted to Exam Room: _____   Time Patient Seen: _____

Appointment Time: _____

Is Patient Being Seen in Relation to:
☐ Motor Vehicle Accident   ☐ Workman's Compensation

Appointment Failure Reason:
☐ Patient Cancel   ☐ No Show   ☐ Walk Out   ☐ PHA Cancel

TYPE OF VISIT

✓	CODE	DESCRIPTION	FEE	✓	CODE	DESCRIPTION	FEE	✓	CODE	DESCRIPTION	FEE	✓	CODE	DESCRIPTION	FE
		OFFICE VISITS-EST.				**OFFICE VISITS-NEW CONT.**				**PREVENTATIVE, NEW**				**COUNSELING**	
	99211	Minimal			99204	Compreh.			99385	E&M 18-39			99401	15 Min.	
	99212	Focused			99205	Comp. & Complex			99386	E&M 40-64			99402	30 Min.	
	99213	Expanded				**NURSE VISIT**			99387	E&M 65 & over			99403	45 Min.	
	99214	Detailed			99211	Minimal				**CONSULTATION**			99404	60 Min.	
	99215	Compreh.				**PREVENTATIVE, EST.**			99241	Focused					
		OFFICE VISITS-NEW			99395	E&M 18-39			99242	Pre-Op Consult					
	99201	Focused			99396	E&M 40-64			99244	2nd Opinion					
	99202	Expanded			99397	E&M 65 & over									
	99203	Detailed													

PROCEDURES

✓	CODE	DESCRIPTION	FEE	✓	CODE	DESCRIPTION	FEE	✓	CODE	DESCRIPTION	FEE	✓	CODE	DESCRIPTION	FE
	88170	Aspiration - Cyst			11200	Skin Tag Removal				**IMMUNIZATIONS/INJECTIONS**				**IMMUNIZATIONS/INJECTIONS CONT**	
	20600	Aspiration - Joint (Small)			20550	Trigger point/Tendon Inj.			G0009	Administration Fee - Pneumovax			J2203	Triamcinolone Inj.	
	20605	Aspiration - Joint (Interm.)							G0010	Administration Fee - Hepatitis B			J3420	Vitamin B₁₂	
	20610	Aspiration - Joint (Large)				**SPECIALTY SERVICES**			95115	Allergy Injection Single				**IN-HOUSE LABORATORY**	
	16020	Burn Dressing			99070	Ace Bandage			95117	Allergy Injection Multiple			89050	Cell Count, except blood	
	69210	Ear Irrigation			E0110	Crutches			90788	Antibiotic IM			89060	Crystalanalysis	
	10120	Foreign Body Removal, Skin			29130	Finger Splint			J2910	Aurothioglucose			82948	Glucose	
	10060	I&D Abscess, simple			29125	Wrist Splint			G0008	Flu Vaccine			85013	HCT	
	90780	IV Infusion Therapy			99080	Form Completion			J1600	Gold Injection			85018	Hemoglobin Screen	
	12001	Laceration Repair, Simple				**TESTING/SCREENING**			90731	Hepatitis B			81025	Pregnancy	
	13160	Laceration Repair, Extens.			95004	Allergy - Skin Test			90741	Immune Globulin			81002	Urinalysis, Dipstick	
	64450	Medial Nerve Infiltration			92557	Audiometry			90724	Influenza			81000	Urinalysis, Full	
	17110	Molluscum/Wart Rmvl			93000	EKG			J9217	Lupron 3.75 mg			G0001	Venipuncture	
	94640	Nebulizer			92506	Hearing Screen			J9217	Lupron 7.5 mg				**OTHER PROCEDURES**	
	82270	Stool for Blood (Hemocult)			86580	PPD			J9250	Methotrexate 2-5 mg					
	12001	Suturing, Superficial			94010	Pulmonary Function			90732	Pneumovax					
	13100	Suturing, Complex			94760	Pulse Oximetry, Single			90718	Td					
	11050	Skin Les./Wart Cautery			45330	Sigmoidoscopy, Flexible			90782	Therapeutic SQ or IM					

P = PRIMARY   S = SECONDARY   S1-S9 = NUMBERED SECONDARY

DIAGNOSIS

✓	CODE	DESCRIPTION	✓	CODE	DESCRIPTION	✓	CODE	DESCRIPTION
	789.0	Abdominal Pain		780.6	Fever		462	Pharyngitis (sore throat)
	879.8	Abrasion/Laceration		704.8	Folliculitis		486	Pneumonia
	995.3	Allergic Reaction		535.5	Gastritis		V70.3	Pre-Marital Testing
	477.9	Allergic Rhinitis		558.9	Gastroenteritis		V72.81	Pre-op Cardiac Exam
	285.9	Anemia		274.9	Gout		V72.83	Pre-op Exam, Other
	413.9	Angina		V72.3	Gyn Exam		601.0	Prostatitis
	300.00	Anxiety		784.0	Headache		600	Prostatism
	716.90	Arthritis		389.9	Hearing Loss		782.1	Rash
	427.9	Arrhythmia		536.8	Heartburn/Indigestion		569.3	Rectal Bleeding
	493.90	Asthma		573.3	Hepatitis		530.81	Reflux
	611.72	Breast Lump		455.6	Hemorrhoids		V81.2	Screening for Cardiac Condition
	490	Bronchitis		553.9	Hernia		780.3	Seizure Disorder
	727.3	Bursitis		401.9	Hypertension (NOS)		473.9	Sinusitis
	354.0	Carpal Tunnel Syndrome		272.4	Hyperlipidemia		848.9	Strain/Sprain
	682.9	Cellulitis		242.00	Hyperthyroidism		438	Stroke
	786.50	Chest Pain		251.2	Hypoglycemia		305.90	Substance Abuse
	575.1	Cholecystitis		380.4	Impacted Cerumen		099.9	STD
	372.3	Conjunctivitis		780.52	Insomnia		727.00	Tenosynovitis, Tendonitis
	496	COPD		564.1	Irritable Bowel Syndrome		451.9	Thrombophlebitis
	414.9	Coronary Artery Disease		719.40	Joint Pain		246.9	Thyroid Disease
	290.9	Dementia		592.0	Kidney Stones		435.9	TIA
	311	Depression		464.0	Laryngitis		463	Tonsilitis
	692.9	Dermatitis		724.2	Low Back Pain		011.90	Tuberculosis
	250.01	Diabetes, IDDM		710.0	Lupus		465.9	Upper Respiratory Infection
	250.00	Diabetes, NIDDM		V70.0	Medical Exam/Physical		599.0	Urinary Tract Infection
	558.9	Diarrhea		346.9	Migraine		V04.8	Vaccination, Flu
	562.10	Diverticular Disease		278.0	Obesity		V03.9	Vaccination, Pneumovax
	780.4	Dizziness		382.9	Otitis Media		616.10	Vaginitis
	995.2	Drug Reaction		614.9	Pelvic Inflammatory Disease		424.9	Valvular Heart Disease
	782.3	Edema		533.9	Peptic Ulcer Disease		079.9	Viral Syndrome
	780.7	Fatigue/Tiredness/Malaise		443.9	Peripheral Vascular Disease			

Comments:

PREVIOUS BALANCE $

TODAY'S CHARGES $

PAYMENT $

BALANCE $

RETURN APPOINTMENT:
_____ Days   _____ Weeks   _____ Months
APPT. LENGTH: _____   PROVIDER: _____

APPT. REASON:

PROVIDER SIGNATURE:

Adult

Philadelphia
Health Associates
Tax ID #23-2350500
PHA Group # PH75923

☐ 3550 Market Street
Philadelphia, PA 191(
(215) 823-8660

☐ The Bourse Building
111 S. Independence
East • 7th Floor
Philadelphia, PA 191(
(215) 625-9100

OTHER DIAGNOSIS

✓	CODE	DESCRIPTION	✓	CODE	DESCRIPTION

FIGURE 14-3.   Sample encounter form and charge slip.

Posting Charges to the Patient's Account

Equipment/Supplies

- Day sheet
- Carbon paper
- Pegboard
- Ledger card
- Charge slip and/or encounter form
- Calculator
- Form
- Pen

Steps	Purpose
1. Take the charge slip from the patient and check to be sure it is complete, signed by the provider, and belongs to the patient whose ledger card or account is in hand.	It is difficult to undo entries to the wrong account. It's best to be accurate the first time. Just as in the clinical area, identify your patient.
2. If using a ledger card, post the total amount of today's charges in the charge column on the ledger card. Each service can be listed in the description column by using abbreviations such as OV, INJ, LAB for office visit, injection, and laboratory services, respectively.	Since the manual billing system uses a copy of the ledger card for a statement, it is important that patients be able to understand your abbreviations. Provide a key at the bottom of the ledger card.
3. If using a computer, post each charge separately on the charge screen. Most programs require a local code for a particular service. When you enable this code or the CPT code, the computer will automatically post the appropriate charge in the proper field.	Proper computer entry allows for accurate financial records to be maintained.

Posting Payments to a Patient's Account

Equipment/Supplies

- Day sheet
- Carbon paper
- Pegboard
- Ledger card
- Charge slip and/or encounter form
- Calculator
- Form
- Pen

Steps

1. Align the patient's ledger card on the day sheet. If the patient is paying for services received by the physician today, the charge slip that shows today's charges should also be in place on the day sheet.

2. Enter the patient's name and previous balance in the appropriate columns. If using a charge slip, make sure you place the charge slip number in the receipt number column. Enter the posting date in the date column.

3. Enter the type of payment being made in the description column, whether personal check (pers. ck.), money order (m. o.), credit card (MC, VISA), or insurance check (ins. ck.). Enter the amount of payment in the payment column and on the deposit section of the day sheet in the cash or checks column.

4. Subtract the payment amount from the previous balance and record the new balance. If only a payment is being posted, no entry is made in the fee area. If an entry has been made in the fee area, you will start with the previous balance, add the charges, subtract the payment, and record the new balance.

Example 1. You receive an insufficient funds (NSF) check from the bank today from a payment made earlier by a patient and posted as such to his account. The previous payment is no longer valid. Therefore, you must eliminate that payment because the patient now owes it again. Because this is not an original charge, you may not use the charge column for this entry. To post this debit adjustment to the patient's account, you will show NSF in the description column and the amount of the NSF check in the adjustment column with brackets.

Example 2. Assume that you have turned over an account to a collection agency and the patient comes in later to pay the amount owed. You must first put the money back on the account, or you will create a credit balance. Place the ledger card on the day sheet and in the description column write "reverse collection." Again, this is not an original or new charge, so you do not use the charge column. Show the amount in the adjustment column in brackets because you are adding the amount to the patient's balance. You may now show the payment in the payment column.

Example 3. Your office requires that you refund all money over $5 to the patient or insurance carrier. You must also post this to eliminate the credit balance on the account. Place the ledger card on the day sheet and in the description column write "refund to patient" (or insurance carrier). To eliminate a credit balance, you must debit the account. You put the amount of the refund in the adjustment column in brackets, indicating that it is a debit, not a credit adjustment.

 Checkpoint Question

4. How does a credit adjustment differ from a debit adjustment?

Posting to Cash-Paid-Out Section of Day Sheet

Sometimes, the physician may take cash from the day's receipts. When this happens, your bank deposit for that day will be short by the amount taken out. The best way to ac-

---

Procedure 14-4

Posting a Credit Adjustment

Equipment/Supplies

- Day sheet
- Carbon
- Pegboard
- Ledger card
- Calculator

Steps	Reason
1. Align the patient's ledger card on the day sheet.	Proper alignment is needed for accurate record keeping.
2. Record the patient's name, previous balance, and the date in the appropriate columns.	Payments and adjustments can be posted at the same time. The payment is recorded in the payment column, and the adjustment is entered in the adjustment column. Both are subtracted from the previous balance, and the new balance is recorded in the new balance column.
3. Record [in brackets][a] the amount of the adjustment in the adjustment column of the ledger card. Enter a description of the adjustment in the professional service column, that is, insurance adjustment or correction adjustment.	A description of the adjustment is needed for proper financial record keeping and quality assurance.
4. Subtract the amount of the adjustment from the previous balance and record the new balance in the balance column.	Knowing the balance of an account is essential for the financial stability and growth of a business.

[a]Brackets indicate that the amount is subtracted.

count for this is to have the physician sign in the cash-paid-out section of the day sheet for the amount. This documents the transaction and prevents anybody else from being able to do this.

Some insurance carriers adjust for money overpaid to your facility by holding that amount out of money they are paying your facility for other patients. Although you are posting the correct amounts in the payment column for each patient, the check amount from the insurance carrier is short the refund or kept-out money. You write this in the cash-paid-out section of the day sheet, explaining, "insurance refund on account of [patient's name]." It is also a good idea to make a copy of the explanation of benefits and staple it to the back of your day sheet for future reference.

COMPUTER ACCOUNTING

Most medical office accounting software available today is easy to use and requires a minimum of computer skills. Computer programs fulfill many of the same functions as a pegboard system but do so much faster. Instead of recording entries on a day sheet, you key entries into a computer. You can print out invoices and receipts for patients and insurance companies. Since most practices have computer stations in several locations, the patient's account can be quickly and easily retrieved in all areas of the office, enabling everyone involved in the patient's care to access information about third-party coverage, co-payments required, and so on.

Computer bookkeeping programs have a variety of advantages over pegboard bookkeeping. Computer programs work as expanded calculators and perform the arithmetic functions, such as balancing individual accounts and the day's totals. Many bookkeeping programs also can write checks. Some programs manage electronic banking between the office and bank. The office may have computerized many functions, including bookkeeping, making appointments, and generating other office reports, such as forms for insurance reimbursement. It is essential that data stored on computer be backed up in a reliable way in case the computer crashes.

Posting to Computer Accounts

If you understand the fundamentals of accounting and how to post entries manually, you will be able to use a computer system with ease. To post payments, first retrieve the patient's account. The software will take you through the process. You enter the source and amount of the payment, the allowed amount for the service, and any necessary adjustments. As in a manual system, this information is provided on the insurance carrier's explanation of benefits (EOB). Calculations are automatic and error free.

When you post charges into the computer database, in most systems you use a local code to indicate a certain procedure or service. For example, you may enter 211 to post a level 2 office visit for a new patient. When the information prints on the claim form, the CPT (current procedural terminology) code 99212 will appear (see Chapter 18).

Computer Accounting Reports

Depending on the software package, you can easily generate daily, monthly, and yearly reports or reports on transactions of an individual physician in a group practice. Daily and weekly reports provide the same information found on the bottom of a day sheet in a manual accounting system. At any given time, you can request a report that displays the practice's period-to-date and year-to-date financial status.

Computer systems record the daily activities described earlier for the manual system, and bookkeeping software enables you to create a closing report that prints a list of the day's financial activities. You may run a trial daily report or a final daily report. In a trial report, the information keyed in that day is printed for review. You correct any errors before running a final report. As on the day sheet, you categorize receipts as cash, check, and so on. A check register report can print the amount of the daily deposit and a list of checks for the day.

BANKING

Banks and Their Services

Besides physical location, several factors are important when choosing a bank for the office business account. These factors include the monthly service fees, overdraft protection programs (protection against bouncing checks), interest-bearing accounts, and returned check fees.

Checking Accounts

A checking account allows you to write checks for funds that are deposited in the account. Each day you will deposit to a checking account the money collected in the office. At the time a new checking account is opened, checks are ordered with a check order form. The administrative medical assistant must maintain the checkbook and ensure that checks are reordered as needed.

Banks offer a variety of options for checking accounts. Variables include monthly service charges, maximum amounts of checks written, minimum balance requirements, and so on. Interest-bearing checking accounts pay interest if the balance is kept above a certain amount. Most banks set the minimum checking account balance at $500 to $2500. The bank pays this interest in exchange for the use of your money for loans and other transactions. If you drop below the minimum balance, however, you will not earn interest. Most banks also charge a monthly service fee and a fee for each check written for the period the balance was below the limit. Some banks waive the monthly service fee if the office agrees to maintain a minimum balance in another account, such as a savings account.

Savings Accounts

The medical practice may use a savings account for money that is put aside for long-term plans or money that is not needed for writing checks. A savings account pays interest at a higher percentage rate than a checking account, allowing the money to grow. Funds can be transferred to the checking account as needed.

Money Market Accounts

Money market accounts are a combination of a savings account and an interest-bearing checking account. The minimum balance is usually much higher than that of a checking account (as much as $2500), but the interest rate also is much higher. These accounts offer limited check-writing privileges, including an initial deposit of $2000 and minimum balance of $500 per check.

Bank Fees

Banks charge fees for services. In an effort to get new business, banks offer special services and plans for small business, including the medical office.

Monthly Service Fees

Bank policies concerning monthly fees or service charges vary widely. A **service charge** is a fee charged monthly for using an account. The charge can be a fixed amount or may be an individual charge for each check written on the account. As discussed, some banks do not levy a service charge if a specific minimum balance is maintained for the account.

Overdraft Protection

Overdraft protection guarantees that checks written against the account will be paid even when there is not enough money in the account at the time. Usually, the bank pays the checks and retrieves the money owed to it when the account balance is restored. Many banks offer overdraft protection only up to a certain dollar amount.

Returned Check Fee

Some banks charge a **returned check fee**, which is a fee charged for any check that is deposited into the checking account but that is later returned to the bank because the account it was issued from had insufficient funds with which to pay the check. Such a check is often referred to as a bounced check. Most facilities charge this amount to the patient. Because this is an original charge, the bad check fee is listed in the charge column of the patient ledger and day sheet, with the amount of the check being recorded as a debit adjustment.

Types of Checks

Most medical offices use the standard business check, but when certain circumstances require, there are other types available:

- Certified checks are stamped and signed by the bank to verify that the amount of the check is being held in the account for payment. The check is written from the customer's account.
- Cashier's checks are sold to a customer for cash or a personal check. The check is written by the bank, giving the recipient the added guarantee that the check is good.
- Traveler's checks are a convenient and safe way to carry cash when traveling. They are available in denominations of $10, $20, and $50, and if lost, they can be replaced. Traveler's checks are signed when bought and are countersigned (signed again) in the presence of the payee.
- Money orders, although not checks, can be purchased with cash from a bank or the U. S. Postal Service. Money orders, which guarantee payment to the recipient, are often used for mailing payments, since it is not safe to mail cash.

Box 14-2 highlights other terms used in the language of banking.

 Checkpoint Question

5. List three types of checks available through banks.

Writing Checks for Accounts Payable

Another financial duty of the medical assistant may be to handle accounts payable, or pay the bills. The accounts payable in a medical office usually include rent, utilities, taxes, salaries,

Receiving Checks and Making Deposits

When checks are received in the office, they are first endorsed. To endorse a check requires writing (or rubber stamping) on the back of the check the name and number of the account into which it will be deposited (Fig. 14-4). This way, if the payments are lost or stolen, no one else can cash them. It also ensures that the bank deposits the payments to the correct account. An endorsement stamp can be purchased from your bank or a stationery store.

After all payments are posted, total all of the checks and all cash received that day. This total should match the totals of the payments column on your day sheet. Detach the deposit sheet from the day sheet and stamp the back with the endorsement check stamp. If a computer program is used, print out a deposit slip. Wrap the deposit slip around the checks and complete a bank deposit slip for the account to which the deposit is made. The deposit can be hand-delivered or mailed to the bank.

A hand-delivered deposit may be taken to a teller, who will issue a deposit receipt, or dropped in a depository. If the deposit is mailed, make sure sufficient postage has been affixed to the envelope. Never include cash payments in a deposit that is mailed or placed in a depository. Cash deposits should always be hand-delivered, and a teller's receipt should always be obtained.

vendors of supplies and services, patient refunds, and petty cash reimbursement. The accounts are usually paid by check. Banks require signature cards for each person authorized to sign checks. In most cases, this is limited to the physician or physicians. Some medical offices require two signatures, especially if the check is over a certain amount. Computer systems allow you to enter information in the proper field and print checks. Software systems also keep track of every transaction using a check. When using a manual system, type or write legibly. Use the current date and write the amount of the payment in both figures and words and the name of the payee. Complete the memo line for reference. Record the date, check number, amount of the check, and payee on the check registry. Post this transaction to the appropriate account in the general ledger or apply it to the proper category in a computer system by entering the type of payment on the proper screen. Recording transactions in the proper account or category is important when preparing the office taxes. Subtract each amount from the check register balance.

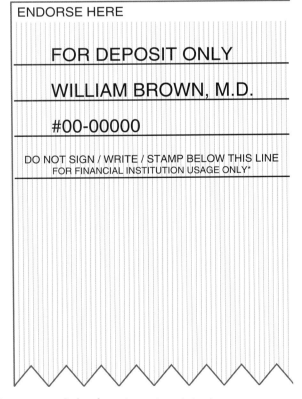

FIGURE 14-4. An endorsed check.

Reconciling Bank Statements

All banks mail monthly statements to account holders on which are listed all transactions since the last closing date. This bank statement must be reconciled, or compared for accuracy, with your records each month.

The statement consists of a list of all checks written and their amounts, all deposits made and their amounts, any electronic transactions, and any service charges. Verify that all checks and deposits are listed correctly. Make a check mark on the checkbook stub of each check that has been paid by the bank. On the back of the statement is a worksheet that explains how to balance the account (Fig. 14-5). Following the steps listed on the worksheet makes balancing the account fairly easy. The steps for reconciling a bank statement are listed in Procedure 14-5.

Checkpoint Question

6. What information is found on a bank statement?

PETTY CASH

A petty cash account is a cash fund kept in the office specifically for small purchases, such as buying postage stamps or office supplies. The value of the petty cash account should always remain the same. A petty cash fund is always a designated sum of money. When money is taken from the fund, a voucher (Fig. 14-6) or receipt is placed in the fund to verify the purchase. The remaining cash and the sum of the vouchers should always equal the designated sum; for example, a petty cash fund of $40 with $13 in actual cash should have receipts that amount to $27.

Petty cash funds should be kept separate from patient cash payments. All cash should be kept in a securely locked area. One person should be designated to maintain the petty cash fund and issue vouchers. A voucher with an attached receipt should always be placed in the petty cash box, both to provide proof of the purchase and to keep the account balanced. The petty cash fund normally is replenished once a month. To replenish the fund, cash a check in the amount of

---

1. Subtract any fees or charges that appear on this statement from your checkbook balance.
2. Add any interest paid on your checking account to your checkbook balance.
3. List the checks you have written that have not been paid (these checks did not yet appear on your bank statement). You can also include in this list any withdrawals you have made since the ending date of the banking statement that do not appear on the statement.

Check Number	Amount
_____	_____
_____	_____
_____	_____
_____	_____
Total	_____

4. If you have entered deposits or other additions to your checkbook that do not appear on the statement, list them there:

Date	Amount
_____	_____
_____	_____
Total	_____

5. Enter the ending balance from your statement here: _____
   Add the total deposits from Step 4:   + _____
   Subtract the total from Step 3:   – _____
   Total (this should equal your checkbook balance):   _____

If these balances do not equal your checkbook balance:
• Check the addition and subtraction in your checkbook
• Check the amount of each transaction in your checkbook with the amount shown on your statement
• Check to see that all transactions from your previous statement have been accounted for
• Call your bank manager for assistance

F I G U R E   1 4 – 5 .   Bank statement reconciling worksheet.

Procedure 14-5

Reconciling a Bank Statement

Equipment/Supplies

- Monthly bank statement
- Check register
- Calculator
- Pen

Steps	Reason
1. Determine which portion of the checkbook is covered on this bank statement.	You must know where your last bank statement ended and where the current one begins.
2. Find the ending balance and the list of checks and deposits on the bank statement.	
3. Check your checkbook register or record of disbursements against the bank statement and place a check mark against each check and deposit on your record that has been recorded on the bank statement.	To balance the account, you must identify which checks or deposits are recorded by the bank and which ones are outstanding.
4. Total all checks not listed on the bank statement. Place this total in the space provided on the back of the bank statement (outstanding checks).	Since there is no standard form, each bank's worksheet may be different, but there will be a space reserved for the total of all outstanding checks and withdrawals.
5. Total all deposits that do no appear on the bank statement and place this total in the space provided on the worksheet (outstanding deposits).	Outstanding deposits must be accounted for to balance the bank statement.
6. Note any additional charges, such as for services, ATM use, or returned checks.	Miscellaneous charges must be taken into account when balancing the checkbook
7. Calculate the correct balance by starting with the ending balance from the bank. Then, add the outstanding deposits to that balance (from Step # 5). Then, subtract the outstanding withdrawals (from Step # 4).	Outstanding deposits and withdrawals must be accounted for to reconcile the bank statement.
8. Verify that the correct balance (from Step # 7) matches with your checking account amount.	This allows verification that, as of today, your checking account balance agrees with your bank statement.
9. If the figure is not the same, recheck your work. If the two numbers still do not match, contact the bank to check for possible bank errors.	This allows you to verify your records with the bank's record. It is easy to transpose numbers or misread figures when using a calculator. You should add the columns again. It is helpful to have a coworker add the columns also.

the total of the vouchers. The money is placed in the fund, and the vouchers are removed and filed.

Some offices keep a petty cash expense record. This record is similar to a checkbook that keeps track of the account balance as checks are written, such as personal checkbook. This expense record also categorizes purchases so that they can be included with the monthly office expenses. Pur-

chases such as stamps and office and medical supplies can be deducted as office expenses and added to the accounts payable expense record.

Checkpoint Question

7. List six guidelines for managing petty cash.

PETTY CASH RECEIPT

_____ 20 _____

To Office Manager:
   Please furnish for_____

Supplies:

Postage:

Travel Expenses:

Other:

Approved

TOTAL

Received Above Amount

_____

FIGURE 14-6.   Petty cash voucher.

CHAPTER SUMMARY

Whether a medical practice uses a manual bookkeeping system, such as the pegboard system, or a computer system, you may be responsible for keeping records of accounts payable, accounts receivable, and petty cash. You may also be responsible for banking functions, such as receiving checks, making deposits, and reconciling monthly bank statements. To carry out these responsibilities effectively, you must record all transactions accurately and promptly. Computers have made the daily bookkeeping practices much easier, but you must understand the principles of accounting applied in the manual system if you are to use the computer system. Using the appropriate banking services will allow the day-to-day financial operations to be efficient, accurate, and secure.

Critical Thinking Challenges

1. Your day sheet deposit slip and your posting proofs do not agree. How do you find the error?
2. An employee is prosecuted for stealing money for more than a year from her physician employer's funds. Investigation reveals that she was stealing any cash payments given to her. How could she do this for so long without being caught? What necessary monthly action would make this crime impossible?
3. Your office is considering going from a pegboard system to a computer bookkeeping system. What features should you look for in the software?

Answers to Checkpoint Questions

1. Five sections of a pegboard day sheet include the distribution columns, adjustment column, deposit slip, payments section, and posting proofs section.
2. Ledger cards provide an overall financial record of a patient; encounter forms provide documentation of today's financial activity.
3. Brackets indicate the opposite of the normal meaning of that column.
4. Generally, a credit adjustment reduces the patient's account balance, whereas a debit adjustment increases the patient's account balance.
5. Three types of checks offered by banks include cashier's checks, certified checks, and traveler's checks.
6. The statement consists of one or more pages that lists all checks written and their amounts, all deposits made and their amounts, any electronic transactions, and any service charges.
7. These are the six guidelines for managing petty cash:
   • Keep petty cash separate from patient cash payments.
   • Keep in a secure, locked area.
   • Designate one person to maintain the petty cash fund and issue vouchers.
   • Place a voucher with an attached receipt in the petty cash fund.
   • Replenish the petty cash fund once a month.
   • Remove and file all vouchers.

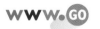 **Websites**

Superbill Forms and Creations
      www.physicianshelp.com
Comptroller of Currency Administrator of National Banks
      www.occ.treas.gov
Maximum Returned Check Fees allowed by state
      www.checkagain.com/statefees.asp

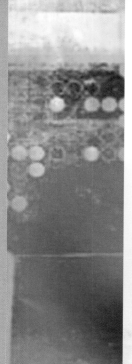

15

Accounts Payable and Payroll

CHAPTER OUTLINE

ACCOUNTING CYCLE

RECORD-KEEPING COMPONENTS

ACCOUNTS PAYABLE
Ordering Goods and Services
Receiving Supplies
Paying Invoices

PAYROLL
Types of Payroll Systems
Employee Records
Tax Withholdings

PREPARATION OF REPORTS

ASSISTING WITH AUDITS

ROLE DELINEATION COMPONENTS

GENERAL: Legal Concepts
- Perform within legal and ethical boundaries

ADMINISTRATIVE: Administrative Procedures
- Perform basic administrative medical assisting functions

ADMINISTRATIVE: Practice Finances
- Apply bookkeeping principles
- Manage accounts receivable
- Manage accounts payable
- Process payroll
- Document and maintain accounting and banking records

CHAPTER COMPETENCIES

LEARNING OBJECTIVES
Upon successfully completing this chapter, you will be able to:
1. Spell and define the key terms
2. Describe the accounting cycle
3. Describe the components of a record-keeping system
4. Explain the process of ordering supplies and paying invoices
5. Discuss the types of payroll records
6. Explain which taxes are withheld from paychecks

PERFORMANCE OBJECTIVES
Upon successfully completing this chapter, you will be able to:
1. Issue a payroll check, using the pegboard system
2. Calculate the amount of an employee's payroll check for a given pay period

KEY TERMS

accounting cycle
audit
check register
check stub
FICA

federal unemployment tax
gross income
Internal Revenue Service (IRS)
invoice

liabilities
net pay
packing slip
payroll
payroll journal

profit-and-loss statement
purchase order
summation report
withholding

ACCOUNTING IS THE compilation of a business's financial records. It is necessary for assessment of the practice's financial history and current financial stakes, which serves as the basis for sound financial management. The medical office, like other businesses, requires strict adherence to sound record-keeping practices. Records must be maintained in an orderly fashion so you can retrieve financial information at any time and to present an organized picture of the business's finances. A system of checks and balances is an integral part of record management. Generally, the check-and-balance status of accounts is examined monthly by comparing the total of all accounts with outstanding balances against the running total taken from the daily logs of all financial transactions. The practice's accountant will also closely scrutinize these records at scheduled intervals for tax-reporting purposes.

Although manual accounting systems are still used widely, computer accounting is available as part of most medical software packages, and the many advantages include efficient tracking and analysis of critical information, improved productivity, and smarter business decisions. General ledger, payables, receivables, inventory, purchasing, cash flow, bank reconciliation, collections, fixed assets, and many other applications integrate with each other so you can manage the office's core processes efficiently and effectively.

ACCOUNTING CYCLE

The finances of medical practices operate in one of two 12-month intervals or durations. The office **accounting cycle** follows either a fiscal year (a consecutive 12-month period starting with a specified date) or a calendar year (January through December). The yearly interval used depends on the way the practice's accountant has structured the business. For example, the medical practice can exist as a sole proprietorship or as a professional corporation.

The federal **Internal Revenue Service** (IRS) examines a business's income statements for the amount of profit and owed tax four times a year by quarterly estimated tax returns. The practice's annual tax return is a summary of the quarterly returns and reports the final year-end profit or loss (income minus expenses equals profit or loss) for the fiscal or calendar reporting period. If financial records are scrupulously maintained all year, preparation of the annual income tax return should merely be a summation of existing accounting facts. Well-maintained office records not only facilitate IRS returns but also provide data that define the practice's business picture.

There are many reasons for a physician along with an accountant to review financial data on a regular basis. Financial records reflect growing expenditures and growth in the business. Conclusions drawn from financial data can affect future financial decisions. For example, analysis of the practice's accounts receivable can predict the amount of salary increases. Tax records must be available in case of an IRS inquiry or **audit** (review of accounts). Records such as receipts should be retained for 7 years, but records such as bank statements, canceled checks, and IRS tax returns should be kept for the duration of the business.

RECORD-KEEPING COMPONENTS

The practice's financial records should include a running record of income, accounts receivable, and total expenditures, including **payroll** (employee salaries), cash on hand, and **liabilities** (amounts the practice owes). Expenditures can be broken down into categories (Box 15-1). This is important because it enables the record keeper to track the practice's expenses and provide the physician and accountant with a cohesive picture of the practice's expenses at tax time.

Categories can be accommodated by several types of bookkeeping systems; a simple business checkbook does not allow this. Pegboard systems allow the bookkeeper to write the check once over the **check register** (a place to record checks) or the ledger sheet and then have multiple pages with columns to distribute an expense into categories, including a back sheet for payroll. These columns are totaled and balanced at the completion of each check register sheet and can be subtotaled monthly, quarterly, and annually (discussed later in the chapter). Keeping a monthly accounts payable disbursement sheet lets the administrative medical assistant easily compare past years' expenses for the same part of the year.

Box 15-1

CATEGORIES OF EXPENDITURES

- Office supplies: items used by the facility's employees, such as paper, pencils, day sheets, ledger cards
- Medical supplies: items used for patients, such as examination gowns, electrocardiograph paper, syringes, tongue depressors
- Drugs: drug purchases, such as injectables; some facilities keep a separate column for these purchases and others put this amount in the medical supplies category
- Payroll: gross amount paid to employees
- Taxes: taxes paid, such as FICA, Medicare, federal withholding, state withholding, listed separately
- Rent: amount paid to rent the facility
- Utilities: gas, electric, telephone
- Maintenance: routine care of the facility, such as cleaning personnel
- Travel: physician's car lease payment, gas mileage if paid to employees, and so on
- Personal: any money used personally by the physician

LEGAL TIP

It is unethical and illegal to falsify any financial documents. Accurate record keeping is essential. The IRS will examine the practice's financial records. You may be held liable for errors or omissions to these documents. If you are not comfortable posting a payment, calculating payroll deductions, always ask your supervisor for clarification. If the employee's W-4 form is illegible, ask the person to complete a new form. W-4 forms should not have any eraser marks or cross-outs. If any do, obtain a new form from that employee.

Software packages offer the most sophisticated way to maintain financial records, not just for the categorization of expenses but also for the rapid formation of financial reports. Automating accounts payable does, however, require a personal computer (PC), software, and the training to use it.

There are advantages and disadvantages to both computer systems and paper records. Each practice should make this decision based on its particular volume and needs. Either system (pegboard or computer) can provide the practice and its accountant with the ability to pay and track expenses and to furnish the financial data necessary to create reports.

Multiple **summation reports**, such as the payroll report, itemized category report, account balances, and the **profit-and-loss statement**, must be prepared for the practice's accountant. If financial data are entered diligently into the bookkeeping system, preparing monthly, quarterly, or yearly reports should not be a daunting task. Income tax accounting cycles are divided into quarters: January through March, April through June, July through September, and October through December. Payroll reports show the amount of taxes being withheld and made monthly, quarterly, or annually. Normally, the practice's accountant will send you necessary reports and have you mail the checks.

ACCOUNTS PAYABLE

Ordering Goods and Services

There are many economical ways to purchase office supplies or equipment. For instance, purchasing cooperatives (co-ops) offer bulk rate discounts by allowing physicians to order in a pool with other purchasers. Vendors may offer discounts for buying in volume or for paying promptly. Large warehouse-type merchandisers and companies with discount catalogs also offer competitive prices. Researching and cost-comparing office products and medical supplies can be time consuming, but it is worth the effort, especially for items used frequently. Compare past invoices with prices in new catalogs.

Besides cost, other considerations come to bear when purchasing office supplies. For example, office supply companies often provide free delivery, but office warehouse chains may charge a fee or require a minimum order for free delivery. Quality also plays a role. Supplies should be of standard quality as well as economical. It is common to use several office supply vendors according to quality or pricing of specific goods.

Office supplies or equipment can be ordered in a number of ways. Once an account is set up, offices can place orders by telephone, fax, mail, or e-mail. These orders can be paid monthly by check or by credit card. It is preferable to pay for supplies by check or credit card rather than by cash, but when cash purchases are necessary, retain a detailed receipt for tax purposes. Credit card purchases can be made over the telephone or by mail, but for security reasons, credit card account numbers should not be faxed.

When placing orders for supplies, give the office's account number to the vendor or write it on the order form. It is a good idea to use a **purchase order** that lists the supplies ordered and their order numbers, so that order numbers for frequently ordered items can be pulled from the previous purchase order; this saves time with subsequent orders. Be sure to record the charges for your order and verify them against the bill later. It is also handy to keep a list of all vendors, telephone numbers, and account numbers.

Checkpoint Question

1. When purchasing office supplies, what factors besides price should you consider?

Receiving Supplies

When goods are delivered to the office, a receipt or **packing slip** listing the enclosed items should always accompany the order. The office staff member who receives the supplies must check the packing slip against the actual contents to ensure that all supplies are in the shipment. The person should initial the packing slip, which shows that all goods were received. When it is time to issue checks for payables, the assistant can then pay the **invoice** or bill. These receipts or packing slips should be placed in a bills pending file, so that they may be compared to the bill when it arrives. If the bill has already been paid by check or credit card, the invoice should be placed in the appropriate accounts paid file; there should be such a file for each fiscal or calendar year.

Paying Invoices

Invoices for supplies and other types of bills payable by the practice should be kept together in a bills pending file to avoid loss or misplacement of a bill. Bills can be paid daily, weekly, biweekly, or monthly.

Manual Payment

Manual payment of bills requires a checkbook and checks. The practice's accountant may recommend use of a log or record book into which is entered information about each check, such as payroll taxes or the breakdown of expenses for a monthly credit card bill. The large checks and checkbooks available from banks and business printers offer more space for writing memos or itemizing a check. Each check, once written, is detached from a **check stub**, which remains in the checkbook. If you make a mistake while writing a check, void the check and stub and staple the voided check to the stub. Never make corrections on the facility's checks. Check stubs should be filed with other fiscal or calendar year records and kept for the life of the practice.

The information recorded on the check stub includes the check number, the date the check was issued, the payee (the party to whom the check was written), and the full amount of the check. Notes should be written on both the memo section of the check and on the check stub. For example, when entering the purchase of a new beeper, the note might read, "payee: Office Communications" or "new beeper for Dr. Smith." The check is then attached to the bill or invoice and signed by an authorized individual.

Memos or notations on check stubs can be referenced later if a question arises concerning payment by a particular check. A log or record book enables the bookkeeper to make entries for each expense, categorize expenses, and maintain detailed payroll records. Unlike one-write (pegboard) or computer systems, multiple entries must be made by hand to track office bill paying. This can seem laborious when compared to other bookkeeping systems, but it may be ideal for smaller practices.

Pegboard Payment

The same pegboard system that is used for accounts receivable (see Chapter 14) may be used for bill paying; it has several advantages over the ordinary manual method of paying bills. Instead of using a day sheet, a **check register** page is used to record the checks that have been written. The check is then aligned on the pegboard over the register page and is filled out as with any other check (Fig. 15-1). Pegboard checks have a carbon or transfer strip, and on this strip is written the date, the payee, the check number, and the amount. The information written on the strip is recorded automatically on the check register. These check-writing systems are referred to as one-write systems for this reason. The check can be addressed directly beneath the payee line and mailed in a window envelope, which saves the time it would take to address an envelope.

The pegboard check register has approximately 20 columns that can be used to categorize expenses, such as rent, insurance, office supplies, utilities, service contracts, postage, and any other applicable categories. All entries on the check register are totaled when the register is completed;

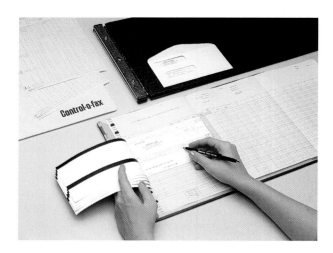

FIGURE 15–1.   Sample pegboard check and check register. (Courtesy of Control-o-fax, Waterloo, IA.)

these totals are carried forward to the new register page. Each fiscal or calendar year begins with a new first page (page 1), and the last check register page will have totals for the entire year. The check register provides a system of checks and balances even before the bank statement arrives because the check register must be balanced, as with a bank statement.

The check register also allows entries for bank deposits, and the back page of the register is used for payroll record keeping. As with pegboard accounts receivable, completed pegboard check registers are filed in a separate binder in chronological order, with the most recent register on top.

Computer Payment

A computer accounts payable system has all the advantages that a pegboard system offers: access at a glance to check registers, itemized categories and their totals, payroll records, and entries for bank deposits. To use such a system, you must have a PC, accounts payable program software, printer, and bank checks that are compatible with the software and printer. The initial expense with a computer system is much higher than that of manual or pegboard systems. Office personnel will need computer training to use the program. Also, since it runs on electricity, a computer may not work during power failures. A good computer accounting program will, however, provide functions for both accounts receivable and accounts payable. Financial data should be recorded in three forms: on the computer's hard drive, on a magnetic tape or floppy disk, and in printout form (hard copy).

Although entering data in the computer at first may be time consuming, this becomes less of a concern with practice. Furthermore, financial reports can be compiled and printed in a fraction of the time required with manual or pegboard systems. The computer program can also perform the record-keeping arithmetic; as a result, mathematical errors are practically nonexistent.

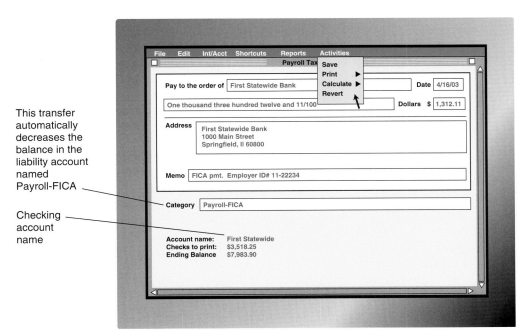

FIGURE 15-2.

Computer screen showing a check for payroll taxes.

This transfer automatically decreases the balance in the liability account named Payroll-FICA

Checking account name

Paying bills by computer requires using the software to open the check-writing file. Checks are presented on the computer screen in the same way that a paper check would normally appear (Fig. 15-2), and the information that is required to appear on the check is entered on the computer keyboard. The information is stored and the check is printed out; the computer program automatically subtracts the amount of the check from the account's balance. The bookkeeper can print one check at a time or a batch of checks together.

The computer can "memorize" checks so that the information on them can be recalled and reprinted without reentering it; this is especially helpful with payroll checks. A good accounting program also allows for bill reminders and disk or magnetic tape backup reminders. Of course, it is essential to back up financial data on magnetic tapes or floppy disks in case of computer problems.

Checkpoint Question

2. Whether using a manual, pegboard, or computer accounts payable system, two steps must always occur when ordering and receiving supplies. What are they?

PAYROLL

Types of Payroll Systems

The medical office will have payroll obligations to its staff, and federal, state, and, possibly, local payroll taxes will be due. The administrative medical assistant may issue payroll checks for the practice's entire staff, including the physician, or just for the office staff. Or an outside payroll service may

be retained to issue the checks and keep the records. These payroll services specialize in computing, withholding, and paying taxes and payroll for businesses. Such a firm can provide all of these services for considerably less than it would cost for office time and personnel or for an accountant. The larger the practice's staff, the more economical a payroll service becomes. Firms that provide payroll services are especially cost effective, in that they are highly accurate, aware of changes in tax laws, and legally liable.

Generally, payroll checks for the medical office will be issued at one of the following intervals:

- Weekly (52 pay periods per year)
- Biweekly (26 pay periods per year)
- Monthly (12 pay periods per year)

The pay period is set up by your employer and is the same for all employees.

There are various ways to record payroll expenditures, depending on what type of bookkeeping system is used by the office.

Manual Payroll Systems

When payroll checks are issued manually without a pegboard system, separate payroll records must be kept. The check stub will indicate to whom the check was issued, in what amount, and on what date. A separate record or log book must be maintained to keep track of gross income and tax withholdings for each employee. These withholdings should be totaled monthly, quarterly, and annually; for this reason, it is advisable to maintain payroll records in a timely manner throughout the year.

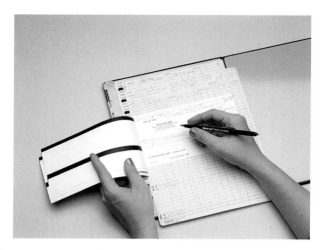

FIGURE 15–3. Sample pegboard payroll journal. (Courtesy of Control-o-fax, Waterloo, IA.)

Pegboard Payroll Systems

The pegboard system allows for payroll entries as well as the accumulation of payroll data by using an employee payroll record form and the correlating back page of each check register, called the **payroll journal** (Fig. 15-3). Procedure 15-1 outlines the steps in issuing a payroll check using the pegboard system.

Computer Payroll Systems

Payroll records can be maintained with various software packages; many such packages integrate payroll with other accounting functions, such as accounts receivable and accounts payable. Computer programs can calculate tax withholdings automatically, record payroll data, and print payroll checks. In most cases, a computer program provides substantial time savings over manual and pegboard payroll systems.

Procedure 15-1

Issuing a Payroll Check Using the Pegboard System

Equipment/Supplies

- Pegboard with checks
- Carbon paper
- Payroll register
- Tax tables
- Calculator
- Time card

Steps	Reason
1. Align the carbon or transfer strip at the top of the check on the employee's payroll record, then align both on the payroll journal.	The write-it-once system will eliminate the need to post information more than one time.
2. Enter the employee's name first, followed by the check number, the payroll period, and the **gross income** (the amount of money an employee earned before taxes are withheld) plus any additional earnings.	The employee's name must be entered to issue a payroll check. The pay period indicates to the employee the time frame of the checks.
3. From the gross income, subtract federal, state, and local taxes and Social Security; this is called tax **withholding**. See Procedure 15-2.	Witholdings must be subtracted from gross income to issue a payroll check.
4. Enter the **net pay** (amount of money an employee is paid after taxes are withheld) on the detachable payroll slip. Fold this slip behind the check.	When the check is placed in the envelope, this information will not be visible, which will protect the employee's privacy.
5. Total the payroll journal as each page is completed.	Total amounts of income and tax withholdings should be accrued for each quarter for tax-reporting purposes.

Employee Records

Regardless of the payroll system used, it is necessary to maintain an individual file for each employee that contains pertinent employment information. The personnel file should include the following information:

- Employee's original résumé or completed job application
- Job references
- Hourly rate or salary at the time of hire
- Dates and amounts of pay raises
- Job evaluations
- All employee withholding authorization forms, such as W-4 forms (discussed later)
- Pension plan, health, and life insurance paperwork
- Vital facts about the employee (e.g., date of birth, name of spouse, Social Security number, address and telephone number, name and daytime phone number of emergency contact person)

Tax Withholdings

Federal, state, and, possibly, local taxes must be withheld from employees' paychecks; for this reason, each employee must complete a W-4 form on the first day of hire. This form must be completed by the employee before the first pay period; otherwise, you are required to withhold taxes at the highest rate, which classifies the person as single with no dependents. The W-4 form lists the employee's name, Social Security number, address, marital status, and the number of exemptions to be used in the calculation of tax withholding. If any of the information contained on an employee's W-4 form changes, the employee must fill out a new form, which is placed in the personnel file.

The federally mandated taxes are Social Security (**FICA**), Medicare, and federal income tax. Each of these taxes is based on a percentage of total gross income; the federal income tax also factors in marital status and the number of withholding exemptions claimed on the W-4 form.

Box 15-2 features the information needed to calculate employee withholding manually by using the combination method found on the IRS website. Procedure 15-2 outlines the steps for calculating the amount of an employee's paycheck.

The employer must match the amount withheld from each employee's paycheck for Social Security and Medicare taxes. For example, if $150 is withheld from an employee's paycheck for Medicare and Social Security taxes, the employer must pay $300 to the IRS ($150 withheld from the employee plus $150 matching amount). The employer does not match federal, state, or local taxes. The practice's accountant should inform the office bookkeeper of tax rates and withholdings. Usually, each pay period or at least monthly you will deposit the federal taxes withheld from all employees plus doubled FICA in an account at a federal depository (normally the facility's bank). Your accountant nor-

Courtesy of the IRS website.

Box 15-2

CALCULATING PAYROLL WITHHOLDING USING THE COMBINATION METHOD

Combined Income Tax, Employee Social Security Tax, and Employee Medicare Tax Withholding Tables

If you want to combine amounts to be withheld as income tax, employee Social Security tax, and employee Medicare tax, you may use the combined tables found in the IRS publications for businesses. Combined withholding tables for single and married taxpayers are provided for weekly, biweekly, semimonthly, monthly, and daily or miscellaneous payroll periods. The payroll period and marital status of the employee determine the table to be used.

If the wages are greater than the highest wage bracket in the applicable table, you must use one of the other methods for figuring income tax withholding described in the publication or in circular E. For wages that do not exceed $84,900, the combined Social Security tax rate and Medicare tax rate is 7.65% each for the employee and the employer for wages paid in 2002. You can figure the employee Social Security tax by multiplying the wages by 6.2%, and you can figure the employee Medicare tax by multiplying the wages by 1.45%.

The combined tables give the correct total withholding only if wages for Social Security and Medicare taxes and income tax withholding are the same. When you have paid more than the maximum amount of wages subject to Social Security tax ($84,900 in 2003) in a calendar year, you may not use the combined tables.

If you use the combined withholding tables, use the following steps to find the amounts to report on your form 941, employer's quarterly federal tax return:

1. Employee Social Security tax withheld: Multiply the wages by 6.2%.
2. Employee Medicare tax withheld: Multiply the wages by 1.45%.
3. Income tax withheld: Subtract the amounts from steps 1 and 2 from the total tax withheld.
4. You can figure the amounts to be shown on form W-2, wage and tax statement, in the same way.

---

mally will send you the estimated federal depository slips for this purpose.

The employer must also pay a **federal unemployment tax** (FUTA) for each employee based on that employee's gross income. The amount of this tax is calculated by the practice's accountant and paid either quarterly or annually. Individual

Procedure 15-2

Calculate the Amount of an Employee's Payroll Check

Equipment/Supplies

- Calculator
- W-4 form

Steps	Reason
1. Calculate the number of hours worked from the employee's time card or record.	The employee's payroll check is based on the number of hours worked.
2. Calculate the employee's annual gross wage using this formula: Hourly wage × number of hours worked per week × 52 (number of weeks in a year) = gross annual wage Assume an employee earns \$7 per hour and works 40 hours per week: \$7 × 40 × 52 = \$14,560 annual gross wage	The annual gross wage must be calculated to determine the employee's payroll check amount.
3. If your pay period is • Biweekly, then ÷ this sum by 26 • Monthly, then ÷ this sum by 12 • Weekly, then ÷ this sum by 52	This converts the gross wage into paycheck amounts.
4. Divide by 52 weeks in a year and then divide by 5 (work days in a week) to get the amount of a day's pay.	Always go to the yearly gross wage when figuring deductions or increases to gross wages; you will get the exact amount.

(continued)

states may levy their own unemployment tax. The practice's accountant calculates this tax.

Other withholdings from an employee's paycheck might include health, life, or disability premiums; pension plan contributions; or court-ordered garnishment of wages owed to a third party.

 Checkpoint Question

3. What taxes must be withheld from an employee's paycheck?

Payment of Taxes

Payroll taxes are paid according to different schedules as determined by the IRS and the state and local tax authorities. Federal taxes, such as Social Security, Medicare, and federal income tax, must be paid monthly, bimonthly, or more frequently, depending on the size of the gross payroll. Always remember to match the Medicare and Social Security payments withheld from the employee's check (the amount withheld × 2). These payments are made on IRS form 941 for deposit requirements; the IRS furnishes these forms free of charge.

If the total federal taxes due are more than \$3000, these payroll taxes must be paid within 3 calendar days of the time the payroll check was issued. State taxes that are withheld from the employee's pay check are usually paid by mail and must be paid and mailed before the tax due date to avoid penalties.

The IRS also requires the employer to file quarterly returns for all federal taxes withheld; these returns are due by April 30, July 31, October 31, and January 31 each year. This quarterly return is a summary of the Social Security, Medicare, and federal wage taxes paid. State quarterly re-

Procedure 15-2 *(continued)*

Steps	Reason
5. Deduct this amount from the gross wage to get the adjusted gross wage from which you will withhold taxes. Using the example above, the calculation would be as follows: $(\$14,560 \div 52) = \$280 =$ week's pay $\$280 \div 5 = \$56 =$ day's pay $\$280 - \$56 = \$224$ (adjusted gross wage)	The adjusted gross wage is needed to calculate withholding taxes.
6. Calculate any overtime worked.	Overtime is defined as hours worked over the normal for the pay period. Overtime is calculated by paying 1.5 times the normal hourly wage. If the employee earns $7 per hour, overtime pay would be calculated by dividing $7 in half ($3.50) and adding that amount to the hourly wage: the hourly pay rate for overtime would be $10.50.
7. Refer to the appropriate tax tables (e.g., federal, FICA, Medicare, state taxes) for the deductions for taxes.	The tax tables will specify the amount of withholdings.
8. Subtract the taxes from the gross or adjusted gross wages to obtain net pay.	The net pay amount is the result of the gross wages minus the withholdings
9. Write the payroll check for this amount.	The net pay is the amount of the payroll check.

turns have the same due dates and are usually paid by mail. Your accountant will keep you informed of taxes due.

W-2 Forms

At the end of the calendar year, all pertinent payroll information should be summarized for each employee and made available to the practice's accountant. The W-2 statement provided to the employee by January 31 of each year should list the following information:

- Total gross income for the previous year
- Total federal, state, and local taxes withheld
- Any taxable fringe benefits
- The employee's total net income

WHAT IF

The medical practice where you work did not pay its payroll taxes. What can happen?

The IRS charges penalties and interest on all unpaid taxes. The IRS can attach the business and its assets and close the business.

Checkpoint Question

4. What information does the employee list on the W-4 form? What happens if this information changes?

PREPARATION OF REPORTS

The bookkeeper must also prepare reports for the practice's accountant or the IRS, based on financial data stored in the office's bookkeeping system. For this reason, care should always be taken when recording financial data.

The manual system, when assisted by the use of a log or record book, should be able to provide monthly, quarterly, and annual summaries for income, expenditures, and payroll. It is advisable to have subtotals and totals for these periods for tax payment purposes.

The pegboard system is also practical for providing summaries of income, expenses, and payroll and can be totaled monthly, quarterly, and yearly. Each day sheet, check register, and payroll journal is individually totaled, with all balances forwarded to the next page. These records are stored in binders and kept for future reference.

A computer system of accounting offers all of the previously mentioned reports along with other more complicated reports that generally require more advanced accounting skills. The great advantage with report generating by com-

ñ Spanish Terminology

Los impuestos deben ser sacados de su cheque.	Taxes must be taken out of your paycheck.
Usted necesita completar estas formas.	You need to complete these forms.
Gracias para su pago.	Thank you for your payment.
Gracias para su cheque.	Thank you for your check.
Esto es su recibo.	This is your receipt.

puter is that the computer will perform all of the mathematical calculations for the time frame requested.

ASSISTING WITH AUDITS

An **audit** may be informal (in-house) and used to assist the practice's accountant with tax preparation, or it may be formal audits by the IRS. If meticulous attention to record keeping has been paid throughout the year, the preparation time needed for such an audit should be minimal. It is important to save all bank statements, copies of annual and quarterly tax returns, and receipts for expenditures. Canceled checks and payroll records should be readily available.

Manual and pegboard systems can provide spending category and payroll summaries in addition to examination of the actual entries for the period being audited. A computer accounting system can provide all of this plus reports such as profit-and-loss statements, which normally would be compiled by an accountant.

CHAPTER SUMMARY

Accounting is a complex process involving many legal issues. As a medical assistant, you must keep neat and well-organized accounting records. You also will be expected to understand how to order goods and services efficiently and economically and how to pay invoices. In addition, you must understand the payroll process. With the computer being used for many administrative medical office functions, it is imperative that you keep abreast of changes and new opportunities to make this process more efficient and up-to-date.

Critical Thinking Challenges

1. Explain the advantages of manual, pegboard, and computer accounting systems. In what instances would each be the preferred method?

2. A vendor continually mixes up your orders, and the physician asks you to look for a new vendor. How do you decide which one to recommend? What factors influence your choice of one office supply vendor over another?

3. An employee gets divorced. She is irate when she gets her W-2 form and discovers that her deductions were still being based on her married filing status. What is your response? What should you do now?

4. The physician asks you, the office manager, how much money is owed to him. How do you gather the information needed to answer his question?

Answers to Checkpoint Questions

1. Besides cost, consider delivery charges and product quality when purchasing office supplies.

2. The bookkeeper must write out a purchase order and compare the packing slip and final invoice to the purchase order.

3. Social Security, Medicare, and federal, state, and local wage taxes must be withheld from an employee's paycheck.

4. The employee provides his or her name, Social Security number, marital status, current address, and number of withholding exemptions. If any of this information changes, the employee must complete a new W-4 form.

 Websites

The Accounting Library (TAL)
        www.accountinglibrary.com
Quickbooks Online
        www.quickbooks.com
Microsoft Business Solutions
        www.microsoft.com/businesssolutions
Internal Revenue Services
        www.irs.gov
Payroll Taxes
        www.payroll.com

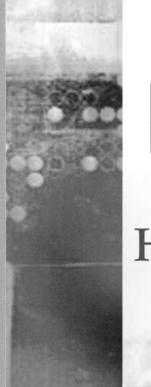

16

Health Insurance

CHAPTER OUTLINE

HEALTH BENEFITS PLANS
Group Health Benefits
Individual Health Benefits
Government-Sponsored (Public)
Health Benefits

MANAGED CARE
Health Maintenance Organizations
Preferred Provider Organizations
Physician Hospital Organizations
Other Managed Care Programsi
The Future of Managed Care

WORKERS' COMPENSATION

FILING CLAIMS
Electronic Claims Submission
Explanation of Benefits

POLICIES IN THE PRACTICE

ROLE DELINEATION COMPONENTS

ADMINISTRATIVE: Administrative Procedures

- Perform basic administrative medical assisting functions
- Understand and apply third-party guidance
- Obtain reimbursement through accurate claims submission
- Monitor third-party reimbursement
- Understand and adhere to managed care policies and procedures

ADMINISTRATIVE: Practice Finances

- Apply bookkeeping principles
- Manage accounts receivable
- Manage accounts payable
- Document and maintain accounting and banking records

CHAPTER COMPETENCIES

LEARNING OBJECTIVES

Upon successfully completing this chapter, you will be able to:

1. Spell and define the key terms
2. Describe group, individual, and government-sponsored (public) health benefits and explain the differences between them
3. Explain the differences between Medicare and Medicaid
4. List the information required on a medical claim form and explain why each piece of information is needed
5. Name two legal issues affecting claims submissions
6. Explain how managed care programs work
7. Explain the differences between health maintenance organizations, preferred provider organizations, and physician hospital organizations

PERFORMANCE OBJECTIVES

Upon successfully completing this chapter, you will be able to:

1. Fill out a CMS-1500 claim form

KEY TERMS

assignment of benefits
balance billing
birthday rule
capitation
carrier
claims
claims administrator
coinsurance
coordination of benefits
co-payments

crossover claim
deductible
dependent
eligibility
employee
explanation of benefits (EOB)
fee-for-service
fee schedule
group member

health maintenance organization (HMO)
independent practice association (IPA)
insurance
insured
managed care
Medicare
peer review organization
physician hospital organization

plan maximum
preexisting condition
preferred provider organization (PPO)
third-party administrator
unbundling
usual, customary, and reasonable (UCR)
utilization review

BEFORE 1930, ACCESS TO medical care in the United States was based on ability to pay. In 1929, Baylor University introduced a plan to provide schoolteachers 21 days of hospital care for $6 per year. The idea quickly spread to other Dallas employers, and the organization known as Blue Cross was born. Health plans were originally designed to protect families from catastrophic financial burdens in the event of a serious illness or accident. By 1939, the Blue Cross symbol was adopted by the American Hospital Association as an endorsement that health plans met guidelines established by its member hospitals.

In the Pacific Northwest, lumber and mining companies wanted to provide outpatient care to their employees as well. They paid monthly fees to groups of physicians to provide care for their employees. This model led to the first Blue Shield plan, founded in California.

Blue Cross and Blue Shield as we know them today are actually a federation of more than 42 independent companies that insure about 30% of the U. S. population.

While the **insurance** industry was developing in the United States, other countries took a different approach to providing health care to their residents. Canada, for example, established publicly funded universal health insurance. This type of coverage provides hospital and physician services with no deductibles, **co-payments,** or dollar limits on coverage for insured services and is funded by tax revenues.

In the United States, health insurance is funded by a combination of employer and employee contributions and tax-funded coverage.

Today, virtually every state has a Blue Cross and a Blue Shield plan. Health benefits also are provided by insurance companies, self-funded group plans, and government plans such as Medicare and Medicaid. The benefits vary with each plan and from state to state. Approximately 80% of Americans are enrolled in health benefits plans of one sort or another. Consequently, most of the patients you will encounter in the physician's office have some type of health insurance. As a medical assistant, you will need to understand the differences in health benefits plans and the requirements of each so that you can complete and file claim forms appropriately. You will also need to learn the special terminology associated with health insurance claims. In addition, you may need to instruct patients about insurance matters.

HEALTH BENEFITS PLANS

Group Health Benefits

Group health benefits are sponsored by an organization, such as an employer, a union, or an association. A person covered by group health benefits is either an **employee** or a **group member**, who by virtue of employment or membership in an organization may participate in and receive benefits from a health plan. Coverage in health plans differs greatly, so you need to know the **eligibility** of the patient for services being provided by your office. For example, birth control is frequently not covered unless there is medical necessity.

Benefits may be either **insured** or self-funded. Commonly, health benefits are referred to as insurance. It is, however, important to distinguish between the actual benefits and the vehicle used to fund and provide them.

With insured benefits, the employer, employee, or both pay a monthly premium to an insurance company. The insurance company, in turn, is obligated to pay for any eligible health benefits. Self-funded benefits on the surface appear the same as insured benefits. They are paid for in the same manner as group health benefits, but instead of the employer paying the insurance company to invest the money to cover payments, they invest it themselves. They pay an insurance company or other agency to process **claims** and make payments on their behalf. Any payment for medical services that are not paid by the patient or physician is said to be paid by a *third-party payer.* In this case, the payer is an agent for the self-funded plan and is, therefore, known as a **third-party administrator** (TPA). Many employers now choose to self-fund their group benefit plans rather than insure them.

You will need to be aware of these funding differences as they relate to state and federal regulations. For instance, insured benefit plans are subject to state regulations. Many states mandate that certain types of benefits be included in any insurance plan. These mandated benefits vary from state to state but often include such medical services as childhood immunizations, routine diagnostic care, and treatment for substance abuse.

Although it would seem that these are routine medical services, many insurance companies consider them outside the scope of treating physical illness. Screening for illness, psychiatric illness, and prevention of illness by immunization are not routinely covered.

For a group benefit plan to cover (pay for) eligible expenses, the patient must meet several criteria, called eligibility requirements. These are defined in the policy or plan document and may include a minimum number of hours worked per week and a waiting period from the date of employment before benefits become effective.

The eligibility of a **dependent** (spouse, children) is based on the employee's eligibility. Certain eligibility limitations apply to dependent children. For example, children are usually eligible until they reach the limiting age defined by the plan. The age limitation is usually extended if the child is a full-time student. Eligibility usually requires that children be the unmarried natural or adopted children of the employee, unmarried stepchildren, or children for whom the employee has legal guardianship.

To confirm a patient's eligibility, call the **claims administrator** for the health benefits plan. A provider inquiry telephone number is commonly included on the patient's identification (ID) card (Fig. 16-1).

Group and individual health benefits describe contractual agreements and how the policies are paid. Both group and in-

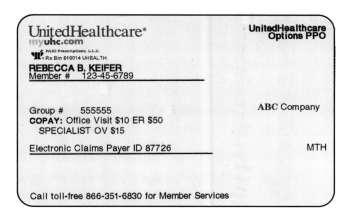

FIGURE 16-1. Sample identification card for a managed care plan.

dividual policies can be many different types of plans, such as traditional, HMO, and PPO. These types are further discussed later in this chapter.

 Checkpoint Question

1. What is the difference between an insured benefits plan and one that is self-funded?

Individual Health Benefits

Individual health benefits policies are purchased by an individual from an insurance company. The individual pays premiums directly to the insurance company, and the insurance company pays either the doctor or the hospital directly if they are a participating provider or reimburses the individual for eligible medical expenses.

For patients with individual health benefits, the criteria for completing and filing claims are the same as for patients with group health benefits. Individual health policies commonly have less generous coverage, however, than group health plans have. An individual policy may also have a rider that limits or eliminates benefits for certain illnesses or injuries, based on the determination of the underwriter at the time the policy was issued. Box 16-1 outlines the requirements of the Health Insurance Portability and Accountability Act of 1996 (HIPAA), which include a provision to protect employees changing jobs from being denied benefits for preexisting conditions.

With the cost of health care skyrocketing and more insurance companies limiting what they will cover, many people have more than one health care insurance policy. It is extremely important that you know which insurance you bill first (primary) and which to bill the remainder of the charges (secondary).

Government-Sponsored (Public) Health Benefits

Government-sponsored benefit programs are funded and regulated by the federal government or individual states. Government programs have been developed over the years to assist persons who do not otherwise have health benefits, such as the elderly, the indigent, and others unable to obtain benefits. Government programs include Medicare, Medicaid, TRICARE/CHAMPVA, and workers' compensation.

Box 16-1

REQUIREMENTS OF HIPAA

As discussed in earlier chapters, the Health Insurance Portability and Accountability Act of 1996 brought about changes in the health care industry that protect patients and health care providers. According to the HIPAA website, **www.cms.gov/hipaa**, the following provisions are now in effect:

- HIPAA contains provisions for insured persons enrolled in employer-sponsored insurance programs without regard to their health status if they change employment.
- HIPAA prohibits the use of genetic testing information to deny health insurance coverage.
- HIPAA provides tax incentives for the purchase of long-term care insurance.
- HIPAA requires the adoption of new standards for financial and administrative electronic transmission of claims, new standards for claims attachments, and standardization of diagnostic and procedure coding.
- HIPAA strengthens existing regulations for fraud and abuse in the system.
- HIPAA Administrative Simplification: These HIPAA requirements, which are separate from the insurance portability requirements, are intended to reduce the costs and administrative burdens of health care by making possible the standardized electronic transmission of many administrative and financial transactions.
- HIPAA adds guidelines for confidentiality issues in electronic medical records, as discussed in Chapter 8.

Medicare

In 1965, the Social Security Act established **Medicare** to provide health insurance for the elderly. Elderly persons were defined as Social Security recipients age 65 or older. In 1972, amendments to the Social Security Act expanded Medicare coverage to two additional high-risk groups: disabled persons who have been receiving Social Security benefits for 24 months and persons suffering from end-stage renal disease.

Medicare Part A covers hospital expenses and is provided at no additional charge to persons eligible for Social Security benefits. Medicare Part B pays for physician fees, both inpatient and outpatient, diagnostic testing, certain immunizations (influenza and pneumonia), and specific screening tests (PSA, mammograms, Pap smears, bone density testing, colorectal screening). Part B Medicare is optional, and the participant is charged a monthly fee. The fee is deducted from the monthly Social Security payment.

Persons signing up for or receiving Social Security benefits are automatically enrolled in both Part A and Part B Medicare when they reach 65. If they do not wish to participate in Part B, they must decline it. Both Part A and Part B of Medicare have deductibles and co-payments, and as with most health insurance policies, these generally increase yearly.

A patient with Medicare coverage who is actively employed and covered by the employer's plan will have secondary Medicare benefits. A retired person age 65 or over who has health insurance in addition to Medicare will have primary Medicare benefits. Physicians are required to submit claims to Medicare on behalf of Medicare patients. These claims must be filed within 1 year of the time the service is incurred. (See section on filing claims for more information.)

After the **deductible** has been met, Medicare Part B reimburses the physician 80% of the Medicare-approved charges. The patient is responsible for the remaining 20% of the Medicare-approved fee. Under certain circumstances, if paying the 20% causes undue financial hardship, the physician may not charge the remaining 20%. The Centers for Medicare & Medicaid Services (CMS) can provide forms with the requirements, and the forms should always be used. In addition to Medicare, the Social Security Act of 1965 established Medicaid, a program of health care coverage for the poor. If patients are financially unable to pay the 20%, they may be eligible for Medicaid. This is referred to as a **crossover claim** because the patient is eligible under both Medicare and Medicaid and the claim crosses over automatically from one coverage to the other. In this situation, Medicare is primary and Medicaid is secondary. Medicare will accept original claims (no copies) filed on CMS-1500 universal claim forms only.

The CMS, which was known as the Health Care Financing Administration (HCFA) prior to July 1, 2001, is a government agency that oversees the financial aspects of health care in the United States (Box 16-2). The CMS has adopted a revised Current Procedural Terminology (CPT) coding system that must be used for Medicare claims. Medicare B claims use the standard CPT codes. For equipment, supplies, and services not listed in the CPT code, the CMS has established the Healthcare Common Procedure Coding System (HCPCS) codes. (See Chapters 17 and 18.)

It is important to inquire of the patient regarding supplemental or secondary coverage. This policy, which patients may purchase on their own, covers charges not covered by Medicare. In this case, filing a second claim is necessary.

 Checkpoint Question

2. What is the difference between parts A and B of Medicare coverage?

Medicaid

Medicaid provides health benefits to low-income or indigent persons of all ages. Often, eligibility for Medicaid is based on a patient's eligibility for other state programs, such as welfare assistance. The federal government provides funds to each state for Medicaid costs; each state is required to provide a Medicaid program. Although the federal government

---

Box 16-2

WHAT IS THE CMS?

In 1977, the administration of the Medicare and Medicaid programs were combined under a single administrative agency. The administrator is appointed by the president of the United States and reports directly to the Secretary of Health and Human Services. Formerly known as HCFA, the CMS has become a big influence in the health care industry.

According to its website, **www.cms.gov**, the CMS is the federal agency that administers Medicare, Medicaid, and the State Children's Health Insurance Program (SCHIP). It provides health insurance for more than 74 million Americans. It also performs quality-focused activities, including regulation of laboratory testing, development of coverage policies, and quality-of-care improvement. The CMS maintains oversight of the survey and certification of nursing homes and continuing care providers, including home health agencies and intermediate-care facilities for the mentally retarded. It makes available to beneficiaries, providers, researchers, and state surveyors information about these activities and nursing home quality.

To ensure public and expert involvement in running their programs, the HCFA maintains a number of chartered advisory committees. These committees, whose meetings are open to the pubic, provide advice or make recommendations on a variety of issues relating to HCFA's responsibilities and activities.

Spanish Terminology

¿Tiene usted seguro médico?	Do you have medical insurance?
¿Qué es el nombre del seguro?	What is the name of the insurance?
¿Qué es el número de su póliza?	What is the number of your policy?
¿Va a pagar el hospital?	Will it pay for the hospital?
¿Tiene Medicare?	Do you have Medicare?
¿Tiene su tarjeta de Medicare?	Do you have your Medicare card?

stipulates the minimum health care coverage, states can provide coverage beyond the minimum. Therefore, Medicaid eligibility and benefits vary from state to state. At a minimum, Medicaid provides 100% coverage for the following:

- Inpatient hospital care
- Outpatient treatment and services
- Diagnostic services
- Family planning
- Skilled nursing facilities
- Diagnostic screenings for children

Many states have gone to a managed care type of Medicaid coverage in which recipients make a co-payment based on their income and are assigned a primary care physician as a gatekeeper.

Since circumstances that make recipients eligible for coverage change from month to month (i.e., employment), Medicaid patients receive a new ID card each month. Make a photocopy of the card for the patient's file on the first visit of each month. Most states require prior authorization by the Medicaid **carrier** before any services are rendered. Because reimbursement is considerably less than other insurances, not all physicians accept Medicaid patients, nor are they required to do so. If Medicaid patients are accepted, you need to be familiar with Medicaid as administered in your state.

Checkpoint Question

3. How often do Medicaid recipients receive a new card?

TRICARE/CHAMPVA

TRICARE, the new name for CHAMPUS, is administered by the U. S. Department of Defense and provides medical coverage for dependents of active service personnel, dependents of service personnel who died during active duty, and retired service personnel. When Congress realized that CHAMPUS costs could be controlled with managed care, they mandated that HMOs and PPOs (discussed later in this chapter) be added to the coverage. This three-part system is now called TRICARE. This system requires that participants

be assigned a primary care manager (PCM). The PCM is named on the beneficiary's card.

If a patient lives within 40 miles of a uniformed services hospital and that facility is unable to handle the needs of patients covered by TRICARE, a statement of unavailability is required for treatment by a physician's office or civilian hospital. Patients who live more than 40 miles from a uniformed services hospital do not need this statement to be treated in a physician's office or civilian hospital and for the physician or hospital to be reimbursed.

The Civilian Health and Medical Program of the Veterans Administration (CHAMPVA) covers dependents of veterans who have total and permanent service-connected disabilities. CHAMPVA is administered by the area Veterans Administration hospital. Once admitted to the CHAMPVA program, patients select their own physician; this allows them the same benefits as private insurance.

MANAGED CARE

Over the past 3 decades, health care costs in the United States have grown at about twice the general rate of inflation. As a result, the United States now spends more for health care services than any other industrialized nation, both as a percentage of gross national product and per person. At the same time, a smaller percentage of our population has health insurance coverage than in other advanced nations.

In the United States, most people obtain health coverage through their employer. The exceptions are Medicare for the

ETHICAL TIP

All patients must be treated equally and fairly. Financial issues regarding the patient's type of insurance or lack of insurance should have no bearing on the care provided. As a medical assistant, you must avoid stereotyping and care for the patient in an objective, professional manner.

elderly, TRICARE for the retired military and their dependents, Medicaid for low-income Americans, and those who do not have access to group coverage and buy coverage directly from insurers. In total, these programs cover fewer people than employment-based health plans.

The rapid rate of health care inflation has encouraged employers to begin offering **managed care** programs, which are typically less costly than traditional insurance coverage systems. Managed care programs vary greatly, but all involve a different relationship between the insurer, health care provider, and covered individual from that of traditional insurance programs. To understand this difference, we first discuss the traditional insurance system.

In traditional insurance systems, the covered patient may seek care from any provider. Normally, the patient and physician decide what care is needed. Then, services are rendered and the insurer pays a portion of the provider's bills (after deductibles and coinsurance). The insurer has no relationship with the provider.

In managed care systems, however, the insurer has a contractual relationship with the provider. The contract usually establishes what prices will be charged for each service and the conditions under which a service would be covered. Most managed care programs contain the following elements:

- *Precertification of hospital admissions* (often also called utilization management [UM] or utilization review [UR]). A patient can be admitted to a hospital for certain conditions only if that admission has been certified (approved) by the insurer. The goal of this requirement is to ensure that a patient's care is provided in the most cost-effective setting. For example, many surgical procedures that used to require an inpatient hospital stay can now be performed in an outpatient setting if proper education and support are available to the patient. Conflict between a UR guideline and the physician's requirements for the patient should be appealed to an impartial **peer review organization** composed of physicians and specialists who will review the case and make the final recommendation.
- *Approved referrals*. In many managed care plans a specialty physician can provide services to a managed care patient only on referral from the patient's primary care physician. The purpose is to ensure that the services provided by the specialist are medically necessary and, again, provided in the most cost-effective setting.
- *Network*. A network consists of providers (physicians, hospitals, pharmacies, and other providers and suppliers) who have signed contracts with the insurer or **health maintenance organization (HMO)** to provide services to covered persons in individual, group, or public health plans. A patient is normally required to use network providers to receive full coverage. The financial penalties (lost coverage) are often very high if a patient does not use these providers.
- *Assignment of benefits.* By contract, the network provider cannot bill the patient for any amounts not paid by the insurer (no **balance billing**) except for co-payments, coinsurance, and deductibles. If payment for a service provided by a network physician or hospital is denied by the insurer because it was not properly authorized, the provider cannot bill the patient for these services unless the contract does not contain a hold-harmless clause for the patient. This puts teeth in the control features of the managed care program.

Most physicians have contracts with more than one managed care program, and each of these programs has it own requirements and reimbursement schedules. So that the physician can provide the patient with needed health care services, while ensuring that the physician is paid for his or her services, it is necessary to consider the requirements of each patient's program. UM or precertification requirements are extremely important. Check the patient's ID card for details. UM requirements may apply to inpatient services or to a variety of outpatient and doctor office services.

Until you are very familiar with the requirements of each of your patient's managed care programs, you should call the number on the ID card before a patient is admitted to a hospital (on a nonemergency basis), referred to another physician, or scheduled for specific laboratory, radiological, or other test or evaluation. For inpatient admissions, the UM firm may ask for the diagnosis, the procedure or procedures to be performed, and other related information before approving the admission. Once the procedure is approved, the UM firm may only approve a specified length of stay in the hospital. Failure to comply with the precertification requirements results in a financial penalty for the patient and possibly also for the physician and the hospital.

It is important to be familiar with physicians within the network. The physician, hospital, laboratory, or other provider you normally refer a patient to may not be in the patient's managed care network. By calling the UM number to check, you can avoid penalties and improve the satisfaction of the patient with your services.

 Checkpoint Question

4. What are the four key elements of a managed care program?

Health Maintenance Organizations

It is easiest to understand how a HMO functions if we contrast it with a traditional health insurance program. In the traditional insurance system, the relationship between the covered individual and the insurer or self-insurer is purely financial. In return for receiving a paid monthly premium, the insurer promises to reimburse (indemnify) the individual if he or she incurs certain types of covered medical expense. There are often limits to coverage (exclusions and limitations), and normally the coverage has a **deductible** (amount below which services are not reimbursable) and **coinsur-**

ance (the patient pays a percentage of the medical expense after the deductible is satisfied). For example, the patient pays the first $200 (deductible) in physician charges each year starting January 1; then insurance pays 80% of covered charges, and the patient must pay the other 20%.

The covered individual seeks medical services and thereby incurs an expense. The individual, not the insurer, must pay for this expense. If the medical treatment is covered as defined in the insurance policy, the insurer will reimburse the patient a portion of the amount incurred after deductibles and coinsurance.

In contrast to traditional insurance companies, a HMO promises to provide covered services rather than pay for them. In this respect, the HMO acts as both an insurer and a provider of service. HMO policies are written differently from insurance policies. The HMO policy lists the medical services that the member is entitled to receive and the physicians and hospitals that will provide these services. The HMO has a contract with both the patient and provider. It must provide covered services to the member either directly from its own physician staff and hospitals or indirectly from physicians and hospitals contracted to provide the services promised to the member. The HMO, rather than the patient, is responsible for the costs of medical services, and providers bill the HMO rather than the patient when a reimbursable service is rendered to a HMO member.

This is one reason HMOs do not normally use deductibles and coinsurance, which are standard features of health insurance programs. A patient does not receive a provider's bill, so deductibles and coinsurance cannot apply. Instead, HMOs use predetermined co-payments (e.g., $10 per physician office visit) to reduce premium prices.

Health maintenance organizations come in many forms. Kaiser Permanente Health Plan is generally recognized as the nation's first HMO (there were earlier organizational forms but none that lasted into the modern era). In the early 1930s, Kaiser Industries needed to provide physician services for its employees in remote areas where no physicians were available. Kaiser sought the services of a physician to build a medical group that would provide the necessary services. Rather than paying for these services on a **fee-for-service** basis, the company paid the physicians per employee (as the company did for workers' compensation coverage).

Over time, the physician group grew and became the Permanente Medical Group. Coverage was expanded first to include non–work-related illness and injury for employees and then services for the dependents and spouses of employees. Finally, the program was expanded to allow other employers to purchase care for their employees from the Permanente Medical Group. The organization was restructured into three mutually dependent entities: Kaiser Permanente Health Plan, Permanente Medical Group (a very large multispecialty group practice), and Kaiser Foundation Hospitals. This company, the best example of the group model HMO, serves more than 6 million members. The HMO contracts with employers to cover their employees. The medical group and hospitals contract with the health plan to provide the services required in the health plan's contract with employers.

Consistent with its history, the health plan does not pay the medical group a fee for each service provided. Instead, it pays each party based on the number of members enrolled in the health plan. This is often called **capitation** because there is one payment per capita. Capitation payments are also used by other types of HMOs.

As group model HMOs developed (they were called prepaid group practices until 1973 federal legislation changed their names), nongroup physicians organized into an entity called an **independent practice association (IPA)**. The early IPA HMOs were often sponsored by a local medical society and were developed to allow independent physicians to compete with prepaid group practices.

IPA HMOs contract with employers in the same manner as group model HMOs, and their members receive covered services from IPA physicians. The HMO's contracts with physicians are different, however, because these physicians are not organized into a single multispecialty group practice. IPA physicians are paid in a number of ways. Some are paid on a capitation basis, and some may be paid on a fee-for-service basis using a **fee schedule** established by the HMO. Often, a portion of any reimbursement is withheld by the HMO and paid only if the HMO's total medical expense is within budget; this encourages the physician to be cost conscious in caring for patients.

In some of these HMOs, the IPA is a separate corporation, often owned by physicians. With this structure (still called an IPA HMO), the IPA contracts with physicians, and the HMO contracts with the IPA instead of directly with each physician.

Over the years, HMOs have continued to evolve, and many are now a mixture of these discussed models. As a medical assistant, you must know what type of relationship the practice has with a HMO before you can determine how the practice is reimbursed. Most HMOs require claims to be submitted even if payment is capitation rather than fee-for-service. Many HMOs also require the collection and transmission of other patient information, which is not required in the traditional insurance industry.

 Checkpoint Question

5. How does a HMO differ from a traditional health insurance program?

Preferred Provider Organizations

Whereas HMOs promise to provide services and have a financial risk in their relationships with subscribers, a **preferred provider organization (PPO)** is a type of health benefit program whose purpose is simply to contract with providers, then lease this network of contracted providers to health care plans. The PPO network is not risk bearing; it does not have any financial involvement in the health plan.

PPOs are typically developed by hospitals and physicians as a vehicle to attract patients, although some are developed and managed by insurance carriers.

PPOs contract with participating providers, including hospitals and physicians. These contracts allow the PPO to contract with insurers and other purchasers of health care services on behalf of the participating providers, who typically accept less than their normal charges and agree to follow the UM and other administrative protocols as specified by the PPO.

Typically, a health plan with a PPO offers benefits at two levels, commonly referred to as in network and out of network. Unlike in a HMO, patients may visit any provider they wish for services. If the provider is in network (a participating provider), the levels of benefits for the patient are greater than if the patient receives services from an out-of-network (nonparticipating) provider.

A typical health plan with a PPO may look like the breakdown shown in Figure 16-2.

As you can see from the example, each time the patient sees an in-network provider, he or she receives significantly better benefits. A primary difference between a HMO and PPO, therefore, is that patients can see any physician of their choice and receive benefits; they simply have an incentive in the form of higher benefits when they see an in-network provider.

As part of your responsibilities, you should identify the PPOs with which the physician has contracted and determine the administrative requirements set forth by each PPO in the contract. To understand the necessary administrative procedures agreed to by the physician, review all managed care contracts carefully. Also be aware that most PPOs have a provider relations representative who works with the contracted providers (physicians) to answer questions and clarify procedures. The PPO is typically operated by a group of hospitals or physicians or by an insurance company or independent organization. Physicians agree to participate in PPOs to serve their existing patients who now have PPO plans and sometimes to gain additional patients who seek the services of a PPO physician.

Participating physicians have agreed to perform certain administrative services for PPO patients. Commonly, the physician's office must accept assignment of benefits and provide claims filing services for the patient. The physician agrees to accept the reimbursement by the claims administrator as payment in full and agrees not to bill the patient for any difference between the physician's usual charge and the PPO-negotiated charge for the service. The participating physician is responsible for collecting any co-pay amount at the time of service. The physician also agrees to comply with any precertification requirements stipulated by the plan.

Checkpoint Question

6. What is the primary difference between a HMO and a PPO?

Physician Hospital Organizations

Physicians and hospitals have become more active in developing managed care alternatives. A **physician hospital organization (PHO)** is a coalition of physicians and a hospital contracting with large employers, insurance carriers, and other benefits groups to provide discounted health services. There are numerous variations of PHOs. A PHO may look much like a PPO with no risk-bearing elements, in which case the network of providers constituting the PHO are under no financial obligation to subscribers. A PHO may be more like a HMO, wherein the participating providers in the PHO do have a risk-bearing contract and assume responsibility for the overall medical budget of subscribing units. Physician organizations (POs) are such groups consisting of physicians only. As with any managed care program, it is important to know and understand the particulars of each managed care contract and requirements of the provider and obligations to patients and the managed care entity.

Other Managed Care Programs

Although HMOs, PPOs, and increasingly PHOs are the most common managed care programs, many others cover patients today and still more are being developed.

Although requirements vary, a gatekeeper provision is common. A gatekeeper is a primary care physician. Participants are required to see a primary care physician for all non-emergency services. That physician will either treat the patient or, if necessary, refer the patient to a specialist. The physician must complete and submit a referral form or call the claims administrator for approval of the referral.

The gatekeeper provision seeks to reduce the plan cost of specialists. For example, without such a provision, a patient might see a specialist first at a more costly fee, even though the condition may have been adequately treated by a less costly primary care physician. The gatekeeper approach also encourages patients to establish a relationship with a primary care physician, who is then in a position to manage the patient's care.

Example of a Health Plan With a PPO		
Benefit	In-network	Out-of-network
Deductible	$100	$300
Coinsurance	90%	70%
Routine care	$200 per calendar year	-0-
Mental health	80%	50%
Office visit	$10 co-pay; no deductible	70%

F I G U R E 1 6 – 2.   A health plan with a PPO.

The Future of Managed Care

Managed care has changed the organizational structure of medicine. To form risk-bearing organizations, physicians and hospitals are combining into new relationships. Hospitals are buying physician practices, and small-group or solo-practice physicians are combining into larger group practices. Some of these are forming public companies and raising investment capital to foster even more rapid growth in size and geographic scope. The size of medical practices is increasing and is expected to continue to increase in the foreseeable future.

The role of primary care physicians is changing relative to subspecialty physicians. In many managed care programs, primary care physicians act as patient care managers. Services authorized by these gatekeepers are covered, whereas those not authorized by the patient's primary physician may be denied or paid at a lower rate. Patients often join managed care organizations only if their primary care physician is a participant in a particular plan.

As coverage changes from an insured fee-for-service system to a managed care system with incentives to decrease the cost of patient care, employers and other purchasers have become much more interested in measuring the quality of care provided by managed care organizations. The very largest employers worked with leading HMOs to develop a report called HEDIS (Healthplan Employer Data Information Set). This uniform data set (reporting many indicators of health care quality, such as immunization rates and cesarean section rates) is now required of any HMO that wishes to serve the largest employers in the nation. HEDIS is upgraded continually and is being adopted by governmental agencies and many smaller employers as a prerequisite for a HMO to cover employees and governmental populations. This is only a start. Demands for increasingly sophisticated medical information will intensify.

The new demands to reduce the cost of care while measuring quality and improving it over time have led many organizations to develop increasingly sophisticated patient care protocols. These require documentation of efficacy and quality using information contained in patients' medical records. These demands are leading to increased automation of medical records. With automated medical records, a patient's medical history can be immediately available to any provider in virtually any location. Not only will it be easier to document quality and measure improvement over time, but a complete medical record that is available to any provider (with the patient's permission) will improve coordination among physicians and reduce illness. This alone can lead to substantial improvement in the quality of care.

Physicians are no longer isolated practitioners but are continuously involved with and accountable to community standards of practice. Protocols for patient care are becoming common and will change further as knowledge increases. Quality measurement and reporting will become more public, and the best medical care systems may be rewarded with higher patient volume for attaining the highest standards of patient care quality and satisfaction.

How does the progression of managed care affect you as a medical assistant? Managed care will continue to evolve and be refined. These trends in managed care will continue to affect individual physician practices as the face of health care continues to change. There will be increasing cooperative efforts by groups of physicians contracting together, with or without hospitals, carriers, or other parties. Family practice physicians will accept expanded responsibilities in managing the total care of a patient, managing specialist care and hospitalizations. These coalitions of providers will result in more uniform protocols of care and the application of outcome measurements in physician practices. The collection of data will become increasingly important to the practice. That collection and the management of the data will be a vital responsibility for you.

WORKERS' COMPENSATION

Employees in every state are covered by a workers' compensation program administered by the state. Workers' compensation benefits were developed to cover the expenses resulting from a work-related illness or injury.

ETHICAL TIP

The following scenario may occur in a medical office:

While you are filing an insurance claim, the physician tells you to "readjust" the laceration length from 4 cm to 9 cm. (The physician can bill more for a 9-cm laceration.) When you question him about this, he says, "Don't worry. The patient isn't paying the difference, the insurance company is, and they have plenty of money." How should you handle this situation?

Ethically and legally, you cannot change the length of a laceration on the medical record or the bill. This is fraud. You must explain to the physician that you are uncomfortable with this request and that you are ethically and legally bound to truthful billing. Any requests to alter or misrepresent the medical records or claims of a patient must be firmly denied.

A physician who operates in an unethical manner should be reported. If he or she is a partner in a practice, alert the other physicians about the suspect actions. You can also contact your state medical association, the American Medical Association, or the institutional review board at the hospital where your physician is affiliated.

PLEASE
DO NOT
STAPLE
IN THIS
AREA

CARRIER

HEALTH INSURANCE CLAIM FORM

PICA   PICA

1. MEDICARE   MEDICAID   CHAMPUS   CHAMPVA   GROUP HEALTH PLAN   FECA BLK LUNG   OTHER   1a. INSURED'S I.D. NUMBER   (FOR PROGRAM IN ITEM 1)

(Medicare #)   (Medicaid #)   (Sponsor's SSN)   (VA File #)   (SSN or ID)   (SSN)   (ID)

2. PATIENT'S NAME (Last Name, First Name, Middle Initial)   3. PATIENT'S BIRTH DATE MM DD YY   SEX   M   F   4. INSURED'S NAME (Last Name, First Name, Middle Initial)

5. PATIENT'S ADDRESS (No., Street)   6. PATIENT RELATIONSHIP TO INSURED   Self   Spouse   Child   Other   7. INSURED'S ADDRESS (No., Street)

CITY   STATE   8. PATIENT STATUS   Single   Married   Other   CITY   STATE

ZIP CODE   TELEPHONE (Include Area Code) ( )   Employed   Full-Time Student   Part-Time Student   ZIP CODE   TELEPHONE (INCLUDE AREA CODE) ( )

9. OTHER INSURED'S NAME (Last Name, First Name, Middle Initial)   10. IS PATIENT'S CONDITION RELATED TO: 11. INSURED'S POLICY GROUP OR FECA NUMBER

a. OTHER INSURED'S POLICY OR GROUP NUMBER   a. EMPLOYMENT? (CURRENT OR PREVIOUS)   YES   NO   a. INSURED'S DATE OF BIRTH MM DD YY   SEX   M   F

b. OTHER INSURED'S DATE OF BIRTH MM DD YY   SEX   M   F   b. AUTO ACCIDENT?   PLACE (State)   YES   NO   b. EMPLOYER'S NAME OR SCHOOL NAME

c. EMPLOYER'S NAME OR SCHOOL NAME   c. OTHER ACCIDENT?   YES   NO   c. INSURANCE PLAN NAME OR PROGRAM NAME

d. INSURANCE PLAN NAME OR PROGRAM NAME   10d. RESERVED FOR LOCAL USE   d. IS THERE ANOTHER HEALTH BENEFIT PLAN?   YES   NO   If yes, return to and complete item 9 a-d.

READ BACK OF FORM BEFORE COMPLETING & SIGNING THIS FORM.
12. PATIENT'S OR AUTHORIZED PERSON'S SIGNATURE I authorize the release of any medical or other information necessary to process this claim. I also request payment of government benefits either to myself or to the party who accepts assignment below.

SIGNED _____   DATE _____

13. INSURED'S OR AUTHORIZED PERSON'S SIGNATURE I authorize payment of medical benefits to the undersigned physician or supplier for services described below.

SIGNED _____

PATIENT AND INSURED INFORMATION

14. DATE OF CURRENT: ILLNESS (First symptom) OR INJURY (Accident) OR PREGNANCY(LMP)   MM DD YY   15. IF PATIENT HAS HAD SAME OR SIMILAR ILLNESS. GIVE FIRST DATE MM DD YY   16. DATES PATIENT UNABLE TO WORK IN CURRENT OCCUPATION   FROM MM DD YY   TO MM DD YY

17. NAME OF REFERRING PHYSICIAN OR OTHER SOURCE   17a. I.D. NUMBER OF REFERRING PHYSICIAN   18. HOSPITALIZATION DATES RELATED TO CURRENT SERVICES   FROM MM DD YY   TO MM DD YY

19. RESERVED FOR LOCAL USE   20. OUTSIDE LAB?   YES   NO $ CHARGES

21. DIAGNOSIS OR NATURE OF ILLNESS OR INJURY. (RELATE ITEMS 1,2,3 OR 4 TO ITEM 24E BY LINE)

1. |___.___| 3. |___.___|
2. |___.___| 4. |___.___|

22. MEDICAID RESUBMISSION CODE   ORIGINAL REF. NO.

23. PRIOR AUTHORIZATION NUMBER

24. A DATE(S) OF SERVICE		B Place of Service	C Type of Service	D PROCEDURES, SERVICES, OR SUPPLIES (Explain Unusual Circumstances)		E DIAGNOSIS CODE	F $ CHARGES	G DAYS OR UNITS	H EPSDT Family Plan	I EMG	J COB	K RESERVED FOR LOCAL USE
From MM DD YY	To MM DD YY			CPT/HCPCS	MODIFIER							
1												
2												
3												
4												
5												
6												

25. FEDERAL TAX I.D. NUMBER   SSN   EIN   26. PATIENT'S ACCOUNT NO.   27. ACCEPT ASSIGNMENT? (For govt. claims, see back)   YES   NO   28. TOTAL CHARGE $ 29. AMOUNT PAID $ 30. BALANCE DUE $

31. SIGNATURE OF PHYSICIAN OR SUPPLIER INCLUDING DEGREES OR CREDENTIALS (I certify that the statements on the reverse apply to this bill and are made a part thereof.)

SIGNED _____   DATE _____

32. NAME AND ADDRESS OF FACILITY WHERE SERVICES WERE RENDERED (If other than home or office)

33. PHYSICIAN'S, SUPPLIER'S BILLING NAME, ADDRESS, ZIP CODE & PHONE #

PIN#   GRP#

PHYSICIAN OR SUPPLIER INFORMATION

(APPROVED BY AMA COUNCIL ON MEDICAL SERVICE 8/88)   **PLEASE PRINT OR TYPE**   APPROVED OMB-0938-0008 FORM CMS-1500 (12-90),   FORM RRB-1500,   APPROVED OMB-1215-0055 FORM OWCP-1500,   APPROVED OMB-0720-0001 (CHAMPUS)

F I G U R E 16-3.   CMS-1500 claim form. This is the most commonly used insurance claim form. On the facing page you will find a detailed list explaining how to complete each line of the form. The form should be clearly and neatly typed.

Box Number	Information to Be Entered	Comments
1	Where the claim is being submitted	Confirm the patient's coverage and accuracy of your file information. A change in the patient's coverage will change how the claim is filed.
1a	The insured's ID number	Important: Enter the ID number of the insured (or employee), not the patient. This frequent filing error will cause rejection of the claim. The ID number is often the SSN, but check the ID card; the ID number may differ from the SSN.
2	Name of patient	The correct order (last, first, middle initial) is important.
3	Patient's date of birth	
4	Name of insured	Again, be sure to enter the name of the insured (or employee), not the patient.
5	Address of patient	
6	Patient's relationship to the insured	
7	Address of the insured	Check and update regularly.
8	Patient's status	Check and update frequently.
	Name of other insured	If the patient is covered under more than one plan, enter second plan here. For example, if a patient's claim is being submitted for her employer but she is also covered under her husband's plan, list the husband's name here.
9	Other insured's name	
9a	Other insured's policy or group number	Husband's policy number
9b	Other insured's date of birth	Husband's date of birth and sex
9c	Employer's name or school	Husband's employer
9d	Insurance plan name or program name	Husband's insurance company
10	Patient's condition	
10a	Patient's condition related to employment?	If yes, claim should be submitted to the workers' compensation carrier.
10b	Related to an auto accident?	If yes, the claim will not be processed unless a police report is attached.
10c	Other accident?	If yes, details of that accident must be attached.
11	Insured's policy group or FECA number	Very important. Some payers automatically return claim if group number is not indicated here. Group number is on patient's ID card.
11a	Insured's date of birth	Again, this is insured person, not patient.
11b	Employer's name	The insured's employer or school.
11c	Insurance plan name or program name	
11d	Is there another health plan?	If the patient is covered under more than one plan, check yes. If yes, the coverage will be coordinated between the plans covering the patient.
12	Patient's or authorized person's signature	This signature authorizes the release of information necessary to process the claim. If the patient's signature is in his or her file in your office, "signature on file" may be entered here.
13	Insured's signature	
14	Date of current	This is not date of service but the date the illness began or accident occurred.
15	If patient has had same or similar illness	If the patient has had this illness before, enter the date of the first occurrence.
16	Is patient unable to work	This information is required for the patient to receive disability payments.
17	Name of referring physician	If this patient was referred by another physician, enter name here.
17a	ID number of referring physician	EIN of the physician who referred the patient
18	Hospitalization dates	If the patient has been hospitalized for this illness or reason for visit, enter dates here.
20	Outside lab	If charges were incurred by an outside lab, check yes and enter amount. If not, check no.
21–24	Codes	Accuracy of this information determines accuracy of reimbursement. Thorough understanding of coding is essential for completing this section. See Chapters 17 and 18.
25	Tax ID number	Enter the EIN of the physician
26	Patient's account number	If you have assigned an account number to the patient, enter it here.
27	Accept assignment?	If you will accept assignment of the benefits, check yes. If not, check no.
28	Total charge	Enter the total amount of charges for this visit or service
29	Amount paid	Enter here any amount paid by the patient.
30	Balance due	Subtract any amount paid from the total charge and enter that amount here.
31	Signature of physician	
32	Name and address of facility where service was rendered	If the service was rendered outside of the physician's office, enter that address here.
33	Physician's billing name, address, zip code, and phone	This information will be used to mail reimbursement. Be sure it is current. The physician's billing name is required; may be a practice or corporate name.

SSN, Social Security number; FECA, Federal Employee Compensation Act; EIN, employer ID number.

In the event of a work-related illness or injury, claims submitted to the group or individual health benefits plan will be returned with instructions to file with the workers' compensation administrator, who determines the validity of the claim and reimburses accordingly. Because your practice will likely be taking care of the patient for both routine medical care and work-related illness or injury, it is important to determine at the time services are rendered whether the illness or injury is work-related and, if so, to account and file for those services separately.

You are responsible for knowing your state's workers' compensation regulations and procedures. Consult your state's office for workers' compensation or your state's designated claims administrator of the workers' compensation program for specific information.

FILING CLAIMS

If the provider requires patients to make full payment at the time of the visit, the physician may still submit a claim on the patient's behalf; however, the patient may need to submit claims to the claims administrator for reimbursement. Most providers accept assignment of benefits, however. To do this, the patient must give written authorization for the claims administrator to reimburse the physician for billed charges. As a medical assistant, you may be responsible for obtaining all necessary claims information from the provider and the patient and then submitting a claim for payment to the claims administrator.

The patient's ID card is a source of information necessary for complete and accurate claims submission. Keep a copy of this card in the patient's file and be sure to update it at least yearly and preferably at each visit, since the patient's employment and eligibility may change.

In addition, a patient may be covered by more than one group plan. For example, a patient may be covered both on an employer's group plan and as a dependent on his or her spouse's group plan. The primary plan—the one that pays first—is the plan provided by the patient's employer. Any unpaid amount is then considered for payment by the spouse's group plan, which is considered secondary. This is called **coordination of benefits**.

Dependent children may be covered under one or two parents' plans. Unless the plans state otherwise, the plan of the parent whose birthday occurs first each calendar year (not necessarily the oldest parent) is the primary plan. This is known as the **birthday rule**. This rule is commonly used by benefit plans and claims administrators to coordinate the benefits of dependent children covered by two plans. If the parents are legally separated or divorced, however, the primary plan is the plan of the parent who has custody or, in some instances, is subject to a court order or divorce decree.

After establishing the primary plan and the claims submission destination, you prepare the claim for filing. The CMS-1500 was developed by the American Medical Association to standardize an acceptable claim form for different plans and different claims administrators. It is the most widely used method of filing a health claim (Fig. 16-3). The CMS-1500 is accepted by most claims administrators, including Blue Shield, Medicare, Medicaid, and TRICARE/CHAMPVA.

Most plans include a clause that excludes coverage for a stated period (usually 12 months) for a condition, called a **preexisting condition**, that existed before the plan's effective date. For example, a patient with a diagnosis of depression before the effective date of his or her plan would be covered for all other conditions from the effective date forward but would not be covered for services related to the diagnosis or treatment of depression for the preexisting exclusion period (in this example, 12 months).

Many pieces of information are necessary for timely and efficient claims processing. The insurance company or managed care plan cannot process claims with incomplete or inaccurate information and will return them to the provider for completion, correction, and resubmission. This lengthens the time the provider must wait for reimbursement, making accurate claims submission a critical aspect of your responsibilities. The most frequent causes for denial of a claim and the corrective actions that you can take are as follows:

1. The patient cannot be identified as a covered person. Confirm that coverage information on file is current, including insurance company and group number, and that the Social Security number is accurate.
2. Coding is deemed inappropriate for services provided. Review provided services and recode as necessary.
3. The patient is no longer covered by the plan. Bill the patient for the charges. The patient may provide confirmation of new coverage.
4. The data are incomplete. Complete the required data and resubmit the claim.
5. Services are not covered by the plan. Bill the patient for the charges unless there is a basis for an appeal.

Electronic Claims Submission

Although some practices continue to submit claims on paper through the mail and most claims administrators continue to accept this practice, most practices submit at least their

WHAT IF

The reason for a rejection or denial of a claim is not clear. What should you do?

If the reasons for denial of the claim are not clear, telephone the claims administrator and ask for clarification. Be sure to have the claim and papers with you when you make the telephone call.

Medicare and Medicaid claims electronically. As of October 2003, HIPAA requires nearly all, with very few exceptions, to be submitted electronically. The physician's office computer software includes the CMS-1500 format for convenient and automated claims filing. With a computer and a modem, health claims can be filed immediately, reducing the time for the reimbursement cycle. You will need to work closely with your practice's software vendor to ensure compatibility with the insurance companies' computer systems

Several regional and national clearinghouses receive health benefits claims and electronically direct them to the appropriate claims administrators. This system allows you to file all electronic claims through one clearinghouse rather than filing separately with each claims administrator.

The system requires that all fields on the electronic claim form be completed and in the required format. If the claim is incomplete or inaccurate, the system will not transmit the form. You can complete or correct the form online, allowing the form to be transmitted. Claims submitted electronically that do not meet the plan's criteria will be rejected by the clearinghouse and must be submitted by mail. In addition, claims that are particularly complicated or cumbersome, have attachments, or are otherwise unsuitable for electronic submission should be filed on paper with the claims administrator.

Explanation of Benefits

When the claims administrator settles a claim, that is, makes a payment, an **explanation of benefits (EOB)** is issued to both the provider and the patient (Fig. 16-4). The EOB tells how the payment was made, including deductible and coinsurance information. Some EOBs include information for several claims on several patients that may have been processed during a particular period. You may be responsible for checking the EOB to be sure that all payments made to the physician are for the appropriate procedures and in the correct amounts.

POLICIES IN THE PRACTICE

Managed care contracts and negotiated services affect many practice policies. You must be knowledgeable and precise in administering practice policies, especially with regard to assignment of benefits and balance billing.

Assignment of benefits is a service the practice may provide. If assignment of benefits is accepted, the patient's signature must be on file, authorizing the claims administrator to reimburse the physician. Managed care plans require physicians to accept assignment, although many physicians do not accept assignment for non–managed care patients. If assignment is not accepted, the patient is responsible for paying all charges and filing a claim with the claims administrator for reimbursement directly to the patient.

Balance billing is prohibited by most managed care contracts. The physician cannot charge the patient the difference between the physician's usual charge and the allowable charge specified by the contract. For other types of plans, however, balance billing is not restricted, and the practice may bill the patient for any difference between the physician's charged fee and the amount allowable by the plan according to **usual, customary, and reasonable (UCR)** tables.

A few national firms provide UCR data to claims administrators who use that information to determine the maximum amount payable for any given service (the **plan maximum**). UCR data are calculated from surveys of the amount physicians charge for each service or procedure. That amount is calculated on a geographic basis to reflect regional variations in health care costs. Non–managed care plan physician reimbursements are based on a maximum allowable charge as specified in the UCR data. The physician may choose to bill the patient for the difference between the amount charged and the UCR amount.

Explanation of Benefits

Employee Name: Joe Doe   Date of Service: 6-15-2004
SSN: 555-55-5555 (1)   Provider: Dr. Jones
Group No. 55555   Provider TIN: 35-5555555
Patient Name: Joe Doe

Date of Service (2)	Comment Code (3)	Amount of Charge (4)	Amount Allowed (5)	At (6)	Amount Paid (7)
6-15-2004	57	87.00	82.00	80%	65.60

Total (8)	65.60
Less Deductible (9)	25.00
Amount Paid (10)	40.60

Payable to: Dr. Jones
               Address

Comment Code:
57 - The amount charged exceeds Usual and Customary

FIGURE 16-4.

Reading the EOB (Explanation of Benefits)

After the claim has been processed, an EOB will be issued. Although each payer has his or her own EOB format, this sample EOB illustrates the key points included in an EOB. The terms used may differ, and the formats differ widely.

(1) The top section typically includes the name of the employee and the Social Security number (SSN) or other identifying number, as well as the name of the patient, the group number, the date of service and provider name, and employer identification number (EIN) (Federal identification number assigned to the physician).

(2) The date of service is included and is shown as the date the service is actually rendered, not the date that was posted or billed.

(3) The Comment Code is a tool used on many EOBs to indicate a coded comment that is either on the bottom as exceeding "Usual and Customary." In this situation, the claim will be processed on the Usual and Customary amount. The difference between the amount charged ($87.00) and the amount allowed ($82.00) is $5.00. Unless the physician is contractually bound by an agreement with a managed care plan that forbids the practice of balance billing, that difference of $5.00 may be billed to the patient.

(4) Amount of Charge shows the amount that the physician's office billed for the service.

(5) Amount Allowed shows the amount of charge upon which the claim processing will be based (in this example, it is the amount of Usual and Customary).

(6) This indicates the percentage of co-insurance payable by the plan.

(7) Amount Paid shows the amount payable by the plan after co-insurance has been applied, but is not necessarily the amount that is actually paid (see #10).

(8) The Total shows the total submitted and payable after the claim has been processed.

(9) After all processing on the claim has been completed, any deductible is applied. In this example, Joe still had $25.00 to be applied to his annual deductible. Therefore, $25.00 is deducted from the amount paid and the actual reimbursement to the physician is $40.60. The amount applied to the deductible should be billed to the patient.

(10) The amount actually reimbursed.

CHAPTER SUMMARY

Most patients in the physician's office have some type of health care plan. Types of plans include group, individual, and government-sponsored health benefits, such as Medicare or Medicaid. Many physicians have contracts with managed care plans, such as HMOs and PPOs. Each type of plan has certain requirements regarding eligibility and claims submission, and you must be knowledgeable about those requirements. In particular, one of your primary duties is to file claims in a timely and accurate manner to ensure appropriate reimbursement for the physician. When filing claims, you must be careful to maintain patient confidentiality and to avoid fraud.

Critical Thinking Challenges

1. Jane and Joe are married, and both are employed and cover themselves and their two children on their health plans. Jane's birthday is July 23 and Joe's birthday is August 9. Joe is 2 years older than Jane. When claims are submitted for their two children, which spouse's plan is primary? Show which plan is primary and secondary for each family member.

	Primary	Secondary
Jane		
Joe		
Child 1		
Child 2		

2. The requirements for Medicaid vary from state to state. How do you determine the Medicaid requirements for your particular state? Locate the name, address, and telephone number of your state's resource.

Answers to Checkpoint Questions

1. With insured benefits, a monthly premium is paid by the employer or organization to an insurance company. The insurance company in turn is obligated to pay for any eligible health benefits. In contrast, self-funded benefits are provided to eligible employees or members by their employer or organization. Claims are processed by a professional claims administrator, such as a third-party administrator.

2. Persons enrolled in Social Security are automatically enrolled in Medicare Part A, which covers hospital services and expenses only, and Medicare Part B, which covers the physician's charges for inpatient or outpatient care as well as diagnostic services. Part B does not cover routine examinations, well care, routine immunizations, or cosmetic surgery. Part A is provided at no charge to Social Security recipients, and Part B caries a monthly fee. If Part B is not wanted, it must be declined.

3. Medicaid patients receive a new ID card each month.

4. The four elements of managed care programs are precertification of hospital admissions (often also called utilization management or **utilization review**—UM or UR), approved referrals, network, and assignment of benefits.

5. In a traditional insurance system, the individual, not the insurer, seeks medical services and thereby incurs the expense. An HMO promises to provide covered services rather than pay for them.

6. A primary difference between a HMO and a PPO is that patients with PPO coverage can see any physician of their choice and receive benefits; they simply have an incentive in the form of higher benefits when they see an in-network provider.

 Websites

Medicare for providers and recipients
   www.CMS.gov
Medicare for recipients
   www.Medicare.gov
Blue Cross Blue Shield
   www.bluecares.com
Local medical review policies
   www.LMRP.net
American Medical Association
   www.AMA-assn.org
All government agencies, federal and state
   www.firstgov.gov

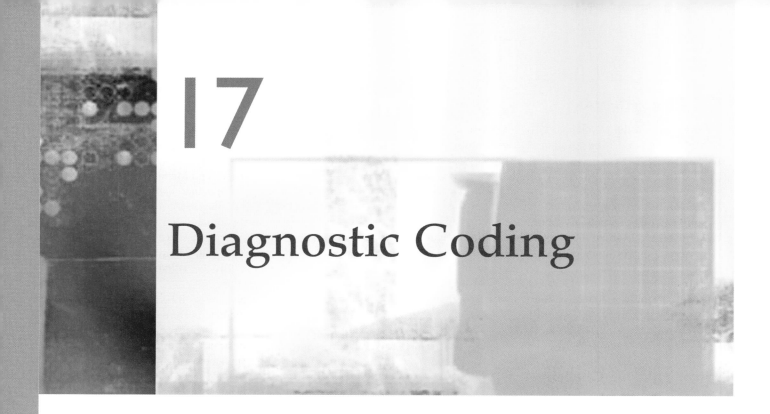

17

Diagnostic Coding

CHAPTER OUTLINE

ROLE DELINEATION COMPONENTS

GENERAL: Legal Concepts
- Perform within legal and ethical boundaries

ADMINISTRATIVE: Administrative Procedures
- Perform basic administrative medical assisting functions

- Obtain reimbursement through accurate claims submission

ADMINISTRATIVE: Practice Finances
- Perform procedural and diagnostic coding

CHAPTER COMPETENCIES

LEARNING OBJECTIVES

Upon successfully completing this chapter, you will be able to:

1. Spell and define the key terms
2. Name and describe the coding system used to describe diseases, injuries, and other reasons for encounters with a medical provider
3. Give four examples of ways diagnostic coding is used
4. Describe the relationship between coding and reimbursement
5. Explain the format of the ICD-9-CM
6. List the steps in identifying a proper code
7. Name common errors in outpatient diagnostic coding

KEY TERMS

advance beneficiary notice
audits
conventions
cross-reference
E-codes
eponym

etiology
inpatient
International Classification of Diseases, Ninth Revision, Clinical Modification

late effects
main terms
medical necessity
outpatient

primary diagnosis
service
specificity
V-codes

CODING, AT ITS SIMPLEST, is the assignment of a number to a verbal statement or description. Medical coding is anything but simple. The *International Classification of Diseases, Ninth Revision, Clinical Modification* is a system for transforming verbal descriptions of disease, injuries, conditions, and procedures into numeric codes. It is essential that the physician and medical assistant work together to achieve accurate documentation, code assignment, and reporting of diagnoses and procedures. Use of standardized codes makes it easier for third-party payers to understand the reason for the patient's encounter with the health care provider and increases the likelihood of timely processing of claims and prompt payment when appropriate.

Coding is a way to standardize medical information for purposes such as collecting health care statistics, performing a medical care review, and indexing medical records. It is also used for health insurance claims processing (see Chapter 16). Because coding is the basis for reimbursement, it is imperative that you code patient visits accurately and precisely. Incorrect, insufficient, or incomplete coding on claims forms can lead to nonpayment for the physician as well as incorrect information in the insurance companies databases, which may effect the patient's insurability. For example, if a patient complaining of chest pain is coded as having "acute myocardial infarction" instead of "chest pain rule out myocardial infarction," that patient may be incorrectly labeled as having heart disease. The Current Procedural Terminology (CPT) codes, used to report services and procedures performed by health care providers, determine the amount paid (see Chapter 18), but the code assigned to the diagnosis or reason for the service or procedure proves the medical necessity for the services or procedures so that claims are paid. The third-party payer needs to know why the service was performed to assess **medical necessity**. Medical necessity means the procedure or service would have been performed by any reasonable physician under the same or similar circumstances. The ICD-9 diagnostic codes convey this information. Is a chest radiograph medically necessary for a patient who has gout? No, but it may be necessary for a patient with acute bronchitis. The diagnosis justifies the procedure.

Since Medicare considers certain procedures medically necessary only at certain intervals, having the patient sign an **advance beneficiary notice** (ABN) will ensure payment of treatments and procedures that will likely be denied by Medicare. An example is a Pap smear for a low-risk woman, which will be paid for once every 2 years. If the physician considers it *not* to be medically necessary, but the patient wants a Pap test, the patient will be responsible for payment and must sign an ABN.

Checkpoint Question

I. What is meant by medical necessity?

DIAGNOSTIC CODING

International Classification of Diseases, Ninth Revision, Clinical Modification (ICD-9-CM) is a statistical classification system based on the *International Classification of Diseases, Ninth Revision* (ICD-9), developed by the World Health Organization (WHO). The CM, which stands for clinical modification, addresses the intent of these codes to describe the clinical picture of the patient. These codes are much more precise than those needed for statistical grouping and trend analysis found in the ICD-9 and used in hospital coding.

The ICD-9-CM, which is now mandated by Health Insurance Portability and Accountability Act of 1996 (HIPAA), is the most current and comprehensive statistical classification of its kind. Containing more than 10,000 diagnostic codes and 1,000 procedure codes, it consists of three volumes:

- Volume 1: Tabular List of Diseases
- Volume 2: Alphabetic Index of Diseases
- Volume 3: Tabular List and Alphabetic Index of Procedures

The ICD-9-CM code books are available from several publishers, and although the presentation of the material may be different, the content must be the same. Depending on the publisher, these three volumes may be included within one book. In the physician's office, only Volumes 1 and 2 are used. Volume 3 is used by hospitals.

The diagnostic classification systems in Volumes 1 and 2 are maintained by a federal government agency, the National Center for Health Statistics (NCHS); the procedure classification (Volume 3) is maintained by the Centers for Medicare & Medicaid Services (CMS), the federal agency that regulates health care financing. All three volumes are updated regularly, with codes being added, revised, and sometimes deleted. Changes in the ICD-9-CM are published by NCHS and CMS with the approval of WHO. Both the American Health Information Management Association (AHIMA) and the American Hospital Association (AHA) advise and assist in keeping the classification system current.

Checkpoint Questions

2. What are the three volumes of the ICD-9-CM system?
3. What organization must approve any changes in the disease classification system?

Inpatient Versus Outpatient Coding

There is a big difference between coding medical claims in a hospital or other inpatient facility and coding for the physician in an outpatient medical practice. The systems and references used to assign codes to third-party claims is only one difference in the coding requirements and practices of the physician and the inpatient medical facility. Volumes 1 and 2 of the ICD-9 CM are used to report the diagnostic code that justifies physician services whether those services are provided in the office or in the hospital. Hospital coders use Volume 3 to report inpatient procedures, services, and supplies, as well as the reasons for the services.

The UB-92 (uniform bill) is used by institutions to report inpatient admissions and outpatient and emergency department services and procedures. These charges are for nursing services, building maintenance, and all costs associated with running the institution. These charges do not include physician services. The CMS-1500 (universal claim form) is used to report physician services, whether the physician sees the patient in the office, emergency department, hospital, or nursing home, because even though the physician may have been in the hospital, it is his **service** for which we are billing in the medical office.

The term **outpatient** is used to describe patients treated in the following places:

- Health care provider's office
- Hospital clinic
- Emergency department
- Hospital same-day surgery unit or ambulatory surgical center that releases the patient within 23 hours
- Observation status in a hospital (the patient is admitted for a short time for observation only, and the physician bills for his or her service during the stay)

The term **inpatient** refers to a patient who is admitted to the hospital for treatment with the expectation that the patient will remain in the hospital for 24 hours or more.

Hospital coders code only services provided by the hospital and hospital employees. Coders who are employed by the physician practice are concerned with the services provided by the physician no matter where the services are provided. For example, the hospital room, meals, and laboratory testing that a patient receives are billed and coded by the hospital billing department. The daily visits the physician makes to the patient are billed and coded by the physician's office.

Since the focus of this textbook is medical assisting, we concentrate on outpatient coding.

Checkpoint Question

4. Define the terms *inpatient* and *outpatient*.

ICD-9-CM: THE CODE BOOK

Coding books are available from several publishers, such as Ingenix and Medicode. The AMA (American Medical Association) Press also publishes coding books and training materials. The classification system is also available as part of a medical software package; one of these packages is CodeManager from the AMA. Although each publisher offers special features and helpful aids, the format remains the same. Some coders become comfortable with certain special features (i.e., AMA publications are spiral bound) and, since the content is the same, can choose among the various publications based on organization, illustrations, tabs, bullets, and color coding.

To become an expert medical coder, you need general knowledge of human anatomy and medical terminology. In addition to using a code book, you will need reference materials such as a medical dictionary and/or medical dictionary software.

To ensure accurate coding, update your ICD-9-CM coding books and software as needed. (Updates and addenda can be purchased from the publisher of your coding book.) You must update codes on superbills (preprinted bills listing a variety of procedures) or any other forms you use. Experts have estimated that millions of dollars in reimbursement have been lost because an incorrect code was taken from a standardized form that had not been updated. New codes are published each October, and most third-party payers require their use after January 1.

Checkpoint Question

5. How often is the ICD-9-CM updated?

Volume 1: Tabular List of Diseases

Volume 1 contains the classification of diseases (conditions) and injuries by code numbers. Figure 17-1 shows the table of contents from this volume. These 17 chapters cover groupings of diseases and injuries by **etiology** or cause (e.g., infectious diseases) and by anatomic system (e.g., digestive, respiratory). Each chapter has a heading or title (e.g., 16, Symptoms, Signs, and Ill-defined Conditions (780–799). Following the title in parentheses is the range of three-digit categories included in that chapter. In each chapter you will find subtitles in large type followed by a range of three-digit categories in parentheses (e.g., 16, Symptoms (780–789). These sections describe general disease. Three-digit codes followed by a title, the category codes, describe specific diseases (e.g., 780, general symptoms). The fourth digit further breaks down the category (e.g., 780.0, alteration of consciousness), and the fifth digit is the highest level of definition (e.g., 780.01, coma). Figure 17-2 is a sample page from the tabular list showing each level of classification.

Volume 1 is always used to code a diagnosis to its highest definition. This volume tells you how many digits are required to code a diagnosis correctly and to a level that most third-party payers will accept. Volume 1 also includes five appendices, outlined in Box 17-1.

Supplementary Classifications

Supplementary classifications in Volume 1 include V- and E-codes.

V-Codes. **V-codes**, which range from V01 to V82, provide a means of indexing the reason for hospital or physician office care for other than current or genuine illness, such as a history of illness, immunizations, or live-born infants according to type of birth. An example of a V-code is V10.04, used for a person with a personal history of a malignant neoplasm of the stomach. Because of this history, it would be

TABLE OF CONTENTS

F I G U R E   1 7 – 1 .   Table of contents from ICD-9-CM, Volume I.

important for this patient to have regular checkups. You would not want to code the visit 230.2, neoplasm of the stomach, because that would imply the patient has the malignant neoplasm at this visit. The ICD-9-CM offers a variety of codes for HIV testing. The patient who is simply afraid carries one V-code, while the patient who has known exposure carries another. V-codes may be used alone if no disease diagnosis is appropriate or as the second or third code to help better explain the reason for the visit.

E-Codes. **E-codes**, which range from E800 to E999, are used to classify external causes of injuries and poisoning. Specificity is limited to the fourth digit level. E-codes are used in conjunction with codes in Chapters 1 to 17. They help to provide information of interest to industrial medicine, insurance underwriters, national safety programs, public health agencies, and others concerned with causes of injuries (e.g., auto accidents, accidents caused by heavy industrial machinery). These codes do not affect reimbursement.

☑5ᵗʰ 780.5 Sleep disturbances

> **EXCLUDES**   *that of nonorganic origin (307.40-307.49)*

780.50 Sleep disturbance, unspecified

780.51 Insomnia with sleep apnea

> DEF: Transient cessation of breathing disturbing sleep.

780.52 Other insomnia

> Insomnia NOS
>
> DEF: Inability to maintain adequate sleep cycle.

780.53 Hypersomnia with sleep apnea

> DEF: Autonomic response inhibited during sleep; causes insufficient oxygen intake, acidosis and pulmonary hypertension.

780.54 Other hypersomnia

> Hypersomnia NOS
>
> DEF: Prolonged sleep cycle.

780.55 Disruptions of 24-hour sleep-wake cycle

> Inversion of sleep rhythm
> Irregular sleep-wake rhythm NOS
> Non-24-hour sleep-wake rhythm

780.56 Dysfunctions associated with sleep stages or arousal from sleep

780.57 Other and unspecified sleep apnea

780.59 Other

☑4ᵗʰ 780 General symptoms

☑5ᵗʰ 780.0 Alteration of consciousness

> **EXCLUDES**   *coma:*
>
> > *diabetic (250.2-250.3)*
> > *hepatic (572.2)*
> > *originating in the perinatal period (779.2)*

780.01 Coma

> DEF: State of unconsciousness from which the patient cannot be awakened.

780.02 Transient alteration of awareness

> DEF: Temporary, recurring spells of reduced consciousness.

780.03 Persistent vegetative state

> DEF: Persistent wakefulness without consciousness due to nonfunctioning cerebral cortex.

780.09 Other

> Drowsiness   Stupor
> Semicoma   Unconsciousness
> Somnolence

780.1 Hallucinations

> Hallucinations: Hallucinations:
> > NOS   olfactory
> > auditory   tactile
> > gustatory
>
> **EXCLUDES**   *those associated with mental disorders, as functional psychoses (295.0-298.9)*
> > *organic brain syndromes (290.0-294.9, 310.0-310.9)*
> > *visual hallucinations (368.16)*
>
> DEF: Perception of external stimulus in absence of stimulus; inability to distinguish between real and imagined.

☑5ᵗʰ 779.8 Other specified conditions originating in the perinatal period

779.81 Neonatal bradycardia

> **EXCLUDES**   *abnormality in fetal heart rate or rhythm complicating labor and delivery (763.81-763.83)*
> > *bradycardia due to birth asphyxia (768.5-768.9)*

779.82 Neonatal tachycardia

> **EXCLUDES**   *abnormality in fetal heart rate or rhythm complicating labor and delivery (763.81-763.83)*

779.89 Other specified conditions originating in the perinatal period

FIGURE 17–2.   Sample page from ICD-9-CM, Volume 1, showing categories, subheadings, and so on.

ICD-9-CM APPENDICES

The following five appendices are found in Volume I
- Appendix A: Morphology of Neoplasms

    This appendix is used in conjunction with Chapter 2 in ICD-9-CM when coding neoplasms. It lists the five-digit alphanumeric codes used to identify the morphology of a neoplasm. For example, in the morphology code M8070/3, the 8070 indicates the morphology is squamous cell carcinoma. The /3 indicates that it is the primary site.
- Appendix B: Glossary of Mental Disorders

    Alphabetic list of mental disorders, including detailed descriptions of each disease.
- Appendix C: Classification of Drugs by American Hospital Formulary Service (AHFS) List Number and the ICD-9-CM Equivalents

    This appendix lists the AHFS list number (e.g., 24:04 for cardiac drugs) and the ICD9-CM code number for each one (e.g., 24.04 cardiac drugs would be equivalent to category 972.9, the ICD9-CM category "other and unspecified agents primarily affecting the cardiovascular system").
- Appendix D: Classification of Industrial Accidents by Agency

    This includes codes that can be used as a supplement to describe types of equipment or materials that may be responsible for an industrial accident or illness.
- Appendix E: List of Three-Digit Categories

    This is a list of all three-digit categories in ICD-9-CM.

    Appendices A through D are not recognized by most government programs, such as Medicare and Medicaid. As previously mentioned, ICD-9-CM has other uses, however, and you may find that you need the appendices to track such things as disorders treated.

Volume 2, Section 3, has a separate index to access E-codes, the Alphabetic Index to External Causes of Injury and Poisoning.

 Checkpoint Question

6. List four reasons for using E-codes.

Volume 2: Alphabetic Index to Diseases

Volume 2, the alphabetic index to diseases, contains many diagnostic terms that do not appear in Volume 1. For example, itch, barbers, beard, and scalp are all listed under *Itch* in

Volume 2. In Volume 1 they are all listed under code 110.0. The index is arranged by condition. Always check all indentations in the index under the condition to ensure that you have the one most appropriate to the diagnosis you intend to code.

The alphabetic index is organized into three sections:

- Section 1, Alphabetic Index to Diseases and Injuries, is organized by **main terms** printed in boldface type. Section 1 is used for reporting the reason for patient encounters for most insurance claims. Following the main term is a code number, which refers you to the tabular listing (Volume 1). You must not accept this number as the correct code without a **cross-reference** or check of the tabular list. Never code directly from the alphabetic index. This could result in an incomplete or incorrect coding assignment. For example, if you have a patient with fluid overload and you look under fluid, it may seem logical to code the first code under fluid, which is abdomen, 789.5, but your patient is generally retaining fluid. If you use the alphabetic index only, you do not know that the correct code is 276.6, fluid overload, which excludes ascites, 789.5, and localized edema, 782.3. Box 17-2 lists several exceptions to the main term rule.
- Section 2, Table of Drugs and Chemicals, includes an extensive listing of drugs, chemical substances, and toxic agents. It also shows E-codes and American Hospital Formulary Service (AHFS) list numbers, which are in the table under the main term *drug*.
- Section 3, Alphabetic Index to External Cases of Injuries and Poisonings, leads you to codes that describe circumstances of injuries, accidents, and violence. These codes are not used for medical diagnoses. Main entries in this section usually are a type of accident or violence (e.g., assault, fall, collision). These codes can supplement the diagnostic code, but they should never be used alone or as principal diagnosis codes. E-codes

EXCEPTIONS TO THE MAIN TERM RULE

Keep in mind the following exceptions to this rule:
1. Obstetric conditions may be found under the main terms *delivery*, *pregnancy*, and *puerperal*.
2. Complications of medical or surgical procedures can be found under *complication*.
3. Late effects are found under *late effect*.
4. V-codes are found under main entries such as *admissions*, *examination*, *history of observation*, *problem* (with), *status*, *vaccination*, *encounter for*, and *follow-up*.

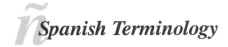

Spanish Terminology

¿Qué son todo estos números?	What are all these numbers? Is that my bill?
No, estos números se utilizan para su seguro.	No, these numbers are used for your insurance.
Estos se llaman los números de codificación.	These are called coding numbers.

are frequently used with these codes. For example, a person who fractured a tibia in a fall off a sidewalk curb would be given a code from chapter 17, Volume 1, in the ICD-9-CM for the injury (e.g., fracture of tibia, closed, is 823.80), and an additional code, E880.0, indicates that the accident was a fall off a sidewalk curb.

Checkpoint Question

7. What are V-codes used for?

Volume 3: Inpatient Coding

Volume 3, the Tabular List and Alphabetic Index of Procedures, is used in inpatient facilities and is based on anatomy, not surgical specialty. There are no alphabetic characters in these procedure codes. The codes are two-digit categories with a maximum of two decimal digits where necessary. Most refer to surgical procedures, and the rest cover miscellaneous diagnostic and therapeutic procedures. An example of a procedure code is 31.61, larynx laceration suture. Volume 3 is used for inpatient coding only.

LOCATING THE APPROPRIATE CODE

Box 17-3 outlines CMS guidelines for diagnostic coding. These are explained next.

Using the ICD-9-CM Conventions

Figure 17-3 lists the conventions used in the ICD-9-CM indexes. **Conventions** are rules that apply to the assignment of the ICD-9 codes. They are found throughout both the Index to Diseases and the Tabular List and include general notes using specific terms, cross-references, abbreviations, punctuation marks, symbols, typeface, and format. They direct and guide the coder to the appropriate code and should be strictly adhered to. Each publisher uses these same conventions, and many add more to assist coders in providing the most complete and accurate reason for the encounter. For example, when you locate the word itch, you will find "see pruritus," the medical term for severe itching. This is a helpful tool for coders who are unfamiliar with medical terminology.

Box 17-3

CMS DIAGNOSTIC CODING GUIDELINES

CMS defines specific guidelines that provide the basic knowledge necessary to apply the correct ICD-9 codes. Although these guidelines were developed for use in submitting government claims, most insurance companies have also adopted them. Many variations exist among the private insurance companies; therefore, care must be taken in recognizing the different requirements for each third-party payer. Most coders operate on the assumption that the government regulations are the strictest, and following those guidelines will satisfy most third-party payers.

1. Identify each service and procedure, or supply with an ICD-9 code from 001.0 through V82.9 to describe the diagnosis, symptom, complaint, condition, or problem.
2. Identify services or visits for circumstances other than disease or injury, such as follow-up care after chemotherapy, with V-codes provided for this purpose.
3. Code the reason for the visit first and code any coexisting conditions that affect the treatment of the patient for that visit or procedure as supplementary information. Do not code a diagnosis that is no longer applicable.
4. Code to the highest degree of specificity. Carry the numeric code to the fourth or fifth digit when necessary.
5. Code a chronic diagnosis as often as it is applicable to the patient's treatment.
6. When only ancillary services are provided, list the appropriate V-code first and the problem second. For example, if a patient is receiving only physical therapy, list the V-code first, followed by the code for the condition on line 24E on the CMS-1500 form.
7. For ambulatory or outpatient surgical procedures, code the diagnosis applicable to the procedure. If the postoperative diagnosis is different from the preoperative diagnosis, use the postoperative diagnosis.

Conventions

Braces { }   These are used in the Tabular List to connect a series of terms to a common stem. Each term on the left of the brace is incomplete without one of the terms to the right of the bracket.

Brackets [ ]   Brackets enclose synonyms, alternate wording, or explanatory phrases

Colon :   A colon is used after an incomplete term that needs one or more of the modifiers that follow to make it assignable to a given category

Parentheses ( )   Parentheses enclose supplementary words that may be present or absent in the statement of a disease or procedure, without affecting the code number to which it is assigned.

NEC (not elsewhere classifiable)   Alerts the coder that the specified form of the condition is classified differently. Codes following NEC should be used only when the coder lacks the information necessary to code the term in a more specific category.

NOS (not otherwise specified)   The coder should continue to look for a more specific code

Note   Used to define terms and give coding instructions. Found most often with list of fifth digits.

"Includes"   Indicates separate terms as adjectives that further modify sites and conditions or to further define or give examples of the content of a certain category.

"Excludes"   A box with "excludes" in italics draws the reader's attention to instructions that direct the coder to the proper code. This convention is found in the Tabular List.

"See," "See Also," and "See Category"   Direct the coder to other terms or sections that should be considered. ALWAYS follow these instructions.

"Use additional code"   This directs the coder to add another code to further explain and give the third-party payer a better understanding of a diagnosis.

"Code First Underlying Disease"   This direction is used in the tabular list when a reason for an encounter results from another disorder. The coder is instructed to indicate the underlying disease that caused the current problem or symptom that brought the patient to the office.

Index to Disease Example

478.1   Other diseases of nasal cavity and sinuses

Abscess
Necrosis   } Of nose (septum)
Ulcer

422.92   Septic myocarditis
Myocarditis, acute or subacute:
Pneumococcal
Staphylococcal
Use additional code to identify infectious organism [e.g., Staphylococcus 041.1]

See above example 478.1 (septum) may or may not be present in the diagnosis given.

Infection
Streptococcal NEC 041.00
Group
A 041.01
B 041.02

As soon as the bacterium is identified, code for specific infection.

At the time of the service, it has not been established whether a neoplasm is benign or secondary, for example. Remember, you are coding for a date of service with the information documented for that date of service.

INCLUDES	Allergic rhinitis (nonseasonal) 477 Allergic rhinitis (seasonal) Hay fever
EXCLUDES	Allergic rhinitis with asthma (bronchial) (493.0)

Itch (see also Pruritus) 698.9

See 422.92 examples above.

362.72   Retinal dystrophy in other systemic disorders and syndromes
Code first underlying disease, as:
Bassen-Kornzweig syndrome (272.5)
Refsum's disease (356.3)

F I G U R E   1 7 – 3 .   Conventions used in ICD-9.

Main Term

When trying to locate a diagnosis with more than one word, look first under the main term or condition. Often, a diagnosis may be an **eponym** (e.g., Ménière's disease or syndrome). These terms can be found under the main term *disease* or *syndrome*. In the diagnosis breast cyst, the main term is *cyst*. Find the condition, not the location. Remember the exceptions to the rules of using the main term.

Fourth and Fifth Digits

In many instances, a fourth digit has been added to a category to provide more detail, or **specificity**. These are subcategory codes. Some codes also have a fifth digit because of the need to code to a higher specificity. For example, diabetes mellitus is category 250. It is necessary to use one of the fourth-digit subcategories to indicate the specific complications that may accompany the diabetes and then add a fifth digit to indicate whether the diabetes is insulin dependent or non–insulin dependent. Those codes requiring a fifth digit are identified in both Volumes 1 and 2. Incomplete coding here affects reimbursement and causes data errors. Figure 17-4 shows samples of fifth-digit classifications from the ICD-9-CM, Volumes 1 and 2. The code 807.1 tells the third-party payer that the patient was seen for an open fracture of a rib. The fifth digit is added to describe how many ribs. A patient who fractured two ribs would be assigned the code 807.12. This gives a more thorough picture of the patient's problem and enables the payer to determine whether the treatment is medically necessary.

Primary Codes

In outpatient coding, the **primary diagnosis** is simply the patient's chief complaint or the reason the patient sought medical attention today. It may be a routine follow-up visit, or there may be a new problem. The primary code is listed first on the CMS-1500 (Box 17-4).

When More Than One Code Is Used

In many cases, more than one code is used for a single patient visit. When patients have more than one diagnosis, it is necessary to convey an accurate picture of the patient's total condition. For example, an elderly patient may have the following diagnoses listed each time she visits the doctor: degenerative arthritis, type II diabetes mellitus, macular degeneration, hypertension, and pernicious anemia. If any of these conditions is related to or affects her treatment, they should be listed as supplementary information. If she visits the doctor because she has influenza and her other diagnoses are not addressed at the visit, it is not necessary to list all the diagnoses given. The primary diagnosis is her reason for coming to the office (symptoms of influenza). But the fact that she is diabetic will affect her treatment and makes her visit medically necessary. Multiple codes should be sequenced with the proper service or procedure code on the proper line of the CMS-1500. Figure 17-5 shows the proper sequencing for another patient's CMS-1500. On line 1 of Section 24 on the CMS-1500 you place the code and charge for the visit. In Block 24E, the diagnosis code for the ankle injury appears first because that is what brought the patient to the office today. One Line 2 of 24A, the laboratory work is listed but is also referenced to the diagnosis on Line 21, Item 2, which is the proper code for the patient's diabetes; this is referenced to Item 2 on Line 24. If the patient did not have diabetes, the laboratory work would not be considered reasonable for a patient with an ankle injury. If this procedure were not followed, the labo-

---

Box 17-4

STEPS IN LOCATING A DIAGNOSTIC CODE

1. Choose the main term within the diagnostic statement.
2. Locate the main term in Volume 2.
3. Refer to all notes and conventions under the main term.
4. Find the appropriate indented subordinate term.
5. Follow any relevant instructions, such as "see also."
6. Confirm the selected code by cross-referencing to Volume 1. Make sure you have added any fourth or fifth digits necessary.
7. Assign the code.

---

ratory work would be seen as medically unnecessary, and the physician would not be reimbursed.

Late Effects

Late effects are symptoms or conditions arising from an acute illness. The effects are present after treatment for the acute illness or injury has ended. Proper coding sequence requires that you list the code number identifying the residual or current condition first, with the code number identifying the cause or original illness or injury listed second. Key words used in the patient's medical records defining late effects include late, due to an old injury, due to a previous illness/injury, due to an illness or injury occurring a year or more ago, sequela of . . . , as a result of . . . , resulting from . . . , and so on. Patients who are status post cerebrovascular accident (CVA) may have residual effects from their original stroke, for example, and may have a diagnosis of left hemiparesis as a result of CVA 3 years ago. Figure 17-6 is a sample listing of a late effect from the ICD-9-CM.

LEGAL TIP

Remember that the ICD-9 codes placed on the CMA-1500 are confidential and should be protected as much as any other medical information. Forms left lying in common areas in the office may be seen by other patients. Keep printers and copies of these forms in a private place and share the diagnosis codes only with those who need the information to carry out their duties. Patients have the right to keep their diagnoses private.

INJURY AND POISONING   807–808.49

☑4ᵗʰ **807 Fracture of rib(s), sternum, larynx, and trachea**

The following fifth-digit subclassification is for use with codes 807.0-807.1:

0 **rib(s), unspecified**
1 **one rib**
2 **two ribs**
3 **three ribs**
4 **four ribs**
5 **five ribs**
6 **six ribs**
7 **seven ribs**
8 **eight or more ribs**
9 **multiple ribs, unspecified**

☑5ᵗʰ **807.0 Rib(s), closed**   `MSP`
☑5ᵗʰ **807.1 Rib(s), open**   `MSP`
    807.2 Sternum, closed   `MSP`
    DEF: Break in flat bone (breast bone) in anterior thorax.

    807.3 Sternum, open   `MSP`
    DEF: Break, with open wound, in flat bone in mid anterior thorax.

    807.4 Flail chest   `MSP`
    807.5 Larynx and trachea, closed   `MSP`
        Hyoid bone   Trachea
        Thyroid cartilage

A   **807.6 Larynx and trachea, open**   `MSP`

Fracture — *continued*
  multiple — *continued*
    skull, specified or unspecified bones, or
      face bone(s) with any other bone(s) —
      continued

> *Note — Use the following fifth-digit subclassification with categories 800, 801, 803, and 804:*
>
> 0   *unspecified state of consciousness*
> 1   *with no loss of consciousness*
> 2   *with brief [less than one hour] loss of consciousness*
> 3   *with moderate [1-24 hours] loss of consciousness*
> 4   *with prolonged [more than 24 hours] loss of consciousness and return to pre-existing conscious level*
> 5   *with prolonged [more than 24 hours] loss of consciousness, without return to pre-existing conscious level*
>
> *Use fifth-digit 5 to designate when a patient is unconscious and dies before regaining consciousness, regardless of the duration of the loss of consciousness*
>
> 6   *with loss of consciousness of unspecified duration*
> 9   *with concussion, unspecified*

    with
      contusion, cerebral 804.1 `5ᵗʰ`
      epidural hemorrhage 804.2 `5ᵗʰ`
      extradural hemorrhage 804.2 `5ᵗʰ`
      hemorrhage (intracranial) NEC
        804.8 `5ᵗʰ`
      intracranial injury NEC 804.4 `5ᵗʰ`
      laceration, cerebral 804.1 `5ᵗʰ`
      subarachnoid hemorrhage 804.2 `5ᵗʰ`
B   subdural hemorrhage 804.2 `5ᵗʰ`

F I G U R E   1 7 – 4 .   Samples of fifth-digit classifications from ICD-9-CM. (A) Volume 1. (B) Volume 2.

PLEASE
DO NOT
STAPLE
IN THIS
AREA

███████████
███████████
███████████
███████████

CARRIER →

□□ PICA **HEALTH INSURANCE CLAIM FORM** PICA □□

1. MEDICARE	MEDICAID	CHAMPUS	CHAMPVA	GROUP HEALTH PLAN	FECA BLK LUNG	OTHER	1a. INSURED'S I.D. NUMBER (FOR PROGRAM IN ITEM 1)
☒ (Medicare #)	□ (Medicaid #)	□ (Sponsor's SSN)	□ (VA File #)	□ (SSN or ID)	□ (SSN)	□ (ID)	000-00-0000A

2. PATIENT'S NAME (Last Name, First Name, Middle Initial)
Naomi A Dishman

3. PATIENT'S BIRTH DATE MM 04 DD 14 YY 24 SEX M □ F ☒

4. INSURED'S NAME (Last Name, First Name, Middle Initial)
Same

5. PATIENT'S ADDRESS (No., Street)
405 Carolina Ave

6. PATIENT RELATIONSHIP TO INSURED
Self □ Spouse □ Child □ Other □

7. INSURED'S ADDRESS (No., Street)

CITY
Danville STATE VA

8. PATIENT STATUS
Single □ Married ☒ Other □

CITY STATE

ZIP CODE 24540 TELEPHONE (Include Area Code) (434) 555-5555

Employed □ Full-Time Student □ Part-Time Student □

ZIP CODE TELEPHONE (INCLUDE AREA CODE) ( )

9. OTHER INSURED'S NAME (Last Name, First Name, Middle Initial)
NONE

10. IS PATIENT'S CONDITION RELATED TO:

11. INSURED'S POLICY GROUP OR FECA NUMBER

a. OTHER INSURED'S POLICY OR GROUP NUMBER

a. EMPLOYMENT? (CURRENT OR PREVIOUS)
□ YES ☒ NO

a. INSURED'S DATE OF BIRTH MM DD YY SEX M □ F □

b. OTHER INSURED'S DATE OF BIRTH MM DD YY SEX M □ F □

b. AUTO ACCIDENT? PLACE (State)
□ YES ☒ NO

b. EMPLOYER'S NAME OR SCHOOL NAME

c. EMPLOYER'S NAME OR SCHOOL NAME

c. OTHER ACCIDENT?
☒ YES □ NO

c. INSURANCE PLAN NAME OR PROGRAM NAME

d. INSURANCE PLAN NAME OR PROGRAM NAME

10d. RESERVED FOR LOCAL USE

d. IS THERE ANOTHER HEALTH BENEFIT PLAN?
□ YES □ NO If yes, return to and complete item 9 a-d.

READ BACK OF FORM BEFORE COMPLETING & SIGNING THIS FORM.
12. PATIENT'S OR AUTHORIZED PERSON'S SIGNATURE I authorize the release of any medical or other information necessary to process this claim. I also request payment of government benefits either to myself or to the party who accepts assignment below.

SIGNED Signature of File DATE 052803

13. INSURED'S OR AUTHORIZED PERSON'S SIGNATURE I authorize payment of medical benefits to the undersigned physician or supplier for services described below.

SIGNED _____

14. DATE OF CURRENT: MM 05 DD 28 YY 03 ◀ ILLNESS (First symptom) OR INJURY (Accident) OR PREGNANCY(LMP)

15. IF PATIENT HAS HAD SAME OR SIMILAR ILLNESS. GIVE FIRST DATE MM DD YY

16. DATES PATIENT UNABLE TO WORK IN CURRENT OCCUPATION MM DD YY FROM TO MM DD YY

17. NAME OF REFERRING PHYSICIAN OR OTHER SOURCE

17a. I.D. NUMBER OF REFERRING PHYSICIAN

18. HOSPITALIZATION DATES RELATED TO CURRENT SERVICES MM DD YY FROM TO MM DD YY

19. RESERVED FOR LOCAL USE

20. OUTSIDE LAB? $ CHARGES
□ YES □ NO

21. DIAGNOSIS OR NATURE OF ILLNESS OR INJURY. (RELATE ITEMS 1,2,3 OR 4 TO ITEM 24E BY LINE)

1. 845.03
2. 250.00
3. L___.___
4. L___.___

22. MEDICAID RESUBMISSION CODE ORIGINAL REF. NO.

23. PRIOR AUTHORIZATION NUMBER

24. A DATE(S) OF SERVICE			B	C	D	E	F	G	H	I	J	K
From MM DD YY	To MM DD YY		Place of Service	Type of Service	PROCEDURES, SERVICES, OR SUPPLIES (Explain Unusual Circumstances) CPT/HCPCS MODIFIER	DIAGNOSIS CODE	$ CHARGES	DAYS OR UNITS	EPSDT Family Plan	EMG	COB	RESERVED FOR LOCAL USE
05 28 03	05 28 03		11		99213	1	100 00	1				
05 28 03	05 28 03		11		82947	2	25 00	1				

25. FEDERAL TAX I.D. NUMBER SSN EIN
54-0000000 □ □

26. PATIENT'S ACCOUNT NO.
1234

27. ACCEPT ASSIGNMENT? (For govt. claims, see back)
☒ YES □ NO

28. TOTAL CHARGE
$ 125 00

29. AMOUNT PAID
$

30. BALANCE DUE
$ 125 00

31. SIGNATURE OF PHYSICIAN OR SUPPLIER INCLUDING DEGREES OR CREDENTIALS (I certify that the statements on the reverse apply to this bill and are made a part thereof.)

SIGNED _____ DATE _____

32. NAME AND ADDRESS OF FACILITY WHERE SERVICES WERE RENDERED (If other than home or office)

33. PHYSICIAN'S, SUPPLIER'S BILLING NAME, ADDRESS, ZIP CODE & PHONE #
JOSEPH G NORTH, MD
1111 GRAYSON STREET
DANVILLE VA
PIN# GRP#

PATIENT AND INSURED INFORMATION

PHYSICIAN OR SUPPLIER INFORMATION

(APPROVED BY AMA COUNCIL ON MEDICAL SERVICE 8/88) **PLEASE PRINT OR TYPE** APPROVED OMB-0938-0008 FORM CMS-1500 (12-90), FORM RRB-1500, APPROVED OMB-1215-0055 FORM OWCP-1500, APPROVED OMB-0720-0001 (CHAMPUS)

FIGURE 17–5. Sample CMS-1500 claim form indicating proper sequencing.

LATE EFFECTS OF INJURIES, POISONINGS, TOXIC EFFECTS, AND OTHER EXTERNAL CAUSES (905-909)

Note: These categories are to be used to indicate conditions classifiable to 800-999 as the cause of late effects, which are themselves classified elsewhere. The "late effects" include those specified as such, or as sequelae, which may occur at any time after the acute injury.

✓4ᵗʰ 905 Late effects of musculoskeletal and connective tissue injuries

905.0   Late effect of fracture of skull and face bones
Late effect of injury classifiable to 800-804

905.1   Late effect of fracture of spine and trunk without mention of spinal cord lesion
Late effect of injury classifiable to 805, 807-809

905.2   Late effect of fracture of upper extremities
Late effect of injury classifiable to 810-819

905.3   Late effect of fracture of neck of femur
Late effect of injury classifiable to 820

905.4   Late effect of fracture of lower extremities
Late effect of injury classifiable to 821-827

905.5   Late effect of fracture of multiple and unspecified bones
Late effect of injury classifiable to 828-829

905.6   Late effect of dislocation
Late effect of injury classifiable to 830-839

905.7   Late effect of sprain and strain without mention of tendon injury
Late effect of injury classifiable to 840-848, except tendon injury

905.8   Late effect of tendon injury
Late effect of tendon injury due to:
  open wound [injury classifiable to 880-884 with .2, 890-894 with .2]
  sprain and strain [injury classifiable to 840-848]

905.9   Late effect of traumatic amputation
Late effect of injury classifiable to 885-887, 895-897
    EXCLUDES   *late amputation stump complication (997.60-997.69)*

A

Late

Late — *continued*
  effect(s) (of) — continued
    tuberculosis — *continued*
      genitourinary (conditions classifiable to 016) 137.2
      pulmonary (conditions classifiable to 010-012) 137.0
      specified organs NEC (conditions classifiable to 014, 017-018) 137.4
    viral encephalitis (conditions classifiable to 049.8, 049.9, 062-064) 139.0
    wound, open
      extremity (injury classifiable to 880-884 and 890-894, except .2) 906.1
      tendon (injury classifiable to 880-884 with .2 and 890-894 with.2) 905.8
      head, neck, and trunk (injury classifiable to 870-879) 906.0

B

FIGURE 17-6.   Sample section of late effects in ICD-9-CM. (A) Volume 1. (B) Volume 2.

Coding Suspected Conditions

In the inpatient setting, coders list conditions after the patient's testing is complete. In other words, they are coding with complete information. In outpatient settings, however, the coder reports the reason for the patient visit as it occurs. When filing claims, the coder is limited by the information and documentation on hand at the time of the patient visit. If at the end of the visit the diagnosis is not confirmed, the physician may indicate "rule out," "suspected," or "probable." For example, a patient who comes in complaining of headache may be sent for magnetic resonance imaging (MRI) of the head because the physician suspects a serious disorder. On the patient's encounter form, the physician may list the diagnosis as "rule out brain tumor." It is not accurate to code the visit as brain tumor before it is confirmed by MRI. On this first visit to the physician's office, the reason for being seen is headache. The patient's symptom

WHAT IF

You need to code a condition described as acute, chronic, or both. What code should you use?

When a particular condition is described as both acute and chronic, code it according to the subentries in the alphabetic index (Volume 2) for the condition. If there are separate entries listed for acute, subacute, and chronic, use both codes. The first code listed should be for the acute condition, the reason the patient came to the office today. Respiratory and orthopedic conditions tend to be acute and chronic. That is, a patient with emphysema will always have underlying symptoms of progressive disease, but during the spring, pollen may aggravate the condition and cause acute breathing problems.

(headache) is the only confirmed reason for the encounter at this point. On the second visit to the doctor, the MRI has confirmed a glioma in the frontal lobe. For the second and all subsequent visits, glioma is coded as the reason for the encounter. Figure 17-2 shows a page from the ICD-9-CM that includes many of the symptom codes.

Checkpoint Question

8. Before a definitive diagnosis is made, what is coded?

Documentation Requirements

As discussed throughout this chapter, you should choose the code assigned to any given claim for a service or procedure based on the documentation available in the patient's record at the time of the service. An **audit** is conducted by the government, a managed care company, and a health care organization to determine compliance and to detect fraud. Remember, if it's not in the chart, it did not happen. Auditors verify the codes used based on information recorded in the chart on the date of service.

THE FUTURE OF DIAGNOSTIC CODING: *INTERNATIONAL CLASSIFICATION OF DISEASES, TENTH REVISION*

A new edition of the ICD, the *International Classification of Diseases, Tenth Revision* (ICD-10), is scheduled to be introduced sometime between 2003 and 2005. The WHO is responsible for revising the ICD to improve the quality of data input into clinical databases. The ICD-10-CM will include

more codes and will be used by every type of health care provider for all encounters, including hospice and home health care. The new codes are alphanumeric, but the format of the index is similar to the ICD-9-CM. Two new chapters relating to disorders of the eye and the ear are being added to the ICD-10. Computer software will be revised, and the ICD-9-CM code books will be obsolete.

Checkpoint Question

9. List two reasons for a chart audit.

CHAPTER SUMMARY

Medical outpatient diagnostic coding involves the use of numbers to describe diseases, injuries, and other reasons for seeking medical care. ICD-9-CM provides an index to report and track diseases. Diagnostic coding is linked to reimbursement because it assures that the physician's service or procedure was medically necessary. As a medical assistant, you must understand the format and guidelines for assigning a code or reason for each encounter, treatment, and/or service.

Critical Thinking Challenges

Tom Barksdale has been seen by the physician for controlled non–insulin-dependent type 2 diabetes mellitus for about 10 years. While being seen for a routine check of his blood sugar, he complains of numbness and tingling in his left lower leg and foot. An x-ray of both legs is performed, since poor circulation in the extremities can be a complication of diabetes. The x-ray confirms the diagnosis of peripheral neuropathy.

1. Which ICD-9 code should be listed with the office visit?
2. Which code indicates the reason for the x-ray?
3. Which code should be placed on the CMA-1500 first as the primary diagnosis or reason for the visit?

Answers:

1. 250.60
2. 337.1
3. 250.60

Answers to Checkpoint Questions

1. Medical necessity means a particular service or procedure is reasonable.
2. The three volumes of ICD-9-CM are Volume 1, the Tabular List of Diseases; Volume 2, the Alphabetic

Index of Diseases; and Volume 3, the Tabular List and Alphabetic Index of Procedures.

3. The World Health Organization must approve any changes in the ICD-9-CM system.

4. Inpatient refers to a patient who is admitted to the hospital for a stay anticipated to be longer than a day. An outpatient is one who is seen in the physician's office or for 1-day surgery and will stay in the inpatient facility for less than 24 hours.

5. ICD-9-CM is updated annually in October.

6. E-codes are used to provide information to (1) industry, (2) insurance underwriters, (3) national safety programs, and (4) public health agencies and others concerned with injuries and poisonings.

7. V-codes are used to report reasons for receiving services other than illness.

8. Before a definitive diagnosis is assigned to a patient, services must be coded with the patient's symptoms at the time he or she was seen.

9. Chart audits are conducted to assess compliance and to detect fraud.

    ## Websites

World Health Organization
www.who.int
Health and Human Services
www.hhs.gov
Centers for Medicare & Medicaid
www.cms.gov
American Health Information Management Association
www.ahima.org
American Hospital Association
www.aha.org

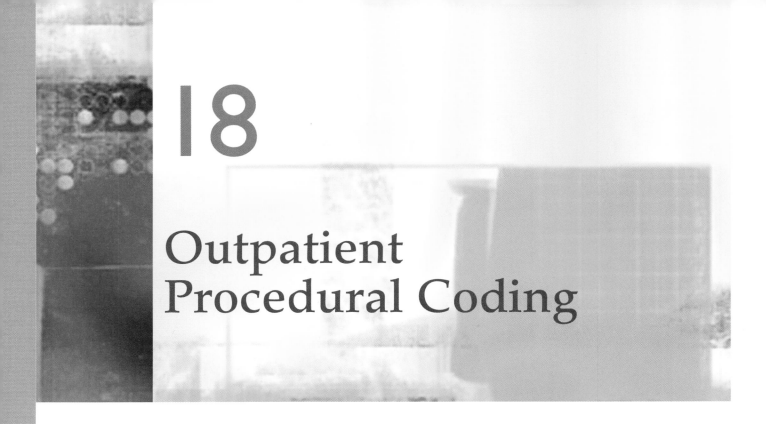

18

Outpatient Procedural Coding

CHAPTER OUTLINE

ROLE DELINEATION COMPONENTS

GENERAL: Legal Concepts
- Perform within legal and ethical boundaries

ADMINISTRATIVE: Administrative Procedures
- Perform basic administrative medical assisting functions.

- Obtain reimbursement through accurate claims submission.

ADMINISTRATIVE: Practice Finances
- Perform procedural and diagnostic coding.

CHAPTER COMPETENCIES

LEARNING OBJECTIVES

Upon successfully completing this chapter, you will be able to:

1. Spell and define the key terms
2. Explain the format of Current Procedural Terminology (CPT-4) and its use
3. Explain the Healthcare Common Procedure Coding System (HCPCS) and level 2 and 3 codes
4. Explain what diagnostic related groups (DRGs) are and how they are used to determine Medicare payments
5. Discuss the goals of resource-based relative value system (RBRVS)
6. Describe the relationship between coding and reimbursement

KEY TERMS

Current Procedural Terminology	Healthcare Common Procedure Coding System	modifiers	resource-based relative value scale
descriptor		outlier	upcoding
diagnostic related group	key component	procedure	

As discussed in Chapter 17, coding is a way to standardize medical information for purposes such as collecting health care statistics, performing a medical care review, and indexing medical records. It is also used for health insurance claims processing (see Chapter 16 for more information). Because coding is linked to reimbursement, you must code accurately and precisely. Incorrect, insufficient, or incomplete coding on claims forms can lead to improper reimbursement for the physician as well as recording and possibly passing along inaccurate patient information.

PHYSICIAN'S CURRENT PROCEDURAL TERMINOLOGY

Physician's **Current Procedural Terminology** (CPT) is a comprehensive listing of medical terms and codes for the uniform coding of procedures and services provided by physicians. First published in 1966 by the American Medical Association (AMA), CPT initially focused mainly on surgical procedures, with a limited number of other codes to describe medical, radiology, laboratory, and pathology procedures. New editions were published in 1970, 1973, and 1977. The fourth edition, CPT-4, contains more than 7000 new codes. Although there has not been a major revision of the CPT since 1977, CPT-4 is updated annually, with the newest version available each December.

CPT-4 contains a listing of all current U. S. Food and Drug Administration–approved physicians' procedures and services. The AMA developed it in collaboration with various other health organizations. In the early 1980s, Congress decided to use CPT-4 to code all physicians' procedures and services for Medicare patients. The aim of CPT-4 was to establish a way in which interested parties would know what procedures and services had been provided to the patient without reading a lengthy report. For example, the CPT-4 allows insurance companies to:

- Communicate easily with one another
- Compare reimbursable amounts for procedures
- Speed claims processing

CPT-4 is a system of five-digit numeric codes and corresponding meanings, as illustrated in Figure 18-1, a sample page from the CPT-4 book.

Every code means something unique and is used only to describe a specific **procedure**, service, or medical supply provided by physicians to their patients. This is true for inpatients and outpatients. Codes and descriptions are updated, revised, or changed yearly. If your physician's office uses a superbill or preprinted routing slip that lists the procedures performed, you must update this form yearly and work with your software vendor to update your computer software. The CPT-4 code selected will be placed on the CMS-1500 universal claim form in Section 24, Box D, along with any modifiers used. Figure 18-2 is a sample universal claim form showing the proper placement of codes for consultation and chest radiography.

The CPT-4 book is divided into six major sections:

1. Evaluation and management
2. Anesthesia
3. Surgery
4. Radiology
5. Pathology and laboratory
6. Medicine

Reading Descriptors

When reading a code's **descriptor**, or description, you will read up to the semicolon and then look down for any indentations using the same words before the semicolon. For example, the code 25065 carries the following descriptor: Biopsy, soft tissue of forearm and/or wrist; superficial. The CPT code for a soft tissue biopsy of the forearm and/or wrist is 25065. If the tissue sample was taken from the superficial skin, 25065 is used. Look at the indented line that bears the code 25066. Because it is indented, you must look at the lines above to find the category. Then read up to the semicolon. The description of this code is Biopsy, soft tissue of forearm and/or wrist; deep superficial or intramuscular. Use of the indentation and the semicolon saves space and keeps the CPT books from becoming too long.

Guidelines

Each section begins with its own specific guidelines and a listing of specific procedures and services applicable in that field. The guidelines contain definitions, explanatory notes, a listing of the previously unlisted procedures found in that particular section, directions on how to file a special report, modifiers for use in that particular section, and definitions to assist the coder.

Unlisted Procedures and Special Reports

Occasionally, a physician will perform a service that is not listed in the CPT-4 book. CPT provides unlisted codes at the beginning of each section for use when an unusual, variable, or new procedure is done. When an unlisted code is used, however, you must submit a copy of the procedure report with the claim. This special report should include the following information:

1. Definition or description of the nature, extent, and need for the procedure
2. Time, effort, and equipment necessary to provide the service
3. Complexity of symptoms
4. Final diagnosis
5. Pertinent physical findings
6. Diagnostic and therapeutic procedures
7. Concurrent problems
8. Follow-up care

27556—27615   Surgery / Musculoskeletal System

(27554 has been deleted. To report, see 27550, 27552, 27556, 27557, 27558)

27556   Open treatment of knee dislocation, with or without internal or external fixation; without primary ligamentous repair or augmentation/ reconstruction

27557   with primary ligamentous repair

27558   with primary ligamentous repair, with augmentation/reconstruction

27560   Closed treatment of patellar dislocation; without anesthesia

(For recurrent dislocation, see 27420-27424)

27562   requiring anesthesia

(27564 has been deleted. To report, see 27560, 27562, 27566)

27566   Open treatment of patellar dislocation, with or without partial or total patellectomy

Manipulation

27570*   Manipulation of knee joint under general anesthesia (includes application of traction or other fixation devices)

Arthrodesis

▲**27580**   Arthrodesis, knee, any techniques

Amputation

27590   Amputation, thigh, through femur, any level;

27591   immediate fitting technique including first cast

27592   open, circular (guillotine)

27594   secondary closure or scar revision

27596   re-amputation

27598   Disarticulation at knee

Other Procedures

27599   Unlisted procedure, femur or knee

Leg (Tibia and Fibula) and Ankle Joint

Incision

27600   Decompression fasciotomy, leg; anterior and/or lateral compartments only

27601   posterior compartment(s) only

27602   anterior and/or lateral, and posterior compartment(s)

(For incision and drainage procedures, superficial, see 10040-10160)

(For decompression fasciotomy with debridement, see 27892-27894)

27603   Incision and drainage, leg or ankle; deep abscess or hematoma

27604   infected bursa

▲**27605***   Tenotomy, percutaneous, Achilles tendon (separate procedure); local anesthesia

27606   general anesthesia

27607   Incision (eg, osteomyelitis or bone abscess) leg or ankle

(27608 has been deleted)

▲**27610**   Arthrotomy, ankle, including exploration, drainage, or removal or foreign body

(27611 has been deleted)

▲**27612**   Arthrotomy, posterior capsular release, ankle, with or without Achilles tendon lengthening

(See also 27685)

Excision

27613   Biopsy, soft tissue of leg or ankle area; superficial

▲**27613**   deep (subfascial or intramuscular)

(For needle biopsy of soft tissue, use 20206)

27615   Radical resection of tumor (eg, malignant neoplasm), soft tissue of leg or ankle area

FIGURE 18–1.   Sample page from CPT 2003.

Evaluation and Management Codes

Evaluation and management (E/M) codes are five-digit numbers that begin with the number 9. These are the most frequently used codes. E/M codes describe various patient histories, examinations, and decisions physicians must make in evaluating and treating patients in various settings (e.g., office, outpatient, hospital). In essence, the E/M codes address what the physician does when interacting with the patient. For this reason, the physician's documentation must meet standards so the physician and coder (medical assistant) can decide which code to use for a specific patient–physician encounter.

To code the services described in the E/M section, you must be sure that the patient's medical record indicates that **key components** are present. Two of three key components are required for established patients and three of three for new patients. These components are the elements that make up the visit. All E/M codes contain the following components:

- History
- Physical examination
- Medical decision making
- Counseling
- Coordination of care

FIGURE 18−2.   Sample insurance claim form for consultation and chest radiography.

- Nature of presenting problem
- Time

History, physical examination, and medical decision making are key components for a visit. The others are contributing elements.

Four classifications of histories and physical examinations are described in CPT-4. These include the following:

- Problem-focused
- Expanded problem-focused

- Detailed
- Comprehensive

Table 18-1 describes these classifications in greater detail. The provider must pick one of these based on information provided by the physician and documented in the patient's record.

The third key component, medical decision making, is defined in CPT-4 as one of the following:

- Straightforward
- Low complexity

Table 18-1 HISTORY AND PHYSICAL EXAMINATIONS

The physician or provider must select which history and physical examination code to use. You, however, should have a basic understanding of each category. It is important to note that there are separate codes for each category and separate codes for both new and established patients.

Type of History and Physical Examination	Patient Problems and Physician Time Required	Examples
Problem focused	Patient problems are self-limited and minor. Physician time: usually 10 minutes	• 9-month-old patient with diaper rash • 40-year-old patient with sunburn • 18-year-old patient with poison ivy • 60-year-old patient with a routine blood pressure check
Expanded problem focused	Patient problems are mild to moderate. Physician time: between 15–20 minutes	• 55-year-old patient with recurrent urinary tract infections • 16-year-old patient with chronic asthma presents with a cold • 76-year-old patient with osteoarthritis • 56-year-old patient with a stomach ulcer
Detailed	Patient problems are moderate to severe. Physician time: usually 30 minutes	• 18-year-old patient with first Pap smear and contraceptive education • 67-year-old patient with new onset of dysuria • 18-month-old patient with delayed motor skill development. • 34-year-old patient with diabetes requiring insulin dose changes
Comprehensive	Patient problems are moderate to severe. Physician time: usually 45 minutes	• 36-year-old patient with infertility • 8-year-old patient with new onset of diabetes • 65-year-old patient with history of left-sided weakness and confusion

• Moderate complexity
• High complexity

Medical decision making refers to the kinds of things the physician must do to establish a diagnosis for the patient (e.g., determine the management options available, the amount and complexity of the data to be reviewed, the risk of complications, or other problems, such as worsening of the illness or death). To qualify for a particular decision-making level, the physician must meet or exceed two of the three elements for an established patient and all three for a new patient.

Time spent with a patient (e.g., counseling or coordinating care) is sometimes the key component in determining E/M codes. When time spent with the patient is more than 50% of the typical time for the visit, time becomes the deciding factor in choosing an E/M code. For example, if a physician spends an additional 15 minutes counseling a patient in what would normally be only a 10-minute expanded problem-focused history and physical examination, the counseling was more than 50% of the typical 25-minute face-to-face time. The appropriate E/M code is one with a 25-minute time frame (10 minutes and an extra 15 minutes for counseling).

There are other special considerations regarding E/M codes. Initial hospital care codes can be used only by the admitting physician. All other physicians must use consultation codes for a first visit and then subsequent hospital care codes. Box 18-1 outlines the difference between a consultation and a referral. Emergency department service codes are to be used only when the service is rendered in a 24-hour hospital-based facility that specializes in providing treatment of unscheduled events.

Checkpoint Question

1. To code for a service in the E/M section, two of the three key components must be present for an established patient, and all three must be present for a new patient. What are the three key elements?

Anesthesia Codes

Anesthesia codes are five-digit codes that begin with 0. Anesthesia codes are divided by anatomic site and by specific type of procedure. For example, head, neck, and thorax

IS IT A REFERRAL OR A CONSULTATION?

There are four subcategories of consultations: office, initial inpatient, follow-up inpatient, and confirmatory (in any setting). Each subcategory has specific reporting instructions. When a physician asks another provider to offer an opinion or advice regarding evaluation and management of a specific problem, the second provider becomes a consultant for the patient. The initial encounter is coded as a consultation, and the documentation must support the encounter. A letter should accompany the patient seeing a consulting physician, and the advising physician should send a letter back to the patient's primary physician outlining the findings. If the consulting physician takes over part or all of the patient's care, follow-up or subsequent visits are coded as regular subsequent visits. A confirmatory consultation is considered a second opinion, and the physician should offer only an opinion or advice. A confirmatory consultant does not take over the treatment of the patient. A referral is defined as passing on a patient to another physician. Referrals are coded as new patients, not consultations. Consider this scenario: A 17-year-old girl sees her family physician for recurrent sore throats. When the family physician realizes that the girl probably needs a tonsillectomy, the patient is *referred* to an otorhinolaryngologist for evaluation and possible surgery. The patient has been referred to the surgeon, who will take over that part of her care. When she has recovered from the procedure, she is discharged from the care of the surgeon and returns to her family physician for continued care.

In another example, a patient may be seen by an orthopedic surgeon for arthritis. When it is determined that the patient's problem may be rheumatoid arthritis, he may be sent to a rheumatologist for consultation. The rheumatologist advises the orthopedic surgeon on a treatment plan, but the orthopedic surgeon continues to see the patient and carries out that plan. Written communications between the two physicians are kept in the chart. The significant difference between a consultation and a referral is whether the patient's treatment is transferred to another physician for that problem.

are anatomic sites, and the codes in each section represent the specific procedure, such as plastic repair of cleft lip. Medical assistants in an anesthesiology practice code anesthesia procedures provided in the hospital setting, even though the office is an outpatient facility.

Two types of **modifiers** (letters or numbers added to a code to add detail to the code) are used in the anesthesia section. One type is the standard modifier that is found in all sections of CPT. The other type is the physical status modifier, a two-digit code beginning with the letter P and ending in a number from 1 to 6. These physical status modifiers indicate the patient's condition at the time of anesthesia and the corresponding complexity of services (e.g., P1 indicates a normal, healthy patient and P5 indicates a patient who is not expected to survive without the procedure).

Surgery Codes

Surgery codes begin with numbers 1 through 6. You need to be aware of the following elements, which are discussed in the guidelines of the surgery section.

Unstarred Codes

The CPT-4 codes in this section that do not have a star (*) refer to codes that include a surgical package. The code that follows identifies the surgical package including normal, uncomplicated follow-up care. The surgical package means that local infiltration, metacarpal, metatarsal, or digital block or topical anesthesia, the operation itself, and normal uncomplicated follow-up care are all included in the code that covers the operation itself.

If there is no star next to the code, it means that you cannot bill separately for preoperative and postoperative components.

The Centers for Medicare & Medicaid Services (CMS) has defined the surgical package for Medicare recipients somewhat differently. According to CPT-4, no complications or problems related to the surgery are included in the surgical package. If additional procedures are performed to correct or alleviate these problems, they should be coded separately. According to CMS, however, complications that do not require a revisit to the operating room are included in the price of surgery.

Some insurance carriers have a set number of follow-up days that is consistent for all unstarred surgical services. Check with your carrier to learn what these are so you can bill for the additional office, outpatient, or hospital visits.

Starred Codes

Codes with a star (*) are for the surgical service itself. The surgical package does not apply. You should code any preoperative anesthesia and postoperative components separately. Figure 18-1 includes several starred codes, for example, of repair—simple superficial wounds of scalp, neck, axilla, external genitalia, and so forth:

12001*—2.5 cm or less
12002*—2.6 cm to 7.5 cm
12004*—7.6 cm to 12.5 cm
12005—12.6 cm to 20.10 cm (notice no star)

If a patient came in for routine follow-up care of a scalp wound coded 12001, 12002, or 12004, the coder could also code for both office visits (99212). There is a corresponding fee for this service. If, however, the patient was returning for routine follow-up care for a wound repair that was originally coded 12005, the code 99024 (postoperative follow-up visit) could be used, but there is no charge for this because the service was already included in the surgical package. Remember, 12005 is not a starred procedure. Third-party payers have different rules about what constitutes a surgery package, so the coder must check with the relevant third-party payers.

Integumentary System

This section has codes for which a measurement is necessary. It is important that both the size of the defect and the size of the specimen be measured before they are sent to the laboratory. All excisions listed in the integumentary section include simple closure.

Repairs

CPT-4 defines three types of repairs: simple, intermediate, and complex. Repairs should be measured and recorded in centimeters to be coded appropriately.

Cast Reapplication

You cannot assign the same code for cast replacement as you did for the original cast application because the code for replacement does not include treatment of the fracture, as the original cast application code did; it, therefore, carries a lower reimbursement rate.

Multiple Procedures Furnished on the Same Day

Unless these are part of the overall service, they should be coded separately and placed on the claims form in order from major to minor.

Checkpoint Question

2. What items are included in a surgical package?

Radiology Codes

The radiology section of CPT-4 is divided into the following four subsections:

- Diagnostic radiology/diagnostic imaging
- Diagnostic ultrasound
- Radiation oncology
- Nuclear medicine

WHAT IF

You need help coding a chart. What should you do?

If you have a question about coding, never guess; find the correct answer. For example, you can ask colleagues, the office manager, or the physician. Insurance companies may have a help line. If you are a member of a professional health care organization, network with fellow members. The American Medical Association (AMA) publishes various books to assist in ICD and CPT coding. The AMA also has a magazine, *CPT Assistant*, that is written by CPT experts. It contains many articles designed to make coding easier. In addition, this magazine will keep you current with updates and changes. For further information on the *CPT Assistant* or other works the AMA publishes on coding, call 800-621-8335 or visit the website at **www.amapress.org**.

All radiology codes are five-digit numbers that begin with 7. They are generally arranged by anatomic site, from the top of the body to the bottom. Many radiology codes indicate the number of views for a particular study. Obviously, the facility must be reimbursed for film, developer, and the radiology technologist's time and service.

Some radiological tests require the administration of a contrast medium that enhances the image. The descriptors for such tests specify "with contrast" or "without contrast." "With contrast" refers to contrast medium that is given intravascularly. If the contrast medium is given orally or rectally, you use the code "without contrast."

If a physician performs the procedure and supervises and interprets a procedure (e.g., injects contrast medium and then supervises and interprets), two codes should be used. A written report in the patient's medical record is necessary for billing these codes. The code for the procedure can be found in the surgery, medicine, or radiology section, and the code for supervision and interpretation is found in the radiology section. If two physicians are participating (e.g., a surgeon and radiologist), the radiology portion is billed by the radiologist.

Pathology and Laboratory Codes

All codes in pathology and laboratory work are five-digit numbers that begin with 8. These codes are divided into sections for panels of tests, drug testing, consultations with pathologists, urinalysis, chemistry testing, antibody testing, cytopathology, and so on. The last part of the pathology and laboratory section includes services and procedures provided by a pathologist, including gross (can be seen by the naked eye) and microscopic examination of tissue removed in surgery. Each tissue specimen is submitted under a different identifying code for diagnosis by the pathologist. The codes represent the level of the physician's work. Postmortem examination or autopsy is performed by a pathologist, and CPT-4 provides codes to report such examinations.

A subsection, automated multichannel tests, deserves a special note. When coding, check that the tests performed are included in the lists under this subsection. For example, the physician may perform the following three tests for a patient: bilirubin, direct; cholesterol; and blood urea nitrogen (BUN). To code this, you assign the code 80003, three clinical chemistry tests, because all of these tests are listed under the automated multichannel test subsection. If the tests performed were bilirubin, direct; cholesterol; and blood acetaldehyde, however, you would code 80002, two clinical chemistry tests, and 82000, blood acetaldehyde. That is because blood acetaldehyde was not on the list of clinical chemistry tests in the automated multichannel test subsections.

Medicine Codes

Like the E/M codes, medicine codes are five-digit numbers that begin with 9. Like the other five sections of the CPT-4, this section includes guidelines for appropriate coding.

Pay particular attention to the information related to the immunization injections subsection, which includes codes from 90701 to 90749. Typically, immunization injections are given when the patient comes to the physician's office for either a routine physical examination or for a minor problem, such as a sore throat. When the injection is given at the time of such a visit, use two codes: one for the service (usually an E/M code) and one for the immunization injection. For example, an established patient may come into the physician's office for a brief examination for a minor problem (e.g., controlled hypertension blood pressure check). The patient may be examined briefly by a nurse or medical assistant while the physician is in the office and may also be given an immunization for poliomyelitis. The coding for this is:

1. 99211, office and other outpatient visit for the evaluation and management of an established patient, which may not require the presence of a physician. Usually, the presenting problems are minimal. Typically, 5 minutes are spent performing or supervising services. (This code is generally used for examination by employees of the practice while a physician is in the office but not performing the examination.)
2. 90713, poliomyelitis vaccine.

For therapeutic or diagnostic injections (codes 90782–90799), you need to specify what was injected (90281–90399). For example, consider the code 90782, therapeutic injection of medication (specify); subcutaneous or intramuscular. This code is the same for a number of injectable therapeutic substances, making the additional, more specific code necessary. A code for administration should also be added (90471–90472). If a significant separately identifiable E/M service is performed, the appropriate E/M service code should be reported in addition to the injection code.

In Medicare claims, the cost of administering injections is included in the price of office and outpatient visits and other procedures furnished on the same day. Supplying the drug is a separate billable service, however, and should be assigned the appropriate code. (This may not be true of other carriers, so you need to check with them.)

Using the most specific codes for different injectable substances and supplies while keeping invoices to document actual cost helps verify charges submitted for these services.

The medicine section also includes cardiac diagnostic testing, such as electrocardiography and echocardiography. This section also lists the codes for performing cardiopulmonary resuscitation and dialysis treatment.

Checkpoint Question

3. A patient comes in for a tetanus booster, and the physician gives the booster and completes a routine physical examination. How many codes do you use for this visit?

CPT-4 Modifiers

CPT-4 provides a way to give additional information about a procedure through the use of additional numbers called modifiers.

There are several ways to write modifiers:

- Write the five-digit code with a hyphen followed by the two-digit modifier (e.g., 28702-22).
- Write the code without a hyphen separating it from the modifier (e.g., 2870222).
- Write the five-digit code that needs multiple modifiers with the first modifier as −99 (multiple modifiers), followed by the additional modifiers (e.g 28702-9922 . . .)

Of course, the modifier can never appear on the claim form by itself because it refers to the procedure and must be directly below it on the claim form (Fig. 18-2).

Box 18-2 provides a few examples of modifiers. A separate listing of available modifiers can be found in Appendix A of CPT-4. Check Appendix A first; then go to the appropriate section to verify that the modifier may be used with the specific CPT code. Failure to use an appropriate modifier causes database and billing errors.

Checkpoint Question

4. Where can a coder find a list of all CPT modifiers?

EXAMPLES OF CPT-4 MODIFIERS

Here are just a few examples of CPT-4 modifiers. A complete list can be found in Appendix A of CPT-4.

- *20 microsurgery or 09920:* This modifier signifies that the surgeon used an operating microscope to perform a procedure.
- *23 unusual anesthesia or 09923:* This modifier signifies that anesthesia was used in a procedure that normally would not require it.
- *26 professional component or 09926:* This modifier signifies that there are two components to the procedure, a professional and a technical one. For example, when a physician requests a radiograph, the radiology technologist takes the radiograph and the physician reads it. This modifier lets the insurance carrier know that the physician did not provide both service components.

HEALTHCARE COMMON PROCEDURE CODING SYSTEM

Because the AMA's CPT-4 codes do not include such items as ambulance service, wheelchairs, or injections, CMS designed another coding system based on the CPT-4. This system is referred to as the **Healthcare Common Procedure Coding System** or HCPCS.

The HCPCS uses codes contained in CPT-4 (now known as HCPCS Level 1) plus expanded codes developed by CMS and fiscal intermediaries to classify physician and nonphysician patient care services on the national level (now known as HCPCS Level 2). Level 2 HCPCS codes are most commonly referred to as the HCPCS codes, and Level 1 HCPCS codes are referred to as CPT. Since 1985, physicians have had to use the HCPCS to bill for services provided to Medicare patients either in the medical office or in the hospital. Since October 1986, physicians also have used the HCPCS to bill for services provided to Medicaid patients.

As of July 1, 1987, federal law requires hospitals to use the HCPCS to report outpatient surgery services to patients receiving health benefits sponsored by the federal government. By October 1, 1987, federal law had extended ambulatory surgical center (ASC) prospective payment methodology to hospital outpatient surgery payments. The purpose of this was twofold:

- To permit identification of ASC procedures so a blended payment rate could be applied to ambulatory surgery performed in the hospital outpatient department
- To provide a database for future payment amounts for all hospital outpatient services

The HCPCS includes three levels of codes, discussed in the following sections.

HCPCS Level 1 Codes

The HCPCS Level 1 codes are in CPT-4. This is a listing of terms and codes that provide a means to report physician procedures and services under both private and government-sponsored health insurance programs.

HCPCS Level 2 Codes: National Codes

The HCPCS Level 2 code listing comes out once a year in the *National Coding Manual*, which can be ordered from the American Hospital Association, American Medical Association, or other publishers of the CPT coding book. It includes codes for the following:

- Chemotherapeutic drugs
- Dental services
- Durable medical equipment
- Injections
- Ophthalmology services
- Orthotics
- Some pathology and laboratory and rehabilitation supplies
- Vision care

National codes are five-digit alphanumeric codes that begin with the letters A to V (e.g., L8100 is elastic support, elastic stocking, below knee, medium weight, each).

HCPCS Level 3 Codes: Local Codes

The HCPCS Level 3 codes were developed to address regional coding—the ability to code something performed or offered in one state that may or may not be performed or offered in another state. These codes, which are produced and made available through your state Medicare carrier, may vary from state to state. Local codes begin with letters W to Z. CMS takes full responsibility for the codes in the *National Coding Manual*, leaving local codes up to Medicare carriers in each state.

Checkpoint Question

5. Where do you find codes for dental services?

REIMBURSEMENT

Diagnostic Related Groups

Diagnostic related groups (DRGs) are categories into which inpatients are placed according to the similarity of their diagnoses, treatment, and length of hospital stay. Initially, these categories were developed by Yale University researchers in the mid 1970s to aid the process of utilization review. Some 13,000 codes were run through a computer and grouped according to their clinical similarities (including similarities in resources used). Today, DRGs are used to determine reimbursement for Medicare patients' inpatient services. The fee attached to each DRG is based on the national average of all Medicare discharges and is adjusted for regional differences in hospital wages and updates. Hospitals are paid a set amount for each DRG regardless of actual costs for treating the patient. For example, if a hospital uses fewer resources to care for a patient and discharges that patient in less time, it may keep the difference between its actual cost and the DRG payment. Conversely, if the patient stays longer than usual and requires more services, the hospital absorbs the loss. A patient who has an unusually long stay or a complicated case is considered an **outlier**, and the hospital may be paid more than the standard DRG rate if the added expenses can be justified. The hospital coder uses ICD-9-CM codes to pick the appropriate DRG. The more information the hospital has prior to admission, the more accurate the coding; for example, for a patient admitted with chest pain, the hospital coder needs to know that the patient also has hypertension and diabetes.

You may be asked to schedule a patient for admission to the hospital. Assigning the correct ICD-9-CM code from the outpatient practice will influence the DRG to which the patient will be assigned. The hospital coder selects the proper DRG based on these factors:

- Principal diagnosis
- Surgeries
- Complications and comorbid conditions

Physicians can help with coding in the following ways:

- Record the appropriate documentation to identify each patient's problems, complaints, or other reasons for the encounter or visit.
- Work with the medical records or the office coding and billing staffs to determine the proper diagnosis to code, using terminology that includes specific diagnoses, symptoms, problems, or reasons for the encounter (ICD-9-CM codes describe all of these).

Resource-Based Relative Value Scale

As part of the 1989 Omnibus Budget Reconciliation Act (OBRA), the U. S. Congress stipulated that reimbursement to physicians for Medicare services is based on a fee schedule. This fee schedule sets a maximal fee for each service based on the **resource-based relative value scale** (RBRVS). The goal of RBRVS is to reduce Medicare Part B costs and to establish national standards for payment based on CPT-4 codes. (Remember, Part B Medicare covers physicians' services; Part A covers hospital expenses.)

Fee calculations are based on the following factors:

- Intensity of the service
- Time required
- Skills needed
- Overhead expenses
- Malpractice premiums

The particular fee is adjusted by a geographical practice cost index (GPCI), which reflects the difference in health care costs in different parts of the country. These determine the relative value unit (RVU). Finally, a national conversion factor is assigned yearly. The formula looks like this:, CPT code 99205 has an RVU of 4.58, and the national conversion factor is 36.7856. The Medicare allowed charge would be $168.48.

 Checkpoint Question

6. Why are DRGs used?

FRAUD AND CODING

Billing for services not performed, using another patient's coverage to receive reimbursement, and falsifying records are examples of blatant fraud. The attorney general of the United States has jurisdiction over such cases, and in most states the Office of the Inspector General investigates reports of possible fraud. Less severe and undeliberate fraudulent practices also cause misuse of health care dollars, and CMS remains vigilant by conducting audits. Even though the physician you work for may already have been paid for a claim, the medical office may still be audited. As a federal program, Medicare has the same authority as the Internal Revenue Service to audit claims and may do so retroactively. This means that an audit can occur even a couple of years after payment has been received for claims. If the medical practice is found to be in error, the physician may be required to repay an amount owed plus interest. Even worse, such errors can jeopardize the physician's ability to participate in Medicare-funded programs. To avoid costly errors, be certain that you can justify your coding:

LEGAL TIP

When submitting Medicare or other insurance claims, do not bill for services the physician has not performed, and do not bill more for a service than it is worth. Billing high is called **upcoding**.

Millions of dollars have been budgeted to investigate fraud and abuse. Fiscal intermediaries (organizations under contract with the U. S. government to handle Medicare claims) randomly review and compare the documentation in the record and report their findings on the particular providers. Peer review organizations have been authorized by CMS to obtain medical records of Medicare beneficiaries for review.

- Keep adequate, accurate, and complete documentation in medical and billing records.
- Use the proper tools to code. Code books are updated yearly. Always use the most recent book.
- Follow the coding rules, becoming familiar with new rules and keeping up-to-date on any changes to existing ones. Medicare has regional updates, usually at no charge, and provides one of the best sources of changes.
- Work closely with the provider, and never code anything about which you are not sure.

CHAPTER SUMMARY

Medical coding involves the use of numbers to describe diseases, injuries, and procedures. It has several purposes, including indexing medical records, performing medical care reviews, deriving health statistics, and reimbursing physicians and hospitals for services. As a medical assistant, you are responsible for knowing the format and usage of CPT-4, the system used to report services and procedures by the physician. Accurate and thorough coding is essential to ensure appropriate reimbursement. You must assist the physician in making sure the proper documentation is available to substantiate the codes used on a claim. Because learning to code is an ongoing process, continuing education is vital. This can be accomplished by attending workshops in your geographic area or by joining a local association of coders, which may also sponsor coding clinics. Two such organizations are the American Academy of Professional Coders (AAPC) and the American Health Information Management Association (AHIMA). Other sources are local medical societies and your school. As in all other aspects of patient contact and care, coding of patients' records is covered by the Health Insurance Portability and Accountability Act of 1996 (HIPAA). Only those with a need to know should have access to patient records.

Critical Thinking Challenges

1. How would you handle a physician who you think overbills for procedures? To whom would you report this? How might you collect documentation of fraud?
2. Create a reminder card to be used when you are to assist with coding.
3. Assume you are working for a family practice physician. Identify three patient problems that you might encounter. Then use the CPT and ICD-9-CM coding books at your school library or the hospital library to find the correct codes.

Answers to Checkpoint Questions

1. The three key elements are history, physical examination, and medical decision making.
2. The surgical package consists of local infiltration, metacarpal, metatarsal, or digital blocks, topical anesthesia, the operation, and normal uncomplicated follow-up care.
3. There are two codes: one for the service and one for the immunization.
4. A list of all modifiers and their meanings is found in Appendix A of CPT-4.
5. Dental codes are found in the HCPCS Level 2 national codes.
6. DRGs are used to determine the reimbursement for Medicare patients' inpatient services.

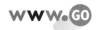 **Websites**

Coding Institute
    www.codinstitute.com
Compliant Billing Service
    www.compliantbilling.com
Medical Billing Association
    www.e-medbill.com

Career Strategies

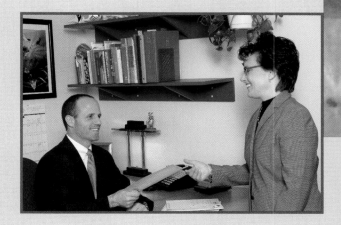

Competing in the Job Market

Congratulations! You have reached a pivotal point in your medical assisting career. This unit prepares you to make the transition from student to employee. Your transition begins with an exciting externship program. Your externship is the springboard to starting your career. The remainder of Chapter 19 focuses on how to acquire the job that you have worked so hard for. You will be prepared to enter this fascinating and exciting career with confidence and professionalism and enjoy the rewards and accept the challenges that face you. Good luck on your new adventure!

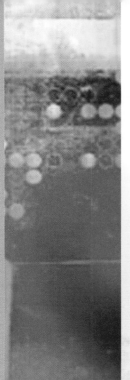

19

Making the Transition: Student to Employee

CHAPTER OUTLINE

EXTERNSHIPS
Types of Facilities
Benefits of Externship
Responsibilities of Externship
Guidelines for a Successful
Externship
Externship Documentation

ESTABLISH THE JOB FOR YOU
Setting Employment Goals
Self-Analysis

FINDING THE RIGHT JOB

APPLYING FOR THE JOB
Answering Newspaper
Advertisements
Preparing Your Résumé
Preparing Your Cover Letter
Completing an Employment
Application

INTERVIEWING
Preparing for the Interview
Crucial Interview Questions

FOLLOW-UP
Why Some Applicants Fail to Get
the Job

KEEP THE JOB OR MOVE ON?

EMPLOYMENT LAWS

ROLE DELINEATION COMPONENTS

GENERAL: Professionalism
- Display a professional manner and image
- Demonstrate initiative and responsibility
- Work as a member of the health care team
- Prioritize and perform multiple tasks
- Adapt to change
- Promote the CMA credential
- Enhance skills through continuing education
- Treat all patients with compassion and empathy
- Promote the practice through positive public relations

GENERAL: Legal Concepts
- Perform within legal and ethical boundaries
- Follow employer's established policies dealing with the health care contract

GENERAL: Communication Skills
- Recognize and respect cultural diversity
- Recognize and respond effectively to verbal, nonverbal, and written communications
- Use medical terminology appropriately
- Serve as a liaison

ADMINISTRATIVE: Administrative Procedures
- Perform basic administrative medical assisting functions

CHAPTER COMPETENCIES

LEARNING OBJECTIVES
Upon successfully completing this chapter, you will be able to:
1. Spell and define the key terms
2. Explain the purpose of the externship experience
3. List your professional responsibilities during externship
4. Understand the evaluation process for the extern student
5. List personal and professional attributes necessary to ensure a successful externship
6. Determine your best career direction based on your skills and strengths
7. Identify the steps necessary to apply for the right position and be able to accomplish those steps
8. Draft an appropriate cover letter
9. List guidelines for an effective interview that will lead to employment
10. Identify the steps that you need to take to ensure proper career advancement

PERFORMANCE OBJECTIVES
Upon successfully completing this chapter, you will be able to:
1. Write a résumé to properly communicate skills and strengths
2. Complete an employment application

KEY TERMS

externship   networking   portfolio   preceptor   résumé

GRADUATION FROM A MEDICAL assisting program is an important milestone in your life. It is normal to have conflicting emotions ranging from excitement to anxiety. The purpose of this chapter is to help you make this transition from student to employee. The first part of the chapter discusses externships. An externship is your first opportunity to use your knowledge in a clinical setting. The chapter also discusses the benefits of externship programs, how to get the most out of your externship, and the documentation that accompanies an externship. The later part of the chapter prepares you to begin searching for employment. Résumé preparation is discussed along with successful interviewing techniques. An introduction to key employment laws is also discussed.

EXTERNSHIPS

Most medical assistant programs provide an **externship** as part of the course requirement. An externship is a training program that gives you the experience of working in a professional medical office under the supervision of a preceptor or supervisor who will help you to apply the theories and procedures you learned during classroom training. This is the opportunity for you to perform and perfect the skills that you have learned during the academic portion of your program.

In an externship you will discover areas of interest in certain types of practices or health care specialties. Rotating through clinical sites will expose you to different offices you may pursue as possible opportunities for future employment. The length and schedule of your externship will depend on your school's curriculum and the medical site where you will be working.

Types of Facilities

The health care industry is diversified, with a wide variety of specialty offices and clinics. As a medical assisting student, you will experience an extensive scope of procedures during an externship in a general or family practice clinic or office. Family practices are generally referred to as primary care providers. Patients range in age from newborns to the elderly and typically have a broad range of complaints and illnesses. General practice facilities provide the best exposure to all types of procedures performed by medical assistants.

Your externship may be more limited in specialty practices. For example, staff members in obstetric offices usually do not perform electrocardiograms, nor do staff members in orthopedic offices perform gynecological examinations. Working in these types of practices, however, will give you experience in special examinations and procedures in areas that you might not observe in a general practice setting. Each specialty has advantages and disadvantages as a site, but all offer invaluable experience that cannot be adequately simulated in the classroom.

Extern Sites

Most schools have extern sites they have used for years. Based on the experience of former students, personnel in these sites know what the student must do to complete the clinical experience. An ideal site should provide a variety of experiences, both in administrative (front office) and clinical (back office) procedures.

A **preceptor** works with externship students the same as the instructor in the classroom. Preceptors typically are graduate medical assistants who have been through a similar externship program.

The school is careful to choose externship sites with preceptors who are willing to work with you and help you feel comfortable in the medical setting. They understand that all of your experience up to this point has been with fellow students in a protected classroom. They understand how nervous you are and will help you to ease the transition from classroom to the medical office. Your clinical sites are usually chosen within easy travel distance.

 Checkpoint Question

1. What is the role of the preceptor?

Benefits of Externship

Benefits to the Student

Externship is a vital part of medical assisting training. You will develop self-confidence and professionalism during the externship portion of your training. No amount of classroom training can compare with the experience of applying skills and knowledge in a medical facility. An externship also allows you to broaden your knowledge base by learning new and different techniques.

Benefits to the Medical Assisting Program

As you gain experience from the externship, the school also benefits from the affiliation, or connection, with the medical community. Many sites have a long history of training students. Schools rely on good training sites to enhance the medical assisting curriculum. Medical assisting programs also rely on the medical profession to aid in updating and revising the curriculum and course content to ensure that the methods and procedures presented to the students from year to year are current.

The school, the program director, and externship preceptors review students' extern experiences to change the program to reflect the needs of the community and the profession as health care constantly changes, such as with new technology. If students are routinely required to perform a procedure or examination that is not a part of the curriculum, for example, this will usually be considered for an addition to future lectures and laboratory sessions. If the accepted practice of a procedure has changed, changes will be made in the way it is taught to ensure that students are kept abreast of health care advances.

Benefits to the Externship Site

The student and the school are not the only ones to benefit from the externship period. The site also gains information about how well different areas of the facility are functioning. Site personnel may discover through the presence and questions of students that they should review certain policies or add others to help the office run more smoothly. Medical facilities must be updated on a continuing basis. Items may be deleted or added to policy, and procedure manuals or parts may have to be revised to provide clearer instructions.

As a student, you will be looking at the office as a newcomer, with a fresh perspective, and you may have many questions for the staff. As you become more familiar with the office routine, you will be more comfortable asking questions without the fear of appearing inexperienced. These questions may help point out to the office personnel things that should be changed or clarified.

Responsibilities of Externship

Responsibilities of the Student

You will develop many attributes, or characteristics, of a professional health care worker during the externship program. You should foster characteristics during this time to ensure that you continue to grow professionally and are an asset to the profession.

You must be dependable. Dependability is a good sign of maturity. Students who are not at the site on time, who take excessive numbers of breaks, or who do not follow through on assignments cannot properly provide for the needs of the patients who rely on the medical staff of the facility.

You must act in a professional manner. All concepts of professionalism include a positive, pleasant, confident attitude with a sincere desire to help the physician, the patient, and the staff.

You must be well groomed and meet the program's dress code. If the medical facility requires clothing that differs from your school's requirements, you are usually asked to comply with the site's requirements.

Checkpoint Question

2. List three responsibilities that you have during your externship.

Responsibilities of the Medical Assisting Program

The primary responsibility of the program is to arrange for the best possible clinical experience for students. The pro-

gram usually has a coordinator who matches students to appropriate sites. Once a site has been chosen, you will meet with the clinical coordinator to discuss the particulars of the medical facility. An interview is sometimes held to acquaint you with your preceptor before the externship begins.

After your site rotation has begun, the program's clinical coordinator will visit or call frequently to follow your progress. If either you or the site has concerns, the coordinator will mediate to eliminate problems or concerns as they arise.

The clinical coordinator will make an evaluation, or appraisal, of your progress at the site. Sites evaluations are usually completed on a form that contains detailed areas to be graded; these are equivalent to grades on a test or examination. These evaluations will be used to determine whether you are prepared for the profession or your skills are deficient and need more reinforcement. The clinical coordinator is responsible for compiling evaluations and keeping you abreast of your progress. Frequent conferences with your coordinator usually help accomplish this.

The school is also responsible for maintaining liability insurance for students during clinical hours. Students are required in most instances to provide proof of general immunizations and vaccination for hepatitis B. Some schools may provide the vaccine for students. Most programs require a current physical examination, a serology profile, and a tuberculin skin test before students are admitted to the program or before they make contact with patients.

Responsibilities of the Externship Site

The medical facility is, of course, responsible for providing opportunities for training. The staff will help orient you to the office and its policies. In some sites, students are allowed only to observe certain procedures but are given permission to perform some basic or routine procedures. Even if you are not allowed to perform specific procedures, the opportunity to observe and ask questions will be useful. In this way, you will become as familiar as possible with all clinical areas and functions.

Guidelines for a Successful Externship

Success in your externship is important for you to obtain employment. Your success in your externship is evaluated according to certain standards, or criteria. The person or persons evaluating you during your externship are professional medical personnel who know the standards for the health care field as they relate to medical assisting. These areas include the following:

- Procedural performance
- Preparedness
- Attendance
- Appearance
- Attitude

Procedural Performance

You will be judged on your ability to measure up to the standard of care for an entry-level medical assistant. This means you are expected to perform at the level of a new employee in the field. Your preceptor is there to assist you, not to teach you the basics that you should have learned in the classroom. Come to your externship prepared. Ask questions, when in doubt, before starting any procedure. Ask questions outside the patient's room. Never perform a procedure alone, unless otherwise directed by your instructor.

Preparedness

Preparation is the best insurance for success, regardless of the goal. Personal preparation for the externship helps prevent losing time because of other extracurricular obligations. Make sure in advance that you have prepared:

- Reliable transportation
- Reliable day care services
- Backup systems for a sick child, snow cancellations of school, or early dismissals from school
- Financial coverage and support for any hours that you are unable to work at your usual job because of your extern site hours.

Attendance

If you have planned well for transportation, family considerations, and finances, you are more likely to attend all sessions at the clinical sites. You must also be healthy. A good diet, regular exercise, and proper rest help you maintain good health. Careful attention to hygiene and medical asepsis help ensure that you do not bring illnesses home from the clinical sites.

If at any time you will be late or will not be able to attend the site for any reason, you must notify both the clinical coordinator and the site preceptor. Never be a no-call or no-show. Almost all sites have an answering service for leaving messages, as do most schools. There is no excuse for not notifying all parties involved if you will be unavoidably late or will not be able to attend the scheduled session.

Office hours vary from site to site; it is always a good practice, however, to arrive a few minutes before the scheduled opening. This allows time to check for telephone messages, arrange the day's appointments, turn on office equipment, and generally get into the routine of the office. Plan your transportation, leaving plenty of time for any problems that may occur. Arriving in a flurry, frustrated by traffic or home problems, with no time to ease into your day causes a high level of tension and anxiety. It is more difficult to have the caring and compassionate attitude necessary to deal with the complex problems in the medical office.

Appearance

You have only one opportunity to make a first impression, which is usually based on appearance. Appearance is much more than looks. A beautiful face on a poorly groomed person is not seen as professional and does not inspire trust and confidence in patients or coworkers. The key to a professional appearance is careful preparation and planning.

If you wear a uniform for your externship, it must be freshly laundered and pressed; clean but wrinkled is not acceptable. Plan your wardrobe for ease of care and a professional appearance. Fad or trendy clothing, suggestive clothing, and flashy clothing are not appropriate for clinical sites. All clothing should be in good repair, with no missing buttons, hanging hems, tears, rips, or stains. Duty shoes should be clean, polished frequently, and kept in good condition. Laced shoes look better with fresh, clean shoelaces. Check nylon hosiery for runs and snags and replace them as needed. You may wear laboratory coats in some programs; uniforms may be worn in others. The clinical preceptor or the clinical coordinator will inform you of the dress code in advance.

Professional appearance includes hair and makeup. Your hair should be conservatively styled, and long hair must be kept away from the face. Wash it frequently so that it is fresh and clean. Makeup should be minimal and tastefully applied. Never use perfume or cologne, which may be irritating to coworkers and patients. Keep fingernails short to avoid transferring pathogens or ripping gloves when you perform procedures.

Wear only minimal, tasteful jewelry. Rings can puncture gloves, possibly causing exposure to a pathogen. Therefore, it is a good idea to avoid wearing them in the clinical site.

 Checkpoint Question

3. Describe the proper attire for your externship.

Attitude

Attitude is also part of appearance. Most patients and coworkers will easily see your emotions revealed by facial expressions and body language. A person who looks eager is usually perceived as a good, diligent worker.

Much attitude is determined by how well you handle change and direction and how adaptable and flexible you are during difficult assignments.

The medical profession is constantly changing, making it imperative for all professionals to stay flexible. In the classroom, you learn generic methods for treatments and procedures. Because of the constantly changing technology, you may have to adjust to other methods in the field. If you learned a procedure one way in the classroom training but find that it is performed differently in the clinical site, the new method must be accepted and performed as well as possible. Frequently, there is more than one right way to do a procedure, and the classroom method you learned may be just one of the accepted methods. The next physician or clinical site may use yet another equally correct procedural method.

Your attitude determines your altitude. Students who work with a positive attitude during their externship are likely to reach higher levels of the profession than those who see the externship as an imposition or a burden. Box 19-1 offers some additional suggestions.

Externship Documentation

Time Records

Most programs use a time sheet or record of some sort to document your hours in the externship (Fig. 19-1). The beginning and ending hours of each day are recorded. How breaks are handled depends on the clinical coordinator, program requirements, and specific site. Some sites allow half an hour for lunch, and others allow an hour; some close for an hour or more midday, while others are open and staffed from morning until evening. Some programs make students responsible for time sheet signatures; others delegate the responsibility to the site preceptor. However the form is handled, it is used to validate your time in the externship and is a requirement for completion of most programs.

Site Evaluation

Most schools use a site evaluation form to gather impressions of the site and externship experience (Fig. 19-2). This form helps determine the effectiveness of the site for training and whether any issues should be addressed before assigning other students. Be objective and honest in your evaluation of the site. When completing a site evaluation, consider these questions:

- Was the overall experience positive or negative?
- Were opportunities for learning abundant and freely offered or hard to obtain?
- Were staff personnel open and caring or unwelcoming?
- Was the preceptor available and easily approachable or preoccupied and distant?

If the site is not providing a positive learning experience, the program should discontinue using it.

Self-Evaluation

The self-evaluation form helps you determine what personal and professional skills you still need to develop or enhance. These forms encourage introspection and personal honesty as you begin a lifelong program of self-improvement. They usually include components that encourage you to outline the things you performed well and are proud of and areas that can use some improvement.

Checkpoint Question

4. What three types of documentation are often required in extern programs?

ESTABLISH THE JOB FOR YOU

Setting Employment Goals

Once your externship is complete, you are one step closer to getting the job that you desire. Before beginning to search for a job, decide what you want and need from a job and make that your goal. People who do not set employment goals too often accept only what is presented to them. They often end up unhappy in their work because they did not choose their job in the first place. The average person approaches the job search with the attitude, "I wonder what is available," rather than, "Here is what I would like to do, and here is the facility where I would like to work." *That* is setting a goal. It is also a positive, proactive approach to the job market rather than a reactive position to what is available. In general, the medical field is looking for proactive people. You will work harder and more enthusiastically if you choose your workplace.

The best way to set a goal and eventually get what you want is to study your strengths and weaknesses and from that self-knowledge design the best job for you. Goal setting means describing the ideal job for you and deciding that this is the job that you will someday have.

On a sheet of paper, describe the best job for you if you had your choice. For example, you might describe these elements:

**CLINICAL EXPERIENCE
STUDENT'S TIME REPORT**

To obtain proper credit, an account of time and days in attendance must be recorded by each intern student. This report must be verified by the job supervisor and attached to the final 55-day roster. This information is kept strictly confidential.

Student's Name: _____   Course No.: _____

Program: _____   Course Title: _____

Minimum Contact Hrs. Required: _____   Quarter/Year: _____

WEEK OF (DATES)	M	T	W	TH	F	S	TOTAL HOURS	SITE SUPERVISOR

TOTAL HOURS FOR QUARTER: _____

I certify that the above time report is a true statement of the hours worked.

I approve this statement of hours in attendance for the quarter covered.

_____   _____
Student's Signature   Date   Curriculum Coordinator's Signature   Date

FIGURE 19–1.   Sample student time report.

- Specialty area (e.g., obstetrics, pediatrics, surgery)
- Duties (clinical or administrative)
- Type of employer and supervisor
- Other employees and coworkers
- Type of facility
- Desired atmosphere (casual or formal)
- Ideal hours
- Availability of flextime (a system of scheduling that allows for a personal choice in hours or days worked)

Next, write down where you expect to be in 2 years and in 5 years, in terms of both position and income. Now you are more focused on where you want to work, what you want to do, and the direction you want to be going. The next question is how to get there.

To win the position you want, you have to learn to sell yourself. Generally, employers will not come looking for you; you will have to go to them. They will compare you with all of the other equally well qualified candidates who are interested in the same position. If 25 people interview for a job, even if you are second best, you still lose. The one who is chosen is the one who interviews best. The one who is best suited for a job does not necessarily get it; instead, frequently the one who performs best in the interview does. To market yourself takes real effort.

Self-Analysis

A good presentation of your qualifications begins with self-analysis. You must know what strengths you have to offer a potential employer as well as your weaknesses. Make an honest list of your strengths and weaknesses. (If you skipped this exercise, one of your weaknesses is likely a failure to follow through, taking short cuts, and perhaps procrastination.)

Each of your strengths presents an opportunity to sell yourself and your value as an employee. When you are interviewing for a position, concentrate on projecting your strengths to the interviewer.

Just as your strengths give you a special advantage, each weakness is a reason someone may not want to offer you the position. Recognize and work to resolve your weaknesses. Recognizing your weaknesses as a threat to securing the position you want will help you develop strategies to eliminate these problems or turn them into strengths. As long as you are aware of your weaknesses, you are better prepared to handle them.

Once you know the type of job you want and have identified your positive and negative qualities, it is time to begin to look for the right job.

 Checkpoint Question

5. What is the purpose of self-analysis?

FINDING THE RIGHT JOB

Everybody begins with the newspaper, and you should too. But other opportunities too might work for you. Keep in

---

CLINICAL SITE EVALUATION
STUDENT QUESTIONNAIRE

Name of Clinical Site: _____

Department/Unit Worked: _____

Dates Worked: From _____   To _____

Name of Preceptor _____

SCALE CODES: 1 = Disagree; 2 = Agree; 3 = No opinion

1. The clinical experience was worthwhile.

    1   2   3

    Comments: _____

2. The objectives of the clinical experience seemed adequately understood and followed by the clinical site.

    1   2   3

    Comments: _____

3. Would you recommend this clinical site for future externs?

    1   2   3

    Comments: _____

4. Was the preceptor helpful?

    1   2   3

    Comments: _____

5. The routines of the department/unit were clearly explained throughout the clinical experience.

    1   2   3

    Comments: _____

6. The clinical site provided sufficient educational experiences.

    1   2   3

    Comments: _____

7. Did you receive constructive feedback, both verbal and written, on your clinical performance?

    1   2   3

    Comments: _____

8. What part of the clinical experience did you like the best?

    Comments: _____

9. What part of the clinical experience did you like the least?

    Comments: _____

10. What changes would you recommend for future clinical experiences at this clinical site?

    Comments: _____

11. Upon completion of your clinical experience, did you feel like a part of the team?

    Comments: _____

12. Were you offered a position at this site?

    Yes _____   No _____

    If yes, fill in the blank spaces.

    FT_____   PT_____   Starting salary _____

Date Completed: _____   Signature: _____

FIGURE 19–2.   Sample site evaluation form.

mind that many of the most desirable job openings are never advertised; they are posted internally and filled from within.

Many studies show that most positions are never advertised in the media. Open positions that are posted internally are often filled with current employees or by referrals from current employees. Any organization that looks within and obtains a recommendation from a current employee to fill an available position accomplishes two things: (1) it saves the cost of advertising, and (2) the recommendation itself is usually a good one because it comes from someone who presumably knows the demands and special needs of that particular organization.

It is important for someone seeking employment in the medical field to build as many contacts within the field as possible. These contacts help you with **networking**. Networking is using friends, family members, and professional colleagues to advance or obtain information in the workplace. It is impossible to have too many contacts. Everyone with whom you associate should know that you are looking for employment. Friends and acquaintances cannot tell you about a job or recommend you for a job if they do not know that you are searching.

Traditional sources of information for job openings:

- *Local, state, or federal government employment offices.* These agencies are designed to find work for the unemployed. They frequently have listings of positions that are not found anywhere else. Rather than calling the office with inquiries, make an appointment to visit. Register with the service. Get to know the contact person with whom you will be contacting frequently.
- *School placement office.* If your school has a placement office, contact the coordinator or personnel officer and outline what you are looking for and where you want to work. Their job is to assist you in securing the position you want. If you establish a working relationship with a contact person, you will probably have better results.
- *Medical facilities.* Do not wait for an advertisement. Go to the office or facility where you would like to work and leave a résumé—a document summarizing your professional qualifications—and a cover letter explaining how much you want to work there. Find out the name of the office manager or personnel officer and call first for an appointment. This shows better planning and foresight and is more professional than dropping by unannounced.
- *Private agencies.* Many medical facilities solicit privately to avoid being swamped by applications from unqualified applicants. A fee is charged for the service but is usually paid by the employer. Call the agency to make an appointment with a representative who will interview you and tell you what steps to follow.
- *Temporary services.* These agencies fill short-term vacancies for medical offices. If you are new in an area, this is a good way to learn which facilities would be good choices for you. You may be assigned for several

days or several weeks. If you work well as a temporary replacement and like the site, leave your résumé and let the appropriate individuals know that you would like to work in this place if an opening occurs. Check with the temporary agency regarding any fees that you may be charged or that the medical office may have to pay if it hires you, often called a finder's fee.

Checkpoint Question

6. List four resources that you may use to identify potential job opportunities.

APPLYING FOR THE JOB

Answering Newspaper Advertisements

When responding to a newspaper advertisement, be sure to do exactly what the advertisement asks you to do; one of the qualities that many interviewers look for is the ability to follow directions. At the same time, try to make your response more distinctive (yet still professional) than others they may receive. The medical profession rarely responds well to those who do not fit its image and almost never accepts someone who does not conform at the entry level. Most employers will require you to submit a résumé. A well-prepared résumé and cover letter are essential to job hunting.

Preparing Your Résumé

Many resources can help you write your **résumé**. Start with your school library. Most schools have books on how to create résumés. Numerous websites also offer this information. Caution: many websites have free information, but some charge fees. Focus on free resources before paying for these services. Many word processing programs have templates for résumés. Put your résumé on a computer disk and be sure to personalize it for the position you are seeking. For example, if you give a career objective, try putting in the title a description of the particular job you are seeking. Keep changing this for every different position so that your résumé is personalized for each interview.

The résumé is a flash picture of yourself; if it is neat and professional, the reviewer will presume that it is a reflection of you. Remember these guidelines as you prepare to capture the reviewer's interest:

1. Evaluate your skills, goals, and what you have to offer. With this list in hand, you can better concentrate on highlighting your strengths.
2. Confine your résumé to one page, selecting carefully what you want to include. The résumé must state just what the reviewer needs to know and no more.
3. Include the following key information:
   - Name, address, and telephone number: Include these at the top of your résumé (usually centered).

Box 19-2

HANDLING CALLS FROM PROSPECTIVE EMPLOYERS

Here are some tips for handling calls from prospective employers:

- Tell family members or other household members that you are expecting important telephone calls.
- Keep a pen and paper with telephone.
- Instruct people to take a complete message. Ask them to write down the person's name, phone number, message, and what time the call was received.
- Leave a professional message on your answering machine. Avoid leaving cute or silly messages.

(Because you are including your telephone number, you should expect calls from prospective employers. Box 19-2 offers some tips for handling such calls.)

- Education: Start with the most recent and work backward.
- Affiliations or volunteer work (if appropriate): If this information shows that you have good organizational skills or have held an office for the group, you should include it.
- Experience: This may be listed in either of two standard forms: functional or chronological. A functional résumé focuses on skills and qualifications rather than employment and works well for those who recently graduated or who are reentering the job market after a period of years (Fig. 19-3). A chronological résumé is useful for those who have an employment history, particularly if the history is relevant to the position be-

FIGURE 19–3. Sample functional résumé.

Tina Elmwood C.M.A.
22 Brandy Drive
Dayton, Ohio 00000
444-777-6666

Employment Objective: To use my medical assisting skills in a challenging position. My goal is to work with children. (*Change this sentence to reflect the type of office that you are applying to.*)

Experience:

Externship (160 hours) at Family Practice Associates, Bayview Drive, Dayton, Ohio (*If you have a positive evaluation from your preceptor, bring it with you to the interview. Do not attach it to the resume.*)

Education:

Medical Assisting Program, Diploma. Graduated June 2003. West County Community College, Dayton Ohio (*Bring a copy of your diploma and transcripts to the interview. Do not attach them unless employer has specifically requested them.*)
Dayton High School, Diploma. Graduated June 2001. Dayton, Ohio

Skills:

Clinical and Laboratory skills listed on Role Delineation for Medical Assisting

Administrative skills listed on Role Delineation for Medical Assisting

Comfortable using all types of standard office equipment

Familiar with XYZ software programs (*List software programs that you are comfortable with. If you know what type of software the office uses, list that as well.*)

Certifications:

Certified Medical Assistant, American Association of Medical Assistants (*Bring copy to interview or attach to résumé.*)
Cardiopulmonary Resuscitation, American Heart Association (*Bring copy to interview or attach to résumé.*)

Beatrice Meza C.M.A.
123 Main Street
West Harford, CT 00000
888-999-6666

Employment Objective: To use my medical assisting skills in a challenging position. My goal is to work in an obstetrical office. (*Change this sentence to reflect the type of office that you are applying to.*)

Education:

2002–2003 Medical Assisting Program; Mountain Laurel Community College, West Hartford, Connecticut (*Bring a copy of your diploma and transcripts to the interview. Do not attach them unless employer has specifically requested them.*)

Externship:

July 2003–(160 hours) Women's Health Care Center, Hartford, Connecticut (*If you have a positive evaluation from your preceptor, bring it with you to the interview. Do not attach it to the résumé.*)

Work Experience:

July 2002–present Receptionist, Dermatology Consultants, West Hartford, Connecticut. Worked part time while I was in school. Answered and triaged telephone calls. Assisted with various other medical administrative responsibilities. (*If you have a reference letter from this employer, bring it with you to the interview. Be prepared to answer questions about why you are leaving this position.*)
May 1999–July 2002 Cashier/Clerk for SuperMarket Grocers, West Hartford, Connecticut. Worked part time. Responsible for training new employees. Promoted to senior cashier.

Skills:

Clinical and Laboratory skills listed on the Role Delineation for Medical Assisting
Administrative skills listed on the Role Delineation for Medical Assisting
Comfortable using all types of standard office equipment
Familiar with XYZ software programs (*List software programs that you are comfortable with. If you know what type of software the office uses, list that as well.*)

Activities/Honors

Student Government representative
Most Improved Medical Assisting Student in 2002

FIGURE 19–4. Sample chronological résumé.

ing sought. Start with the most recent employment and work backward. Include your title, position, and a few of your key responsibilities (Fig. 19-4). Explain any gaps such as pregnancy, schooling, relocations, and so on.

- References: You may or may not include your references on a separate sheet. When you have chosen the people you want to use as references, be sure to ask their permission. Start by asking your instructors if you can use them as references. Other medical professionals (physicians or nurses) will also make strong references. Previous employers also make very good references. You should have a minimum of three references. Do not bring a list of more than five people. Prospective employers are not interested in your

neighbors or pastor and are certainly not interested in your relatives as references.

4. Do not include hobbies and personal interests unrelated to work. It is not relevant that you play the guitar, but it would be impressive to know that you volunteer at a free clinic.

5. Use action words (Box 19-3).

6. Center the résumé on white or off-white heavy bond or high rag content paper, 8.5 by 11 inches. (Colors are not acceptable, and cheap paper will not convey the professional impression you hope to make.) Keep a 1-inch margin around the text. Single-space within the sections of information but leave a blank line between the sections.

7. Use regular type. Avoid fonts that are cute or fancy. Use black ink. Do not print your résumé in color.

Box 19-3

ACTION WORDS

Achieved	Established	Planned
Attained	Filed	Prepared
Assisted	Handled	Processed
Conducted	Generated	Scheduled
Completed	Implemented	Selected
Composed	Maintained	Systemized
Created	Organized	Screened
Developed	Operated	Solved
Directed	Participated	Wrote
Ensured	Performed	

8. Have someone proofread your work. It is difficult to find your own errors or see areas that are not clearly worded.
9. Print your résumé on a letter-quality printer. A dot matrix printer is not acceptable.
10. Mail the résumé in an 8.5 by 11 inch manila envelope. This will present the interviewer with a résumé and cover letter that are smooth, with no fold lines. Many prefer to work with résumés that have not been folded for an envelope.
11. **Be honest.** Do not embellish your résumé or add fictional information. This could get you fired.

Checkpoint Question

7. What is the difference between a functional and a chronological résumé?

Preparing Your Cover Letter

When contacting a prospective employer about a job, you need to send a résumé along with a cover letter. Keep your cover letter brief and meaningful. You want it to be read, and you want the reader to be impressed by what it says. Be sure that you mention the job itself in your letter. You may even consider a statement such as, "This is the type of position I would prefer." If you are applying to a pediatrician's office, you may write, "My goal is work with children." If you know something favorable about the facility, include that in your letter. If you know anyone who works for the company, mention it. *Do not* mention the person by name unless you have secured his or her permission.

Make sure you address your letter to the right person. Call the personnel department or office manager and ask the name of the person handling the applications. Determine the correct spelling of the name and the preferred honorific, such as Mr., Ms., or Mrs.

The standard form for a cover letter has three brief paragraphs:

- First paragraph: State the position for which you are applying.
- Second paragraph: Stress your skills. Do not be redundant, since you will also send a résumé, but mention or highlight specifically the skills needed for this job.
- Third paragraph: Request an interview. Offer to call in a week to set up an interview (then do so). Keep a copy of your letter to refer to when calling.

Use the same good quality paper for the cover letter that you use for your résumé. Include your name, address, and telephone number at the top of the page, centered or in block form. Single-space the letter and double-space between paragraphs. Either block or modified block form is acceptable.

Completing an Employment Application

Some sites will have you fill out an employment application while you wait for your interview; others may mail one to you to be filled out and taken to the interview. Although résumés have their place and are indispensable, many facilities rely more on an application form.

Follow these guidelines when completing an application:

1. Read through completely before beginning.
2. Follow the instructions exactly. Prospective employers notice neatness, erasures, evasions, and indecision.
3. Answer every question. If the question does not apply to you, draw a line or write N/A so that the interviewer will know that you did not overlook the question.
4. In the line for wage or salary desired, write "negotiable" or find out before the interview what is usual for the area for this type of position.
5. In spaces requesting your reason for leaving a previous position, try to sound positive. Answers such as "to explore a new career direction" are general enough to fill many needs. If the reason for leaving was relocation, schooling, or pregnancy, say so.
6. Write your very best, being as neat as possible.
7. Use a black or blue pen. Never use a pencil or colored pen (red, green, purple) to complete the application. It does not portray a professional image.

You may attach your résumé to the application if you did not mail one already.

INTERVIEWING

Interviewing well is a skill that takes effort to develop. As with any skill, if you want to stay proficient and keep your skills in good working order, you have to practice. Ask friends or family members to work with you to develop a relaxed approach to answering the questions most often asked during an interview. Have them try to trip you up or confuse you by throwing in tricky questions. Although the effect will not be the same with a friend or family member as with an interviewer, this practice can make a difference between getting the job and losing the chance. You can also rehearse in front of a mirror.

Usually, the person who interviews best is hired for the position. An excellent interview is absolutely crucial for obtaining any job. It is highly unlikely that you will get the job you want without doing well in the interview.

Preparing for the Interview

Before the day of the interview, find out all you can about the facility. What is its reputation? Does it have a big turnover of employees? Review your textbooks that cover the specialty so that you can ask informed questions about procedures performed at the site. Think of questions to ask and write them down. Anticipate questions that might be asked of you. Find out the name of the interviewer; if it is a difficult name, practice saying it. Go to the site ahead of time to be sure of its location and time the trip so that you will not be late for your appointment. Do this ideally at the same time of day as your appointment to judge traffic delays, parking problems, and so on.

Dress appropriately for the interview. The general rule is to dress one step above what is required for the job. Do not overdress, as if for a party; make sure your outfit is professional. Your personal hygiene must be above reproach. If you normally smoke, avoid smoking before the interview. Those who do not smoke are acutely aware of the odor of smoke on one's clothes and breath. Avoid large jewelry and apply makeup carefully. Avoid perfumes; some people are very sensitive to scents.

Arrive on time or a few minutes early. Go alone; do not take a friend or family member for moral support. When you are introduced to the interviewer, offer your hand for a handshake and sit only when and where you are directed. Do not fidget, swing your foot, play with your hair, or tap your fingers on the chair arm. Make eye contact when the interviewer speaks with you and when you respond to the questions (Fig. 19-5). Sit up straight but relaxed, with your portfolio on your lap. A **portfolio** is a folder containing all of the information you will need to impress the interviewer. If you do not have a special folder or briefcase, a neat, new manila folder will be adequate. This folder or portfolio will contain items crucial to your interview (Box 19-4.)

Crucial Interview Questions

Every interviewer must have the answers to three basic questions. When you respond to the interviewer's questions, keep these in mind:

1. Do you have the necessary skills to do the job? (Don't forget to include any foreign language skills (Box19-5)).

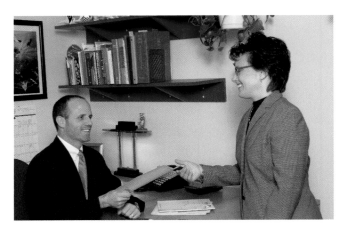

FIGURE 19–5.   During an interview, be sure to use correct posture and to make eye contact with the interviewer.

Box 19-4

PORTFOLIO BOX

Take these items with you to the interview:
- Two pens
- A notepad
- Your Social Security card
- Verification or at least the dates of immunizations (hepatitis B, TB test)
- Two copies of your résumé
- Two letters of reference
- Copies of awards received
- Typed list of three references including names, phone numbers, and addresses
- Documentation of any special projects

Box 19-5

KNOWLEDGE OF A FOREIGN LANGUAGE

If you are applying for a position that encourages bilingual applicants, be prepared for questions during the interview regarding your ability to speak another language. Know what languages are commonly spoken in your community. Whether it is Spanish, Polish, Italian, or any other language, take the time to become familiar with simple greetings: "Hello." "What is your name?" "Can I help you?" Tell the interviewer that you know a few words but are not fluent. It is not fair to the employer or to the patients to pretend otherwise if you are unable to communicate effectively. Most community colleges offer language courses. A local hospital may offer these courses with a focus on medical terms. Finally, the best way to learn a new language is to use it. If your classmates speak another language, ask them to tutor you. Being bilingual in the medical profession is always an asset.

2. Do you have the necessary drive, energy, and commitment to get the job done?

3. Will you work well with the rest of the team?

A positive answer to all of these questions is not a guarantee that you will be offered the job, but a negative answer to any one of these will most assuredly mean that you will *not* get the job. Make sure that your comments make a positive impression regarding these three questions. In the medical field, the interviewer will need to establish your professionalism and ability to keep confidentiality. The interviewer will also want to know how interested you are in increasing and continuing your education and skills. Be sure that your answers will satisfy the interviewer.

Many interviewers use a prepared list of questions to direct the flow of the interview. Table 19-1 contains some commonly asked interview questions and guidance for responses. Be prepared with answers that will reflect well on your professionalism and qualifications.

When the interviewer finishes asking questions, he or she will usually ask if you have any questions. Refer to your notepad, on which you have listed questions such as these:

- What are the responsibilities of the position offered?
- If it is not personal, why is the current employee leaving?
- What are the opportunities for future advancement?
- How long is the training or probation period?

Table 19-1 INTERVIEW QUESTIONS AND RESPONSES

Common Interview Questions	Possible Responses and Points to Mention
1. Tell me about yourself.	"I enjoy working with other people." Stress the good points you wrote on your self-analysis. Keep the comments professional. Do not give long explanations about personal topics. ("I have three brothers." "I like basketball.")
2. What are your strengths?	"My strengths are honesty and dependability." List any clinical or administrative skills that you excel at.
3. What are your weaknesses?	Be honest; everyone has a weakness. "My weakness is phlebotomy skills," and add, "but I have improved my skills by reading magazine articles about blood drawing and by practicing in the school laboratory." Do not say, "I am perfect" or "I have no weaknesses." State one weakness and explain how you are trying to improve it.
4. Why do you want this position?	"I like this office setting." "I always wanted to work for [as an example] a cardiologist." Mention that you are aware of the office's good reputation in the community, and if the location of the office is convenient, say so.
5. What are your goals?	List two or three immediate goals: "My priority is to acquire a medical assisting position that will be challenging and rewarding." Have at least two goals in your mind for where you want to be in 5 years.
6. Why did you leave your last position?	Always place a positive spin on why you left: "Looking for new challenge." Never criticize past employers, their offices, or your coworkers.
7. What salary rate are you looking for?	Know the average pay in your area. Check with your placement office if you are unsure of the typical salaries. Never demand a certain pay rate.
8. How do you handle pressure?	Possible explanations can include, "I set priorities" and "I remain calm and well organized." Avoid comments such as "I hate stress" or "I panic when I feel pressured."
9. Do you work better alone or as a team?	Stress that you can work as a team member but that you can also function independently.
10. Who was your best supervisor and why?	Possible remarks may include phrases such as "always fair," "supportive," and "encouraging." Avoid comments such as "She gave us long lunch breaks" or "She didn't make us work hard."
11. How do you handle conflict?	Indicate that you begin trying to resolve any problems in a professional manner. Indicate that you are always open to constructive criticism.
12. How would your classmates describe you?	Include remarks such as "good student," "team worker," and "helpful."
13. I noticed your grades in computer class were poor. Why?	Be honest: " It was a tough course" or "Although my grade was poor, I have restudied the course material, and my computer skills have improved." If you have taken any additional studies or tutoring to help in this subject area, mention that. Never say the teacher was unfair, the class was boring, or you didn't care about the class.
14. Describe the term *confidentiality* and how you would use it in our office.	Review the term. Stress to the interviewer that you know how important patient confidentiality is from a legal and ethical viewpoint.

- How does the facility feel about continuing education? Is time off offered to employees to upgrade their skills? Does the facility subsidize the expense?
- Is there a job performance or evaluation process?
- What is the benefit package? Is there access to a 401(k) plan or other retirement plan? Health insurance? Life insurance?

Make notes of the answers for future reference. Avoid asking about time off or vacations during the interview. These questions imply that you are more interested in being paid to avoid work than you are in contributing to the work at hand.

Make sure the interviewer knows how important continuing education is to you. Talk about the types of continuing education courses you would like to attend and the subjects you would like to study. Show that you realize that the only constant in medicine is change and that you expect to keep abreast of the information in your area. Thank the interviewer for the opportunity to apply for the position and ask the time frame for a decision. As you leave, offer your hand for a handshake and ask if you may call again before the decision date to clear up any questions that the interviewer may have during the decision-making process.

FOLLOW-UP

The day of the interview or no later than the day after, write a short thank-you note for the opportunity to be interviewed and restate how interested you are in the job (Fig. 19-6). Remind the interviewer that you are available for additional questions.

Call several days after the interview. Reintroduce yourself politely and add any new information or ask any questions

FIGURE 19–6. Sample follow-up letter.

Maria Sefferin C.M.A.
11 Jersey Road
Fredericksburg, VA 00000
888-555-4444

Ms. Joan Brown
Office Manager
Middletown Cardiology Consultants
24 Main Street
Williamsburg, VA 00000

October 22, 2003

Dear Ms. Brown:

Thank you for giving me the opportunity to interview for the position of Medical Assistant in your office. I enjoyed meeting you and touring your facility.

I feel I would be an asset to your office for many reasons. I have a strong knowledge of medical terminology, anatomy and physiology, and cardiac diseases. I have solid clinical and administrative skills. I believe that this position will offer me an opportunity to use the education and training that I have received in my medical assisting courses.

I am very interested in this position. This is the type of career opportunity that I had hoped to find. If you have any questions, please feel free to call me at 888-555-4444.

Sincerely,

Maria Sefferin, C.M.A.

WHAT IF

You become tongue-tied during an interview. What should you do?

It's not unusual to feel nervous during the interview. To stay calm, take a deep breath and count to three before answering a question. Doing this also gives you time to think before you speak. Remember: Believe in yourself and your skills. Say to yourself, "I am going to get this job." Rehearse your answers to the common interview questions. Doing this exercise in front of a mirror is beneficial. Visit the websites listed in this chapter. Some of these sites offer virtual interviewing skills and have excellent tips for interviewing. Finally, arrive prepared and relaxed. Avoid excessive caffeine ingestion before the interview. Caffeine will increase your anxiety level.

that might have occurred to you after the interview. Thank the interviewer again for this opportunity.

Why Some Applicants Fail to Get the Job

The first reason not to be hired is simple: lack of the necessary abilities (Box 19-6). Every employer is looking for something special from each employee. Medicine has special needs. The employer must believe that you possess a number of skills necessary to do the job:

- *Technical skills.* You must have the necessary proficiency to get the job done.
- *Confidentiality.* In medicine you are exposed to sensitive information about patients. Is the interviewer convinced that you can be relied on to keep those confidences?
- *Human relations skills.* Will you get along with the others in the workplace?
- *Communication skills.* Do you have the verbal and writing skills that the job demands? Remember the importance of correct English. You will not be hired if your English and grammar are not exemplary.

If you fail to impress the interviewer with your grasp of these skills, you will never be considered for the position.

Another major reason an applicant is not hired is lack of professionalism. Watch the way you dress and speak. The interviewer knows that whatever you display in the interview will also be displayed to the patients.

KEEP THE JOB OR MOVE ON?

Almost everyone comes to this question at some point in his or her career. Should I look for a new place to work and leave this place where I am safe and comfortable? Would another job be better or more satisfying? Would benefits be better?

An important factor in many relocations is salary. In addition to the financial aspects, however, employees today are looking for other elements that contribute to job satisfaction:

- A sense of achievement
- Recognition
- Opportunity for growth and advancement
- Harmonious peer group relationships
- A good working relationship with supervisors
- Status
- Job security
- Comfortable working conditions
- Fair company policies

If you are no longer happy in your job, the reason probably lies in one or more of these elements. Before you make the decision to change jobs, do some internal soul searching to determine exactly what type of position would make you happy. If you decide to leave, you must leave with positive feelings all around. Box 19-7 offers some guidelines for leaving your job.

EMPLOYMENT LAWS

Many state and federal laws regulate employers. The U. S. Equal Employment Opportunity Commission (EEOC) enforces many of these laws. Under Title VII, Americans with Disabilities Act (ADA), and the Age Discrimination in Employment Act (ADEA), it is illegal to discriminate in any as-

---

Box 19-6

NO HIRE

Here are several reasons a person may not be hired:
- Poor personal appearance
- Inappropriate demeanor, such as unenthusiastic, overly aggressive
- Displayed lack of purpose or direction
- Lack of tact and diplomacy
- Inappropriate humor
- Failure to research the type of office setting or practice
- Failure to make eye contact
- Poorly completed application, messy application, spelling errors on application
- Overemphasis on need for time off or higher wages

Box 19-7

LEAVING A JOB

Always follow these steps when you decide to leave your position:

- Always give adequate notice (minimum 2 weeks, optimal a month).
- Write a resignation letter. Keep the letter positive: "I am leaving this position to explore new opportunities." This is often the last item in your personnel file.
- Be positive during your exit interview. Do not criticize employees or the position.
- Clean and empty your locker, desk, and any other assigned space.
- Return your pager and any other equipment that has been assigned to you.
- Finish all duties and tie up any loose ends.
- Alert your supervisor to any unfinished business.
- Ask for a letter of reference.

CHAPTER SUMMARY

Your externship is the transition from classroom to employment. A successful externship helps lead to your ultimate goal—employment. During your externship you will work with a preceptor who will help you perform your skills in the workplace. After your externship is complete, do a self-analysis and write your résumé. Many resources can help you locate job openings. A job should be fulfilling and rewarding in ways beyond just the income. Learn how to promote yourself and earn the position you want. Know the laws that protect your rights as an employee. You will work hard, but there are many rewards. Welcome to the world of medical assisting!

pect of employment. For example, it is illegal to discriminate in areas such as hiring, firing, transfers, promotion, recruitment, training, benefits, pay, retirement plans, and disability leave of employees. All employees must be treated fairly in all areas.

It is illegal to discriminate against an employee for any of these reasons:

- Race
- Color
- National origin
- Religion or religious beliefs
- Sex
- Age (age limits can be specified only when there is a bona fide occupational qualification)
- Disability
- Martial status
- Political affiliation
- Sexual orientation
- Pregnancy

The Equal Pay Act prohibits pay discrepancies on the basis of sex. In other words, a man and a woman who perform the same job with the same experience level must be paid the same and have the same benefits. The law also protects you against sexual harassment in the workplace. If you feel that you are being discriminated against in the workplace, you should contact your local EEOC district office.

Critical Thinking Challenges

1. You notice that your preceptor does not follow standard precautions on several occasions. Why is this dangerous? Whom should you tell? Would you tell your instructor at school? Why or why not? How would you discuss this with your preceptor?
2. Read the classified section of the Sunday newspaper and select a job advertisement that interests you. Write a cover letter and résumé tailored to this position. Assume you have been called for an interview. What questions do you ask the prospective employer? What questions do you expect to be asked? Explain your responses.
3. Obtain two employee application forms from the human resources department of your local hospital. Complete one application form yourself and invite a fellow student to complete the other. Swap applications and evaluate each other's work. Determine which areas are appropriately addressed and which need further attention.
4. Visit the EEOC website. What is the purpose of the EEOC? Where is your nearest EEOC district office? Would you talk to your supervisor if you felt that you were discriminated against? Why or why not?
5. Suppose you were just hired into your dream position. On day 2, you overhear your supervisor telling another employee, "Don't report that billing error to Medicare. They won't catch us." What would you do? Whom would you tell, or would you pretend you didn't hear it? Would you report to Medicare? Why or why not?

Answers to Checkpoint Questions

1. The preceptor acts as the instructor in the clinical site, providing supervision and technical direction to medical assisting students.
2. You must be dependable, professional, and well groomed.
3. The proper attire includes a freshly laundered uniform, clean shoes, neatly groomed hair, limited makeup, and jewelry kept to a minimum.
4. Documentation includes times sheets, a site evaluation, and a self-evaluation.
5. A self-analysis helps you identify your strengths and weaknesses.
6. Sources of job information include government employment offices, your school placement office, medical facilities, private agencies, and temporary services.
7. A functional résumé stresses skills and qualifications rather than employment history. A chronological résumé lists positions held, starting with the most recent and working backward.

 Websites

Careerspan.com
Resume.com
Resumewriters.com
Seekingsuccess.com
10minuteresume.com
U. S. Equal Employment Opportunity Commission
www.eeoc.gov

Appendices

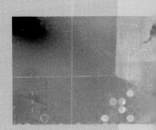

APPENDIX A

MEDICAL ASSISTING ROLE DELINEATION CHART

Administrative

Administrative Procedures
- Perform basic administrative medical assisting functions
- Schedule, coordinate, and monitor appointments
- Schedule inpatient/outpatient admissions and procedures
- Understand and apply third-party guidance
- Obtain reimbursement through accurate claims submission
- Monitor third-party reimbursement
- Understand and adhere to manage care policies and procedures
  —*Negotiate managed care contracts*

Practice Finances
- Perform procedural and diagnostic coding
- Apply bookkeeping principles
- Manage accounts receivable
  —*Manage accounts payable*
  —*Process payroll*
  —*Document and maintain accounting and banking records*
  —*Develop and maintain fee schedules*
  —*Manage renewals of business and professional insurance policies*
  —*Manage personnel benefits and maintain records*
  —*Perform marketing, financial, and strategic planning*

Clinical

Fundamental Principles
- Apply principles of aseptic technique and infection control
- Comply with quality assurance practices
- Screen and follow up patient test results

Diagnostic Orders
- Collect and process specimens
- Perform diagnostic tests

Patient Care
- Adhere to established patient screening procedures
- Obtain patient history and vital signs
- Prepare and maintain examination and treatment areas
- Prepare patient for examinations, procedures, and treatments
- Assist with examinations, procedures, and treatments
- Prepare and administer medications and immunizations
- Maintain medication and immunization records
- Recognize and respond to emergencies
- Coordinate patient care information with other health care providers
- Initiate IVs and administer IV medications with appropriate training and as permitted by state law

General

Professionalism
- Display a professional manner and image
- Demonstrate initiative and responsibility
- Work as a member of the health care team
- Prioritize and perform multiple tasks
- Adapt to change
- Promote the CMA credential
- Enhance skills through continuing education
- Treat all patients with compassion and empathy
- Promote the practice through positive public relations

Communication Skills
- Recognize and respect cultural diversity
- Adapt communications to individual's ability to understand
- Use professional telephone technique
- Recognize and respond effectively to verbal, nonverbal, and written communications
- Use medical terminology appropriately
- Utilize electronic technology to receive, organize, prioritize and transmit information
- Serve as a liaison

Legal Concepts
- Perform within legal and ethical boundaries
- Prepare and maintain medical records
- Document accurately
- Follow employer's established policies dealing with the health care contract
- Implement and maintain federal and state health care legislation and regulations
- Comply with established risk management and safety procedures
- Recognize professional credentialing criteria
  - *Develop and maintain personnel, policy, and procedures manuals*

Instruction
- Instruct individuals according to their needs
- Explain office policies and procedures
- Teach methods of health promotion and disease prevention
- Locate community resources and disseminate information
  - *Develop educational materials*
  - *Conduct continuing education activities*

Operational Functions
- Perform inventory of supplies and equipment
- Perform routine maintenance of administrative and clinical equipment
- Apply computer techniques to support office operations
  - *Perform personnel management functions*
  - *Negotiate leases and prices for equipment and supply contracts*

APPENDIX B

KEY ENGLISH-TO-SPANISH HEALTH CARE PHRASES

Although English is the major language spoken in North America, a variety of languages are used in certain areas. Prominent among them is Spanish, representing Spain, the Caribbean Islands, Central and South America, and the Philippines. Rapport can be more easily established, and the patient and family will be at ease and feel more relaxed, if someone on the staff speaks their language. Some health care facilities, especially in areas with a large population of Spanish-speaking people, provide interpreters. In smaller hospitals or smaller communities this may not be possible.

It is to your advantage to learn the second most prominent language in your community. For this reason, the following table of English-to-Spanish phrases has been prepared. Instructions for using it are simple. Look for the phrase in English in the first column of the table. The second column gives the phrase in Spanish. You can write this or point to it. The third column gives a phonetic pronunciation. The syllable in each word to be accented is printed in italic type. Even if you are not proficient in English-to-Spanish, your Spanish-speaking patients will appreciate your trying to converse in their language. Begin with "Buenos días. ¿Cómo se siente?" And remember "por favor."[a]

Introductory Phrases

please[a]	por favor	por fah-*vor*
thank you	gracias	*grah*-see-ahs
good morning	buenos días	*bway*-nos *dee*-ahs
good afternoon	buenas tárdes	*bway*-nas *tar*-days
good evening	buenas noches	*bway*-nas *noh*-chays
my name is	mi nombre es	me *nohm*-bray ays
yes/no	si/no	see/no
What is your name?	¿Cómo se llama?	¿Koh-moh say *jah*-mah?
How old are you?	¿Cuántos años tienes?	¿*Kwan*-tohs ahn-yos tee-*ayn*jays?
Do you understand me?	¿Me entiende?	¿Me ayn-tee-*ayn*-day?
Speak slower.	Habla más despacio.	*Ah*-blah mahs days-*pah*-see-oh
Say it once again.	Repítalo, por favor.	Ray-*pee*-tah-loh, por fah-*vor*
How do you feel?	¿Cómo se siente?	¿*Koh*-moh say see-*ayn*-tay?
good	bien	bee-ayn
bad	mal	*mahl*
physician	médico	*may*-dee-koh
hospital	hospital	*ooh*-spee-tall
midwife	comadre	koh-*mah*-dray
native healer	curandero	ku-ren-*day*-roh

General

zero	cero	*se*-roh
one	uno	*oo*-noh
two	dos	dohs
three	tres	trays

From Rosdahl, C.B. [1995]. Textbook of Basic Nursing. 6th ed. Philadelphia: J.B. Lippincott.
[a]You should begin or end any request with the word PLEASE (POR FAVOR).

four	cuatro	*kwah*-troh
five	cinco	*sin*-koh
six	seis	says
seven	siete	see-*ay*-tay
eight	ocho	oh-choh
nine	nueve	new-*ay*-vay
ten	diez	*dee*-ays
hundred	ciento, cien	see-*en*-toh, see-*en*
hundred and one	ciento uno	see-*en*-toh *oo*-noh
Sunday	domingo	doh-*ming*-goh
Monday	lunes	*loo*-nays
Tuesday	martes	*mar*-tays
Wednesday	miércoles	mee-*er*-cohl-ays
Thursday	jueves	*hway*-vays
Friday	viernes	vee-*ayr*-nays
Saturday	sábado	*sah*-bah-doh
right	derecho	day-*ray*-choh
left	izqierdo	ees-kee-*ayr*-doh
early in the morning	temprano por la mañana	tehm-*prah*-noh por lah mah-*nyah*-na
in the daytime	en el día	ayn el *dee*-ah
at noon	a mediodía	ah meh-dee-oh-*dee*-ah
at bedtime	al acostarse	al ah-kos-*tar*-say
at night	por la noche	por la *noh*-chay
today	hoy	oy
tomorrow	mañana	mah-*nyah*-nah
yesterday	ayer	ai-*yer*
week	semana	say-*may*-nah
month	mes	mace

Parts of the Body

the head	la cabeza	lah kah-*bay*-sah
the eye	el ojo	el *o*-hoh
the ears	los oídos	lohs o-*ee*-dohs
the nose	la nariz	lah nah-*reez*
the mouth	la boca	lah *boh*-kah
the tongue	la lengua	la *len*-gwah
the neck	el cuello	el koo-*eh*-joh
the throat	la garganta	lah gar-*gan*-tah
the skin	la piel	lah pee-el
the bones	los huesos	lohs hoo-*ay*-sos
the muscles	los músculos	lohs *moos*-koo-lohs
the nerves	los nervios	lohs *nayhr*-vee-ohs
the shoulder blades	las paletillas	lahs pah-lay-*tee*-jahs
the arm	el brazo	el *brah*-soh
the elbow	el codo	el *koh*-doh
the wrist	la muñeca	lah moon-*yeh*-kah
the hand	la mano	lah *mah*-noh
the chest	el pecho	el *pay*-choh
the lungs	los pulmones	lohs puhl-*moh*-nays
the heart	el corazón	el koh-rah-*son*
the ribs	las costillas	lahs kohs-*tee*-jahs
the side	el flanco	el *flahn*-koh
the back	la espalda	lay ays-*pahl*-dah
the abdomen	el abdomen	el ahb-*doh*-men

the stomach	el estómago	el ays-*toh*-mah-goh
the leg	la pierna	lah pee-ehr-nah
the thigh	el muslo	el *moos*-loh
the ankle	el tobillo	el toh-*bee*-joh
the foot	el pie	el *pee*-ay
urine	urino	u-*re*-noh

Diseases

allergy	alergia	ah-*layr*-hee-ah
anemia	anemia	ah-*nay*-mee-ah
cancer	cancer	kahn-sayr
chickenpox	varicela	vah-ree-*say*-lah
diabetes	diabetes	dee-ah-bay-tees
diphtheria	difteria	deef-*tay*-ree-ah
German measles	rubéola	roo-*bay*-oh-lah
gonorrhea	gonorrea	gun-noh-*ree*-ah
heart disease	enfermedad del corazón	ayn-*fayr*-may-*dahd* dayl koh-rah-*sohn*
high blood pressure	presión alta	pray-see-*ohn al*-ta
influenza	gripe	*gree*-pay
lead poisoning	envenenamiento con plomo	ayn-vay-nay-nah-mee-*ayn*-toh kohn *ploh*-moh
liver disease	enfermedad del hígado	ayn-*fayr* may-dahd del *ee*-gah-doh
measles	sarampión	sah-rahm-pee-*ohn*
mumps	paperas	pah-*pay*-rahs
nervous disease	enfermedades nerviosa	ayn-fayr-may-*dahd*-days nayr-vee-*oh*-sah
pleurisy	pleuresía	play-oo-ray-*see*-ah
pneumonia	pulmonía	pool-moh-*nee*-ah
rheumatic fever	reumatismo (fiebre reumatica)	ray-oo-mah-*tees*-moh (fee-*ay*-bray ray-oo-*mah*-tee-kah)
scarlet fever	escarlatina	ays-kahr-lah-*tee*-nah
syphilis	sífilis	*see*-fee-lees
tuberculosis	tuberculosis	too-*bayr*-koo-lohs-sees

Signs and Symptoms

Do you have stomach cramps?	¿Tiene calambres en el estómago?	¿Tee-*ay*-nay kah-*lahm*-brays ayn el ays-*toh*-mah-goh?
chills?	escalofrios?	ays-kah-loh-*free*-ohs?
an attack of fever?	un ataque de fiebre?	oon ah-*tah*-kay day fee-*ay*-bray?
hemorrhage?	hemoragia?	ay-moh-*rah*-hee-ah?
nosebleeds?	hemoragia por la nariz?	ay-moh-*rah*-hee-ah por-lah nah-*rees*?
unusual vaginal bleeding?	hemoragia vaginal fuera de los periodos?	ay-moh-*rah*-hee-ah *vah*-hee-nahl foo-*ay*-rah day lohs pay-ree-*oh*-dohs?
hoarseness?	ronquera?	rohn-*kay*-rah?
a sore throat?	le duele la garganta?	lay doo-*ay*-lay lah gahr-*gahn*-tah?
Does it hurt to swallow?	¿Le duele al tragar?	¿Lay doo-ay-lay ahl trah-gar?
Have you any difficulty in breathing?	¿Tiene difficultad al respirar?	¿Tee-*ay*-nay dee-fee-kool-*tahd* ahl rays-*pee*-rahr?
Does it pain you to breathe?	¿Le duele al respirar?	¿Lay doo-*ay*-lay ahl rays-*pee*-rahr?
How does your head feel?	¿Cómo siente la cabeza?	¿*Koh*-moh see-*ayn*-tay lah kah-*bay*-sah?
Is your memory good?	¿Es buena su memoria?	¿Ays *bway*-nah soo may-*moh*-ree-ah?
Have you any pain in the head?	¿Le duele la cabeza?	¿Lay doo-*ay*-lay lah Kah-*bay*-sah?
Do you feel dizzy?	¿Tiene usted vértigo?	¿Tee-*ay*-nay ood-*stayd* vehr-tee-goh?
Are you tired?	¿Está usted cansado?	¿Ay-stah ood-*stayd* kahn-*sah*-doh?
Can you eat?	¿Puede comer?	¿*Pway*-day koh-*mer*?

Have you a good appetite?	¿Tiene usted buen apetito?	¿Tee-*ay*-nay ood-*stayd* bwayn ah-pay-*tee*-toh?
How are your stools?	¿Cómo son sus heces fecales?	¿*Kog*-moh sohn soos *bay*-says fay-*kal*-ays?
Are they regular?	¿Son regulares?	¿Sohn ray-goo-*lah*-rays?
Are you constipated?	¿Está estreñido?	¿Ay-*stah* ays-trayn-*yee*-do?
Do you have diarrhea?	¿Tiene diarrea?	¿Tee-*ay*-nay dee-ah-*ray*-ah?
Have you any difficulty passing water?	¿Tiene dificultad en orinar?	¿Tee-*ay*-nay dee-fee-kool-*tahd* ayn oh-ree-*nahr*?
Do you pass water involuntarily?	¿Orina sin querer?	¿Oh-*ree*-nah seen kay-rayr?
How long have you felt this way?	¿Desde cuándo se siente asi?	¿*Days*-day *Kwan*-doh say see-*ayn*-tay ah-see?
What diseases have you had?	¿Qué enfermedades ha tenido?	¿Kay ayn-fer-may-*dah*-days hah tay-*nee*-doh?
Do you hear voices?	¿Tiene los voces?	¿Tee-*ay*-nay los *vo*-ses?

Examination

Remove your clothing.	Quítese su ropa.	*Key*-tay-say soo *roh*-pah.
Put on this gown.	Pongáse la bata.	Pohn-*gah*-say lah *bah*-tah.
We need a urine specimen.	Es necesário una muestra de su orina.	Ays nay-say-*sar*-ee-oh oo-nah moo-*ay*-strah day oh-*ree*-nah.
Be seated.	Siéntese.	See-*ayn*-tay-say.
Recline.	Acuestése.	Ah-*cways*-tay-say.
Sit up.	Siéntese.	See-*ayn*-tay-say.
Stand.	Parése.	*Pah*-ray-say.
Bend your knees.	Doble las rodíllas.	*Doh*-blay lahs roh-*dee*-yahs.
Relax your muscles.	Reláje los músculos.	Ray-*lah*-hay lohs *moos*-koo-lohs.
Try to . . .	Atente . . .	Ah-*tayn*-tay . . .
Try again.	Atente ótra vez.	Ah-*tayn*-tay *oh*-tra vays.
Do not move.	No se muéva.	Noh say moo-*ay*-vah.
Turn on (or to) your left side.	Voltese a su lado izquierdo.	Vohl-*tay*-say ah soo *lah*-doh is-key-*ayr*-doh.
Turn on (or to) your right side.	Voltése a su ládo derécho.	Vohl-*tay*-say ah soo *lah*-doh day-*ray*-choh.
Take a deep breath.	Respíra profúndo.	Ray-*speer*-rah pro-*foon*-doh.
Hold your breath.	Deténga su respiración.	Day-*tayn*-gah soo ray-speer-ah-see-*ohn*.
Don't hold your breath.	No deténga su respiración.	Noh day-*tayn*-gah soo ray-speer-ah-see-*ohn*.
Cough.	Tosa.	*Toh*-sah.
Open your mouth.	Abra la boca.	*Ah*-brah lah *boh*-kah.
Show me . . .	Enséñeme . . .	Ayn-*sayn*-yay-may . . .
Here?	¿Aqui?	¿Ah-*kee*?
There?	¿Allí?	¿Ah-*jee*?
Which side?	¿En qué lado?	¿Ayn kay *lah*-doh?
Let me see your hand.	Enséñeme la mano.	Ayn-*sehn*-yay-may lah *mah*-noh.
Grasp my hand.	Apriete mi mano.	Ah-*pree*-it-tay mee *mah*-noh.
Raise your arm.	Levante el brazo.	Lay-*vahn*-tay el *brah*-soh.
Raise it more.	Más alto.	Mahs *ahl*-toh.
Now the other.	Ahora el otro.	Ah-*oh*-rah el *oh*-troh.

Treatment

It is necessary.	Es necesario.	Ays neh-say-*sah*-ree-oh.
An operation is necessary.	Una operación es necesaria.	Oo-nah oh-peh-rah-see-*ohn* ays neh-say-*sah*-ree-ah.
a prescription	una receta	*oo*-na ray-*say*-tah
Use it regularly.	Tómelo con regularidad.	*Toh*-may-loh kohn ray-goo-*lah*-ree-dad.
Take one teaspoonful three times daily (in water).	Toma una cucharadita tres veces al dia, con agua.	*Toh*-may oo-na koo-chah-rah-*dee*-tah trays *vay*-says ahl *dee*-ah, kohn ah-gwah.
Gargle.	Haga gargaras.	*Ah*-gah gar-*gah*-rahs.
Use injection.	Use una inyección.	*Oo*-say *oo*-nah in-*yek*-see-ohn.

oral contraceptives	una pildora	*oo*-nah peel-*doh*-rah
a pill	una pastilla	*oo*-nah pahs-*tee*-yah
a powder	un polvo	oon *pohl*-voh
before meals	antes de las comidas	*ahn*-tays day lahs koh-*mee*-dahs
after meals	despues de las comidas	*days*-poo-ehs day lahs koh-mee-dahs
every day	todos los día	*toh*-dohs lohs *dee*-ah
every hour	cada hora	*kah*-dah *oh*-rah
Breathe slowly—like this (in this manner).	Respire despacio—asi.	Rays-*pee*-ray days-*pah*-see-oh—ah-*see*.
Remain on a diet.	Estar a dieta.	Ays-*tar* a dee-*ay*-tah.

General

How do you feel?	¿Cómo se siénte?	*¿Koh*-moh say see-*ayn*-tay?
Do you have pain?	¿Tiéne dolor?	¿Tee-*ay*-nay doh-*lorh*?
Where is the pain?	¿Adónde es el dolor?	¿Ah-*dohn*-day ays ayl doh-*lorh*?
Do you want medication for your pain?	¿Quiére medicación para su dolor?	¿Kay-*ay*-ray may-dee-kah see-*ohn pak*-rah soo doh-*lorh*?
Are you comfortable?	¿Está confortáble?	¿Ay-*stah* kohn-for-*tah*-blay?
Are you thirsty?	¿Tiene sed?	¿Tee-*ay*-nay sayd?
You may not eat/drink.	No cóma/béba.	Noh *koh*-mah/bay-*bah*.
You can only drink water.	Solo puede tomar agua.	Soh-loh *pway*-day toh-mar *ah*-gwah.
Apply bandage to . . .	Ponga una vendaje a . . .	*Pohn*-gah *oo*-nah vehn-*dah*-hay ah . . .
Apply ointment.	Aplíquese unguento.	Ah-*plee*-kay-say oon-goo-*ayn*-toh.
Keep very quiet.	Estese muy quieto.	Ays-*tay*-say moo-ay key-*ay*-toh.
You must not speak.	No debe hablar.	Noh *day*-bay ha-*blahr*
It will be uncomfortable.	Séra incomódo.	*Say*-rah een-koh-*moh*-doh.
It will sting.	Va ardér.	Vah ahr-*dayr*.
You will feel pressure.	Vá a sentír presión.	Vah ah sayn-*teer* pray-see-*ohn*.
I am going to . . .	Voy a . . .	Voy ah . . .
Count (take) your pulse.	Tomár su púlso.	Toh-*marh* soo *pool*-soh.
Take your temperature.	Tomár su temperatúra.	Toh-*marh* soo taym-pay-rah-*too*-rah.
Take your blood pressure.	Tomar su presión.	Toh-*mahr* soo pray-see-*ohn*.
Give you pain medicine.	Dárle medicación para dolór.	*Dahr*-lay may-dee-kah-see-*ohn* pah-rah doh-*lohr*.
You should (try to) . . .	Trate de . . .	*Trah*-tay day . . .
Call for help/assistance.	Llamar para asisténcia.	Yah-*marh* pah-rah ah-sees-*tayn*-see-ah.
Empty your bladder.	Orinar.	Oh-ree-*narh*.
Do you still feel very weak?	¿Se siente muy débil todavía?	¿Say see-*ayn*-tay moo-ee *day*-beel toh-dah-*vee*-ah?
It is important to . . .	Es importánte que . . .	Ays eem-por-*tahn*-tay day . . .
Walk (ambulate).	Caminar.	Kah-mee-*narh*.
Drink fluids.	Beber líquidos.	Bay-*bayr lee*-kay-dohs.

APPENDIX C

TWO-LETTER POSTAL ZIP CODE ABBREVIATIONS

Alabama	AL	Nebraska	NE
Alaska	AK	Nevada	NV
Arizona	AZ	New Hampshire	NH
Arkansas	AR	New Jersey	NJ
American Samoa	AS	New Mexico	NM
California	CA	New York	NY
Colorado	CO	North Carolina	NC
Connecticut	CT	North Dakota	ND
Delaware	DE	Northern Mariana Islands	MP
District of Columbia	DC	Ohio	OH
Federated States of Micronesia	FM	Oklahoma	OK
Florida	FL	Oregon	OR
Georgia	GA	Palau	PW
Guam	GU	Pennsylvania	PA
Hawaii	HI	Puerto Rico	PR
Idaho	ID	Rhode Island	RI
Illinois	IL	South Carolina	SC
Indiana	IN	South Dakota	SD
Iowa	IA	Tennessee	TN
Kansas	KS	Texas	TX
Kentucky	KY	Utah	UT
Louisiana	LA	Vermont	VT
Maine	ME	Virginia	VA
Marshall Islands	MH	Virgin Islands	VI
Maryland	MD	Washington	WA
Massachusetts	MA	West Virginia	WV
Michigan	MI	Wisconsin	WI
Minnesota	MN	Wyoming	WY
Mississippi	MS	Armed Forces of the Americas	AA
Missouri	MO	Armed Forces Europe	AE
Montana	MT	Armed Forces Pacific	AP

APPENDIX D

ABBREVIATIONS COMMONLY USED IN DOCUMENTATION

Abbreviation	Meaning	Abbreviation	Meaning
$\bar{a}$	before	ml, mL	milliliter (1 mL = 1 cc)
abd	abdomen	NAD	no apparent distress
ac	before meals	NG	nasogastric
ADL	activities of daily living	NKDA	no known drug allergies
ad lib	as needed	noct.	nocturnal
adm	admitted, admission	NPO	nothing by mouth
amp	ampule	os	mouth
ant.	anterior	OOB	out of bed
AP	anterior-posterior	oz	ounce
ax.	axillary	$\bar{p}$	after
b.i.d.	twice a day	p.c.	after meals
BP	blood pressure	post	posterior
BR	bed rest	prep	preparation
BRP	bathroom privileges	pm	when necessary
C	Celsius	p.r.n.	as needed
$\bar{c}$	with	pt.	patient
caps	capsule	$\bar{q}$, q	every
CC	chief complaint	$\bar{q}$ 2 (3, 4, etc.) hours	every 2 (3, 4, etc.) hours
cc	cubic centimeter (1 cc = 1 mL)	qd	every day
c/o	complains of	qh	every hour
CVP	central venous pressure	q.i.d.	four times a day
CPX	complete physical examination	q.o.d.	every other day
Cx	canceled	q.s.	quantity sufficient
D/C	discontinue	R	right
disch; DC	discharge	R/O	rule out
drsg	dressing	ROM	range of motion
dr	dram	r/s	rescheduled
elix	elixir	$\bar{s}$	without
ext	extract or external	SBA	stand by assistance
F	Fahrenheit	SC	subcutaneous
Fx	fracture, fractional	SL	sublingual
gm	gram	SOB	shortness of breath
gr	grain	sol, soln	solution
gt/gtt	drop/drops	spec	specimen
"H," SC, or sub q	hypodermic or subcutaneous	s/p	status post
h	hour	sp. gr.	specific gravity
HOB	head of bed	S.S.E.	soapsuds enema
h.s.	bedtime (hour of sleep)	ss	one-half
Hx	history	STAT	immediately
I & O	intake & output	tab	tablet
IM	intramuscular	t.i.d.	three times a day
IV	intravenous	tinct or tr.	tincture
kg	kilogram	TKO	to keep open
KVO	keep vein open	TPN	total parenteral nutrition hyperalimentation
L	left, liter		
lat	lateral	TPR	temperature, pulse, respiration
MAE	moves all extremities	tsp	teaspoon
mg	milligram	TO	telephone order

Abbreviation	Meaning	Abbreviation	Meaning
TWE	tap water enema	Ortho	orthopedics
VO	verbal order	OT	occupational therapy
VS	vital signs	PE	physical examination
VSS	vital signs stable	PERRLA	pupils equal, round, & react to light and accommodation
W/C	wheelchair		
WNL	within normal limits	PID	pelvic inflammatory disease
		PI	present illness

Selected Abbreviations Used for Specific Descriptions

Abbreviation	Meaning
AKA	above-knee amputation
ASCVD	arteriosclerotic cardiovascular disease
ASHD	arteriosclerotic heart disease
BKA	below-knee amputation
ca	cancer
chest clear to A & P	chest clear to auscultation &* percussion
CMS	circulation movement sensation
CNS	central nervous system
DJD	degenerative joint disease
DOE	dyspnea on exertion
DTs	delirium tremens
D$_5$W	5% dextrose in water
FUO	fever of unknown origin
GB	gallbladder
GI	gastrointestinal
GYN	gynecology
H$_2$O$_2$	hydrogen peroxide
HA	hyperalimentation headache
HCVD	hypertensive cardiovascular disease
HEENT	head, ear, eye, nose, throat
HVD	hypertensive vascular disease
ICU	intensive care unit
I & D	incision and drainage
LLE	left lower extremity
LLQ	left lower quadrant
LOC	level of consciousness; laxatives of choice
LMP	last menstrual period
LUE	left upper extremity
LUQ	left upper quadrant
MI	myocaridal infarction
Neuro	neurology; neurosurgery
NS	normal saline
Nys.	nursery
NWB	non–weight-bearing
O.D.	right eye
O.S.	left eye
O.U.	each eye
OPD	outpatient department
ORIF	open reduction internal fixation

Abbreviation	Meaning
PM & R	physical medicine & rehabilitation
Psych	psychology; psychiatric
PT	physical therapy
RL (or LR)	Ringer's lactate; lactated Ringer's
RLE	right lower extremity
RLQ	right lower quadrant
RR, PAR, PACU	recovery room, post-anesthesia room, post-anesthesia care unit
RUE	right upper extremity
RUQ	right upper quadrant
Rx	prescription
SOB	short of breath
STD	sexually transmitted disease
STSG	split-thickness skin graft
Surg	surgery, surgical
T & A	tonsillectomy & adenoidectomy
THR, TJR	total hip replacement; total joint replacement
URI	upper respiratory infection
UTI	urinary tract infection
vag	vaginal
WNWD	well-nourished, well-developed

Selected Abbreviations Related to Common Diagnostic Tests

Abbreviation	Meaning
BE	barium enema
B.M.R.	basal metabolism rate
Ca^{++}	calcium
CAT	computed axial tomography
CBC	complete blood count
Cl$^-$	chloride
C & S	culture & sensitivity
Dx	diagnosis
ECG, EKG	electrocardiogram
EEG	electroencephalogram
FBS	fasting blood sugar
hct	hematocrit
Hgb	hemoglobin
IVP	intravenous pyelogram
K$^+$	potassium
LP	lumbar puncture
MRI	magnetic resonance imaging
Na$^+$	sodium
RBC	red blood cell

Abbreviation	Meaning	Abbreviation	Meaning
UGI	upper gastrointestinal x-ray	°	degree
UA	urinalysis	#	number or pound
WBC	white blood cell	$\times$	times
		@	at
		+	positive
Commonly Used Symbols		−	negative
		±	positive or negative
>	greater than	F_1	first filial generation
<	less than	F_2	second filial generation
=	equal to	PO_2	partial pressure of oxygen
$\simeq$	approximately equal to	PCO_2	partial pressure of carbon dioxide
$\leq$	equal to or less than	:	ratio
$\geq$	equal to or greater than	∴	therefore
↑	increased	%	percent
↓	decreased	2°	secondary to
♀	female	△	change
♂	male		

From Craven, R.F., and Hirnle, C.J. (1996). Human Health and Function, 2nd ed. Philadelphia: Lippincott-Raven.

APPENDIX E

COMMONLY MISUSED WORDS

Because these words have similar spellings and pronunciation, they can easily be confused or misused. Watch your spelling carefully! Always proofread all business letters for accuracy and grammar.

Word	Example of Correct Use
adverse (harmful) averse (opposed to)	Some adverse reactions can be life threatening. I am not averse to working on Mondays.
affect (verb, to influence, change) effect (noun, result)	The protesters will not affect the outcome. The effect of the antibiotics has been beneficial.
already (previously) all ready (prepared, all set)	We already tried that approach. Are we all ready to go?
anoxia (without oxygen) anorexia (without appetite)	Anoxia will cause the brain cells to die quickly. Anorexia is a serious illness that faces teenagers.
aphagia (without swallowing) aphasia (without speech)	A feeding tube is needed because of her aphagia. Her stroke caused aphasia.
appendices (end of book) appendicitis (inflammation of appendix)	There are five appendices at the end of book. The patient was treated for appendicitis.
biannual (twice a year) biennial (occurring every 2 years)	Productivity reports are printed on a biannual basis. Staff contracts are renewed on a biennial basis.
bite (grip with teeth) byte (character)	The patient's bite is poorly aligned. Buy a computer with enough bytes for future growth.
bowl (container) bowel (intestines, colon)	The jelly beans are in the bowl. Instruct the patient to complete the bowel preparation.
emphysema (chronic lung disease) empyema (accumulation of pus)	Smoking causes emphysema. Empyema most commonly occurs in the pleural cavity.
ensure (be certain) insure (protect against risk) assure (provide confidence)	Call this patient to ensure that he comprehends the instructions. Please insure this package for $200. I assure you that he is getting the correct treatment.
everyday (adjective, routine, ordinary) every day (adverbial phrase, each day)	Quality checks are an everyday procedure. There can be legal ramifications if this is not done every day.
except (exclude) expect (anticipate) accept (agree)	All antibiotics except penicillin will work. I expect this work to be completed by noon. I accept this challenge.

Word	Example of Correct Use
farther (greater distance) further (greater degree)	It is 1 mile farther down the road. The process needs further refinement.
fundus (pertains to hollow organ) fungus (organism that can lead to infection)	The fundus was firm after the baby's delivery. A fungus was growing under her nails.
its (possessive pronoun) it's (contraction of it and is)	The pharmacy must protect its supply of opioids. It's time to take a break.
lactose (type of sugar in milk) lactase (enzyme)	I have a lactose allergy. Lactase is responsible for dissolving lactose.
libel (written defamatory statement) liable (legally responsible)	The statements about John Roberts were libel. You are liable for your actions.
may be (compound verb) maybe (adverb, perhaps)	Dr. Rogers may be in surgery this afternoon. Maybe it will snow tomorrow.
metatarsals (bones in foot) metacarpals (bones in palm)	Crutches are often needed when the metatarsals are fractured. Typing is difficult for patients with a metacarpal fracture.
mucus (substance that is secreted) mucous (membrane that secretes)	The patient had a mucus plug. The mucous membrane secretes the mucus.
parental (pertaining to parent) parenteral (not by mouth)	Follow parental guidelines for TV use. Parenteral feedings will start on Monday.
postnatal (after birth) postnasal (behind nose)	Complications can occur in the postnatal period. Postnasal drainage can be uncomfortable.
principle (noun, law) principal (noun, leader; adjective, most important)	A key principle of economics is understanding cash flow. The principal's name is Tina Sefferin; her experience is the principal reason she was hired.
rubella (German measles) rubeola (14-day measles)	You need a rubella vaccination. There is a outbreak of rubeola at the middle school.
serum (watery component of blood) sebum (oily substance secreted by the sebaceous glands)	The patient's serum is used for various tests. Sebum helps to lubricate the skin surface.
tact (behavior) tack (different direction)	He handled his child with great tact. A new tack may be needed for us to win that bid.
than (to show comparison) then (next)	Salaries are higher now than they were a year ago. Clean room 2; then go to lunch.
there (place, point) their (possessive pronoun) they're (pronoun plus verb)	You need to be there at 2 PM. Leaving their bikes on the road caused the accident. They're going to be late.
uvula (soft tissue at back of palate) vulva (external female organ)	The patient's uvula was swollen. A laceration of the vulva was noted during the gynecological examination.
weather (climate) whether (indicating a possibility)	The weather is unpredictable. I wonder whether it will rain or snow.

GLOSSARY OF KEY TERMS

Chapter 1

accreditation a nongovernmental professional peer review process that provides technical assistance and evaluates educational programs for quality based on preestablished academic and administrative standards.

administrative pertaining to office management (e.g., office procedures and nonclinical tasks that a medical assistant performs)

caduceus a symbol of a wand or staff with two serpents coiled around it; sometimes used as the sign of the medical profession (the more appropriate symbol has only one snake).

certification voluntary testing to prove an individual's baseline competency in a particular area; or official recognition that the testing was successful.

clinical pertaining to direct patient care.

cloning genetically identical replication of cells, an organ, or an organism in the laboratory.

continuing education units credits awarded for attendance at approved local and state AAMA meetings and seminars, completion of guided study courses, and journal articles designed to submit a posttest for CEU credit.

externship an educational course that allows the student to obtain hands-on experience.

inpatient a residential medical setting for diagnostic, radiographic, or treatment purposes; a patient in such a setting.

laboratory a place where research, investigation, or scientific testing takes place.

medical assistant a multiskilled health professional who performs a variety of clinical and administrative tasks in a medical setting.

multidisciplinary involving many disciplines; describes a group of health care professionals from various specialties brought together to meet the patient's needs.

multiskilled health professional an individual with training in more than one discipline in health care.

outpatient a medical setting where patients receive care but do not reside; also, such a patient.

recertification certification renewed either by taking the examination again or by completing a specified number of continuing education units in a 5-year period.

role delineation chart a list of the areas of competence expected of the graduate

specialty a subcategory of medicine, such as pediatrics, studied after completion of medical school.

Chapter 2

abandonment withdrawal by a physician from a contractual relationship with a patient without proper notification while the patient still needs treatment.

advance directive a statement of a patient's wishes regarding health care prior to a critical medical event.

age of majority age at which an individual is considered to be an adult, usually 18 to 21 years.

appeal process by which a higher court reviews the decision of a lower court.

artificial insemination the insertion of sperm into a vagina by artificial means.

assault an attempt or threat to touch another person without his or her consent.

battery physical touching of a patient without consent.

bench trial trial in which the judge hears the case and renders a verdict; no jury is present.

bioethics moral issues and concerns that affect a person's life.

blood-borne pathogens viruses that can be spread through direct contact with blood or body fluids from an infected person.

breach an infraction, such as breach of contract, in which the agreed-on terms are violated.

censure a verbal or written reprimand from a professional organization regarding a specific incident.

certification voluntary testing to prove an individual's baseline competency in a particular area; or official recognition that the testing was successful.

civil law a branch of law that focuses on issues between private citizens.

coerce to force or compel a person to do something against his or her wishes.

common law a group of laws originating in England, established by tradition and the courts rather than by statute.

comparative negligence a percentage of damage awards based on the contribution of negligence between two parties.

confidentiality protection of information about patients from unauthorized personnel.

consent an agreement between a patient and physician to do a given medical procedure.

consideration the exchange of fees for a service.

contract an agreement between two or more parties for a given act.

contributory negligence a defense strategy in which the defendant admits to negligence but claims that the plaintiff assisted in promoting the damages.

cross-examination questioning of a witness by the opposing attorney.

damages injury or suffering compensated for with an award of money.

defamation of character making false or malicious statements about a person's character or reputation.

defendant the party that is accused of wrongdoing.

depositions processes in which one party questions another party under oath.

direct examination questioning of a witness by the attorney for the individual the witness is representing.

durable power of attorney a legal document, not time limited, giving another person the authority to act in one's behalf.

duress the act of compelling or forcing someone to do something that he or she does not want to do.

emancipated minor a patent under the age of majority who is legally considered to be an adult.

ethics guidelines for moral behavior that are enforced by peer groups.

expert witness a professional who testifies on the standard of care in a trial.

expressed consent a statement of approval from the patient for the physician to perform a given procedure after the patient has been informed about the risks and benefits of the particular procedure; also referred to as informed consent.

expressed contracts formal agreements between two or more people.

fee splitting sharing fees for the referral of patients to certain colleagues.

fraud a deceitful act with the intention of concealing the truth

implied consent an informal agreement of approval from the patient to perform a given task.

implied contracts contracts between physician and patient not written but assumed by the actions of the parties.

informed consent a statement of approval from the patient for the physician to perform a given procedure after the patient has been told about the risks and benefits of the procedure; also referred to as expressed consent.

intentional tort an act that takes place with malice and with the intent of causing harm; a deliberate violation of another person's legal rights.

legally required disclosure reporting of certain events to governmental agencies without the patient's consent.

libel written statement that defames a person's reputation or character.

licensure the strictest form of professional accreditation.

litigation process of filing or contesting a lawsuit.

locum tenens a substitute physician.

malpractice a tort in which the patient is harmed by the actions of a health care worker.

negligence performance of an act that a reasonable health care worker would not have done; omission of an act that a reasonable person would have done.

noncompliant describes a patient who refuses or is unable to follow prescribed orders.

plaintiff the party who initiates a lawsuit.

precedents previous court decisions used as a legal foundation.

protocol a code of proper conduct; a treatment plan.

registered indicates that a professional has met basic requirements, usually for education; has passed standard testing; and has been approved by a governing body to perform given tasks within a state.

res ipsa loquitur "the thing speaks for itself."

res judicata "the thing has been decided."

respondeat superior "let the master answer."

slander oral statement that defames a person's reputation or character.

stare decisis "the previous decision stands."

statutes laws written by federal, state, or local legislators.

statute of limitations a time limit on legal action; e.g., the period during which a patient may file a lawsuit.

tort wrongdoing or misdeeds resulting from a breach of legal duty.

unintentional tort describes an honest mistake by a person operating in good faith.

verdict a decision of guilty or not guilty based on evidence presented in a trial.

Chapter 3

anacusis complete hearing loss.

bias the formation of an opinion without foundation or reason; prejudice.

clarification explanation; removal of confusion or uncertainty.

cultures societies; customary beliefs, values, or religious traits of a group of people.

demeanor the way a person looks, behaves, and conducts the self.

discrimination making a difference in favor of or against someone.

dysphasia impairment of speech; difficulty speaking.

dysphonia impairment of voice; hoarseness.

feedback the response to an input during communication.

grief great sadness caused by loss.

messages communications sent from one person to another though words, body language, or in writing.

mourning to demonstrate signs of grief; grieving.

nonlanguage communication that is expressed not in spoken language but through laughing, sobbing, grunting, and sighing.

paralanguage factors connected with language, such as voice, volume, pitch.

paraphrasing restating what you heard using your own words.

presbyacusis   loss of hearing associated with aging.

reflecting   repeat what one heard using open-ended questions.

stereotyping   an opinion of a particular group, culture, or age that is based on negative perception.

summarizing   briefly review the information discussed to determine the patient's comprehension.

therapeutic   having to do with treating or curing a disease; describes a task that can cure or help a patient.

Chapter 4

alternative   an option or substitute to the standard medical treatment plan, e.g. herbal therapies, acupuncture, hypnosis.

assessment   gathering information about the patient, such as by touching, talking, taking vital signs.

carbohydrates   chemical elements in food that convert to sugar, providing energy.

coping mechanisms   unconscious methods of relieving intense stress.

detoxification   clearing of drugs from the body and treating the withdrawal symptoms.

documentation   written evidence of a task or procedure done.

evaluation   determining whether a patient is reaching a given goal or objective; if the goal has not been met, reassessment begins.

implementation   initiating and carrying out a procedure or task.

learning objectives   procedures or tasks that the learner will achieve.

noncompliance   patient's inability or refusal to follow a recommended plan of care.

nutrition   the study of food and how it used for growth, nourishment, and repair.

placebo   the power of believing that something will make you better without any chemical reaction that warrants improvement, e.g., sugar pills.

planning   the process of using information gathered during assessment of a patient to organize the approach to teaching a patient; setting goals and objectives.

psychomotor   describes a physical task.

range-of-motion   the amount or degree to which a joint can be extended or flexed.

stress   a factor that induces body tension; can be positive or negative.

Chapter 5

attitude   a state of mind; how a person feels about a given subject or at a given time.

closed captioning   printed words displayed on a television screen to help people with hearing disabilities or impairments.

diction   speech and pronunciation.

diplomacy   the art of handling people with genuine care and concern.

emergency medical service (EMS)   a group of health care providers working as a team to care for sick or injured patients before they arrive at the hospital.

ergonomic   describes a workstation designed to prevent work-related injuries and to promote work efficiency.

receptionist   a person who greets patients as they arrive at a medical office and performs various administrative tasks.

teletypewriter (TTY)   a special machine that allows communication on a telephone with a hearing-impaired person.

triage   sorting of patients into categories based on their level of sickness or injury; to ensure that life-threatening medical conditions are treated immediately.

Chapter 6

acute   abrupt in onset

buffer   extra time to accommodate emergencies, walk-ins, and other demands on the provider's daily time schedule that are not considered direct patient care

chronic   long-standing.

clustering   grouping patients with similar problems or needs.

consultation   request for assistance from one physician to another.

constellation of symptoms   a group of clinical signs indicating a particular disease process.

double booking   the practice of booking two patients for the same period with the same physician

matrix   a system for blocking off unavailable patient appointment times.

precertification   approved documentation prior to referrals to specialists and other facilities

providers   a health care worker who delivers medical care.

referral   instruction to transfer a patient's care to a specialist

STAT   immediately.

streaming   a method of allotting time for appointments based on the needs of the individual patient to minimize gaps in time and backups

tickler file   a file that provides a reminder to do a given task at a particular date and time.

wave scheduling system   a flexible scheduling method that allows time for procedures of varying lengths and the addition of unscheduled patients, as needed.

Chapter 7

agenda   a brief outline of the topics to be discussed at a meeting.

annotation   the process of reading and highlighting key points in a document.

BiCaps   words or phrases with unusual capitalization.

block   letter format in which the date, salutation, subject line, and closing are flush right, all others flush left.

enclosure   an indication to the reader of a letter that a document has been included with the letter.

font   a typeface; affects the way written messages look.

full block letter format in which each line is flush left; most commonly used format for business letters.

intercaps words or phrases with unusual capitalization.

margin the blank space around the edges of a piece of paper, such as a letter or page of a book.

memorandum written interoffice communication.

proofread to read text and check for accuracy.

salutation an introductory phrase that greets the reader of a letter.

semiblock letter format in which the first word of each paragraph is indented; also refereed to as modified block.

template a skeleton of a letter or document with preset and prespaced elements.

Chapter 8

alphabetic filing arranging of names or titles according to the sequence of letters in the alphabet.

chief complaint a description of the symptoms that led the patient to seek the physician's care.

chronological order time-ordered; usually the most recent item is foremost.

cross-reference verification to another source.

demographic data statistical characteristics of populations.

electronic medical records (EMR) information about patients that is recorded and stored on computer

flow sheet color-coded sheets that allow information to be recorded in graphic or tabular form for easy retrieval.

medical history forms record containing information about a patient's complete past and present health status.

microfiche sheets of microfilm.

microfilm photographs of records in a reduced size.

narrative a paragraph indicating the contact with the patient, what was done for the patient, and the outcome of any action.

numeric filing arranging files in number order.

present illness a specific account of the chief complaint, including time frames and characteristics.

problem-oriented medical record (POMR) a common method of compiling information that lists each problem of the patient, usually at the beginning of the folder, and references each problem with a number throughout the folder.

reverse chronological order items placed with oldest first.

SOAP a style of chanting that includes subjective, objective, assessment, and planning notes.

subject filing arranging files according to their title, grouping similar subjects together.

workers' compensation employer insurance for treatment of an employee's injury or illness related to the job.

Chapter 9

analogue pertains to use of dictation machine with a handheld microphone to tape a report of a patient encounter or other correspondence.

digital pertaining to, resembling, or performed with a finger; expressed in digits (0–9).

transcription the process of typing a dictated message.

Chapter 10

cookies tiny files that are left on your computer's hard drive by a website without your permission.

downloading transferring information from an outside location to your computer.

encryption scrambling E-mail messages as they leave one site and unscrambling them when they arrive at the designated address.

Ethernet system that allows the computer to be connected to a cable or DSL system.

Internet global system used to connect one computer to another.

intranet a private network system of computers.

literary search finding professional journal articles on a given subject.

search engine program that allows you to find information on the Internet rapidly and effectively.

surfing navigating the Internet.

virus a harmful invader that can damage your computer.

virtual a paperless system or chart on your computer.

Chapter 11

Centers for Medicare & Medicaid federal agency that regulates Medicare and Medicaid along with the Clinical Laboratory Improvement Amendments Act and Health Insurance Portability and Accountability Act.

Clinical Laboratory Improvement Amendments Act federal law that aims to reduce errors made in laboratories and set standards for laboratories.

expected threshold a numerical goal.

incident reports written documentation of a negative or untoward patient, staff, or visitor event.

Health Insurance Portability and Accountability Act federal law that requires all health care settings to ensure privacy and security of patient information. Also requires health insurance to be accessible for working Americans and available when changing employment.

Joint Commission on Accreditation of Healthcare Organizations a nationally recognized agency focused on setting health care standards and accrediting settings that meet these standards.

Occupational Safety and Health Administration a federal agency with a mission to protect employees from work related hazards.

outcomes final results of patient care.

quality improvement a commitment or plan to provide patients with the best medicine and health care possible.

sentinel event an unexpected occurrence or event that results in death or serious physical or psychological injury.

task force   a group of employees working together to resolve a problem.

Chapter 12

Americans with Disabilities Act   a law designed to meet the needs of people with physical and mental challenges.

budget   financial planning tool that helps an organization estimate its anticipated expenditures and revenues.

compliance officer   person charged with ensuring that a facility follows laws, policies, and protocols.

Family and Medical Leave Act   a law designed to allow an employee up to 12 weeks of unpaid leave from his or her job to meet family needs.

job description   a statement that informs an employee about the duties and expectations for a given job.

mission statement   a statement describing the goals of the medical office and those it serves.

organizational chart   a flow sheet depicting the members of a team in a structured or hierarchical manner.

policy   a statement that reflects an organization's rules on a given topic.

procedure   a series of steps required to perform a given task.

Chapter 13

adjustment   change in a posted account.

aging schedule   a form used to track outstanding balances.

collections   acquiring payments that are due.

credit   balance in one's favor on an account; promise to pay a bill at a later date.

installment   partial payment of a bill.

participating providers   those who agree to participate with managed care contracts and other third-party payers in exchange for building a solid patient base.

patient co-payment   the part of an insured service that the patient must pay.

professional courtesy   a discount fee given to health care professionals.

write-off   cancel an unpaid debt.

Chapter 14

accounts payable   amounts owed to others.

accounts receivable   amounts due from others.

adjustment   entry to change an account, often to include a discount.

balance   equality between the debit and credit sides of an accounting equation; that which is left over after additions and subtractions have been made to an account.

bookkeeping   organized and accurate record keeping for financial transactions.

charge slip   a preprinted three-part form that can be placed on a day sheet to record the patient's charges and payments along with other information in an encounter form.

credit   record of a payment received.

day sheet   record of daily financial transactions in a pegboard bookkeeping system.

debit   record of a debt.

encounter form   a preprinted statement that lists codes for basic office charges and has sections to record charges incurred in an office visit, the patient's current balance, and next appointment.

ledger card   a card used to record financial transactions on a particular patient's account.

posting   transferring information from one account to another.

returned check fee   amount of money a bank or business charges for a check written with insufficient funds.

service charge   amount of money a bank charges for certain transactions.

Chapter 15

accounting cycle   a consecutive 12-month period for financial record keeping following either a fiscal year (starting on a specified date) or the calendar year (January to December).

audit   a review of an account.

check register   place to record checks as they are written.

check stub   part of a check that is retained; indicates to whom it was issued, in what amount, and on what date.

FICA   Federal Insurance Contributions Act; the law that established Social Security and that mandates Social Security tax payments and benefits.

federal unemployment tax   tax is used to finance all administrative expenses of the federal/state unemployment insurance system and the federal costs involved in extended benefits.

gross income   the amount of money earned by an employee before taxes are withheld.

Internal Revenue Service (IRS)   a federal agency that collects taxes and enforces various tax laws.

invoice   a statement of debt owed; a bill.

liabilities   amounts the practice owes.

net pay   the amount of money an employee is paid after all taxes and co-payments are withheld.

packing slip   a document that accompanies a supply order and lists the enclosed items.

payroll   the process of calculating employee salary.

payroll journal   a method of keeping payroll data using the pegboard system.

profit-and-loss statement   statement of income and expenditures; shows whether in a given period a business made or lost money and how much.

purchase order   a document that lists items to be purchased and authorization to make the expenditure.

summation report   any report that provides a summary of activities, such as a payroll report or a profit-and-loss statement.

withholding   moneys held back (not paid to employee) for federal, state, and local taxes and for Social Security.

Chapter 16

assignment of benefits   transfer of the patient's legal right to collect third-party benefits for medical expenses to the provider of the services.

balance billing   billing the patient for the balance or difference between the physician's charges and the Medicare-approved charges; prohibited by most managed care contracts.

birthday rule   determination of which policyholder's insurance is the first to pay when a patient is covered by two policies. The policyholder whose birth month and day comes first in the calendar is primary.

capitation   managed care plan that pays a certain amount to a provider over a specific time for caring for the patients in the plan regardless of what or how many services are performed.

carrier   a company that assumes the risk of an insurance company.

claims   requests to an insurance company for reimbursement of costs.

claims administrator   an individual who manages the third-party reimbursement policies for a medical practice.

coinsurance   the agreed-upon amount paid to the provider by a policyholder. Also called co-payment.

coordination of benefits   the method of designating the order in which multiple carriers pay benefits to avoid duplication of payment.

co-payments   that part of an insured service the patient must pay.

crossover claim   a claim that crosses over automatically from one coverage to another for payment.

deductible   a specified amount paid by the policyholder before the carrier begins paying.

dependent   spouse, children, and sometimes other individuals designated by the insured who are covered under a health care plan.

eligibility   the determination of an insured's right to receive benefits from a third-party payer based on such criteria as payment of premiums and date of start of coverage.

employee   a person hired to perform given duties in return for financial compensation.

explanation of benefits (EOB)   a statement that accompanies a payment from an insurance carrier and outlines which dates and services are being paid.

fee-for-service   an established set of fees charged for specific services and paid by the patient or insurance carrier.

fee schedule   a list of preestablished fee allowances set for specific services and procedures performed by a provider.

group member   a policyholder who is a member of a group and covered by the group's insurance carrier.

health maintenance organization (HMO)   an organization that provides a wide range of services through a contract with a specified group at a predetermined payment.

independent practice association (IPA)   several independently practicing physicians contracted with a health maintenance organization to provide services to HMO members.

insurance   a policy that promises to pay some or all of a customer's medical bills.

insured   an individual who owns a policy that promises to pay some or all of his or her medical bills.

managed care   the practice of third-party payers to control costs by requiring physicians to adhere to specific rules as a condition of payment.

Medicare   Social Security–established health insurance for the elderly.

peer review organization   a group of physicians and specialists that conducts a review of a disputed case and makes a final recommendation.

physician hospital organization   a coalition of physicians and a hospital contracting with large employers, insurance carriers, and other benefits groups to provide discounted health services.

plan maximum   the highest amount paid by a third-party payer for any given service.

preexisting condition   medical problem treated by a physician before an insurance plan's effective date. A third-party payer may exclude coverage for preexisting conditions.

preferred provider organization (PPO)   an organization whose purpose is to contract with providers, then lease this network of contracted providers to health care plans.

third-party administrator   administrator who processes claims for the sponsor of self-funded benefit planning.

unbundling   the practice of submitting a claim with several separate procedure codes rather than a single code that represents the services performed.

usual, customary, and reasonable (UCR)   the basis of a physician's fee schedule, the usual and customary cost of the same service or procedure in a similar geographic area and under the same or similar circumstances.

utilization review   an analysis of individual cases by a committee to make sure services and procedures being billed to a third-party payer are medically necessary and to ensure compliance with its rules and regulations regarding reimbursement.

Chapter 17

advance beneficiary notice   document that informs covered patients that Medicare may not cover a certain service and the patient will be responsible for the bill.

audits   inspection of records to determine compliance and to detect fraud.

conventions   general notes, symbols, typeface, format, and punctuation that direct and guide the coder to the most complete and accurate ICD-9 code.

cross-reference   checking the tabular list against the alphabetic list in ICD-9 coding.

E-codes   codes indicating the external cause or reason for an injury or illness.

eponym   word derived from a personal name, e.g., *Alzheimer* disease.

etiology   cause of an illness or injury.

inpatient   a patient who is admitted to a medical facility for an overnight stay.

International Classification of Diseases, Ninth Revision, Clinical Modification   a system for transforming verbal descriptions of disease, injuries, conditions, and procedures to numeric codes.

late effects   conditions that result from another condition. For example, left-sided paralysis may be a *late effect* of a stroke.

main terms   words in a multiple-word diagnosis that a coder should locate in the alphabetic listing. They represent the condition (not the location) to be coded.

medical necessity   a determination made by a third party that a certain service or procedure was necessary based on sound medical practice.

outpatient   a patient who is treated by a physician in the office or a hospital but is not admitted for an overnight stay.

primary diagnosis   the condition or chief complaint that brings a person to a medical facility for treatment.

service   medical interventions completed by a provider.

specificity   the amount of detail in an explanation of a diagnosis.

V-codes   codes assigned to patients who receive service but have no illness, injury, or disorder, e.g., a vaccination or a screening mammogram.

Chapter 18

Current Procedural Terminology (CPT)   a comprehensive listing of medical terms and codes for the uniform coding of procedures and services provided by physicians.

descriptor   description of a service listed with its code number.

diagnostic related group   category in which inpatients are sorted according to the similarity of their diagnoses, treatment, and length of stay.

Healthcare Common Procedure Coding System   AMA's coding system based on CPT-4; assigns alphabetic and numeric codes to items such as ambulance service, wheelchairs, and injections.

key component   the criteria or factors on which the selection of a CPT-4 evaluation and management is based.

modifiers   letters or numbers added to a code to clarify the service or procedure.

outlier   a patient who has an unusually long stay in the hospital or a complicated case.

procedure   a medical service or test that is coded for reimbursement.

resource-based relative value scale   a schedule that sets a maximal fee for each service based on the reduction of Medicare Part B costs—the establishment of national standards for payment based on CPT-4 codes.

upcoding   coding a claim that pays more than the actual procedure or service performed.

Chapter 19

externship   a training program that allows students close to graduating to work in a clinical setting under the direct supervision of an experienced medical assistant.

networking   use of friends, family members, or professional colleagues to advance or obtain information in the workplace.

portfolio   a folder containing pertinent documentation and supplies that may be needed during an interview.

preceptor   an experienced medical assistant who works with new medical assisting students to ease their transition from student to employee.

résumé   written account of an individual's education and work experience.

ESL GLOSSARY

This textbook was reviewed by an English as a second language (ESL) learning expert to ensure that the language is appropriate and understandable for all students. While the structure, grammar, and active voice used in this text will help you better understand the content, some words and phrases may be difficult or confusing. This glossary defines the terminology by first identifying it as a noun, verb, adverb, adjective, or phrase and then explaining the meaning of the term as it is used in the textbook.

Term	Part of Speech	Meaning
Acutely	adverb	sharply, severely
Adhere	verb	stick to, follow completely
Adhere	verb	stay with, stick
Advent	noun	coming, arrival
Adverse	adjective	negative, bad, undesirable
Allay	verb	do away with (fears), calm
Alleged	adjective	said to have happened but not proved
Allied	adjective	joined, united
Alter	verb	change
Angled (at an angle)	adjective	not directly facing
Appropriate	adjective	right, correct
Arise	verb	come up
Arrears	noun	overdue payment or debt not settled
Assault	noun, verb	attack
Asset	noun	advantage, highly valued person
Attuned	adjective	sensitive to or aware of
Batch	noun	group
Belittle	verb	disparage; make a person feel unimportant
Bias	noun	prejudice, personal opinion
Blatant	adjective	obvious
Blurred	adjective	not clear
Breach	noun	break, split
Bruise	noun	contusion; dark mark on the skin from an injury

Term	Part of Speech	Meaning
Burden	noun	trouble, problem
Buzz	noun	sound of zzzzzz, as a bee makes
Carcinogen	noun	substance that causes cancer
Cast	verb	throw, as cast a glance at
Cessation	noun	a stopping
Charge	noun	accusation
Cliché	noun	a saying that is so generally understood to be true that it is unnecessary to repeat it
Complexity	noun	amount of complication
Compliance	noun	the act of following the rules
Compromise	verb	find middle ground in a dispute or conflict
Conglomerate	noun	very large company with many products, services, and locations
Consensus	noun	general agreement
Contamination	noun	presence of unclean substances
Convey	verb	literally transport; explain, make clear
Core	adjective	basic, most important
Countersue	verb	respond to a lawsuit with lawsuit
Creed	noun	a statement of beliefs
Crutches	noun	supports used by people with leg or foot injuries to help them walk
Daunting	adjective	frightening
Deem	verb	decide, conclude
Demeanor	noun	behavior
Denigrate	verb	make someone feel unimportant, lower
Dereliction	noun	failure to carry out a duty or responsibility
Deterrent	noun	action or object that stops a person from doing something
Discard	verb	throw away
Distort	verb	make appear different from reality, change
Distraction	noun	thing that takes the attention from what the person is doing
Distressed	adjective	upset, not calm
Doubt	noun	uncertainty; lack of belief
Dressing	noun	bandage, protective cover on wound
Drive	verb	power, transport by car or bus
Efficacy	noun	level of efficiency or usefulness

Term	Part of Speech	Meaning
Elderly	adjective	old
Elective	noun	a choice, the thing chosen
Elicit	verb	bring out, encourage
Enhance	verb	make better
Enlightenment	noun	the awakening of new ideas
Entitled	adjective	allowed, authorized
Enunciate (well)	verb	say words very clearly
Escalate	verb	to become greater
Euphoria	noun	a feeling that everything is great
Evolve	verb	develop
Exacerbation	noun	thing that makes something worse
Extraneous	adjective	extra, unnecessary
Felon	noun	person guilty of one or more major crimes
Fidget	verb	move parts of the body, such as hands, feet, indicating nervousness
Fine	noun	money the government demands in payment from a person who has done something wrong
Fiscal	adjective	related to money management, especially governmental spending
Flight of ideas	phrase	many ideas spoken quickly
Flow (of traffic)	noun	the pattern people walk through an office area
Foster	verb	support or encourage
Fraudulent	adjective	deceptive and illegal
Freestanding	adjective	not connected to a larger institution
Gatekeeper	noun	a controller
Gather	verb	to collect into one place
Gear (up)	verb	equip, prepare
Germicide	noun	something that kills germs
Grimace	noun	movement of the face that indicates dislike or pain
Given (a given)	noun	something definite and expected, taken for granted
Gross breach	noun	very serious illegal act
Grossly	adverb	greatly
Grunt	verb	make a sound deep in the throat that can show hard work, disgust, or boredom
Hacker	noun	person who finds a way into a private computer system to take information or cause damage

Term	Part of Speech	Meaning
Hailed	adjective	praised as something good
Halt	verb	stop
Handle	verb	take care of
Harsh	adjective	irritating, as *bright, harsh light*
Higher	adjective	more powerful
Hinder	verb	to slow or stop an action or idea
Hose	noun	stockings, pantyhose
Hospice	noun	a center or program to care for people who are dying
Immunity	noun	protection from punishment
Impairment	noun	malfunction, handicap, diminished ability as a result of an injury
Impartial	adjective	having no opinion or preference before the action
Impassive	adjective	not showing emotion
Inappropriate	adjective	not right or correct for the situation
Incur	verb	cause, bring on oneself
Indigent	noun	poor, in poverty
Infraction	noun	breach of a rule or law
Insanity	noun	mental illness
Integrity	noun	honesty, steadfast morality, trustworthiness
Intermediary	noun	person or organization that communicates between two groups
Intermingled	adjective	mixed
Intimidating	adjective	causing fear
Introspection	noun	thoughts about oneself
Invasive	adjective	entering or cutting into the body
Irate	verb	angry
Jargon	noun	slang; special words understood by specific group of people, as *medical jargon*
Jeopardize	noun	put in danger
Jump start	noun	a quick beginning
Kin	noun	family, relatives
Lethal	adjective	deadly, causing death
Levy	verb	ask for, require
Liable	noun	responsible
Likelihood	noun	probability

Term	Part of Speech	Meaning
Lot	noun	group; large amount
Lower	adjective	less powerful
Low-key	adjective	not exciting or loud
Malicious	adjective	causing pain, injury, or distress
Malpractice suit	noun, verb	a legal action saying a doctor or medical facility did something wrong
Mandate	verb	command, as in a law
Manslaughter	noun	killing someone by accident
Meticulous	adjective	careful
Mound	noun	a large quantity; literally a heap
Mute	adjective	not able to talk
Omit	verb	leave out, not do
Open-ended	adjective	with no definite answer or choice of answers
Opt	verb	choose
Optimal	noun	the best, most nearly perfect
Options	noun	possibilities
Outburst	noun	a sudden loud expression or action
Outlay	noun	money spent
Outline	verb	describe, especially in a list
Perceived	adjective	understood
Perceive	verb	see, understand
Pertinent	adjective	related to, relevant
Phone tag	noun	sequence of unanswered phone calls between two people who keep leaving messages
Physically challenged	adjective	having physical problems making it hard to walk or perform other activities of daily living
Piece	noun	part, fragment of a whole
Pitch	noun	the way the voice goes up and down
Pleasant	adjective	nice
Polarized	adjective	opposite; having opposite opinions or ideas
Pose (a question)	verb	ask, raise
Potential	noun	the possibility of an act or event
Prelude	noun	something that comes before the main event
Prerequisite	noun	requirement before doing something

Term	Part of Speech	Meaning
Prescription	noun	a paper from a doctor that you take to the pharmacy to get medicine; an order for treatment
Procrastination	noun	waiting to do something instead of doing it immediately
Protocol	noun	the right way to do something
Range	noun	how high or how low a voice goes
Rape	verb	to force someone to have sex
Red flag	noun	sign that something is wrong, not good
Reimburse	verb	pay money owed
Relay	verb	tell, pass on to another person
Render	verb	provide
Repel	verb	force away
Residency	adjective	the final hospital training for a doctor
Restitution	noun	payment to someone for harm or damage
Retain	verb	keep
Retrievable	adjective	able to get or obtain again
Retroactive	adjective	going back in time
Review	noun	the process of checking something
Risk	noun	danger
Run the spectrum	phrase	go from one extreme to the other
Good Samaritan	noun	someone who takes care of people in need
Sanction	noun	a law that punishes for not following the rules
Scope	noun	range; set of limitations
Scribble over	verb	make marks on paper, not words, to cover incorrect information; cross out heavily
Scrupulously	adverb	very carefully
Scrutinize	verb	look very carefully
Sequential	adjective	in order
Setback	noun	thing or action that stops progress
Shift	verb	change
Shift	noun	time of day when a person works, such as day shift
Sibling	noun	brother or sister
Sigh	verb	let air out of the mouth, meaning the person is tired or feeling a strong emotion
Simulate	verb	imitate, fake

Term	Part of Speech	Meaning
Skyrocket	verb	go up quickly
Sluggish	adjective	slow moving, not alert
Snapshot	noun	a quick look or understanding, like a photograph taken casually
Snap	noun	a quick, strong reaction, usually negative
Soar	verb	go up quickly
Sob	verb	cry, weep
Sole	adjective	only
Solid	adjective	firm, hard
Sophisticated	adjective	very complex or complicated
Spatial	adjective	related to space, room, area
Stake	noun	interest
Stalled	adjective	stopped by something
Stark	adjective	bare, blunt, extreme
Stat.	adverb, abbreviation	immediately; from Latin *statim*
Statute	noun	law
Stipulate	verb	say what is required
Stirrups	noun	set of foot rests used to keep legs up and apart for female internal examination
Stoic	adjective	not showing emotion or reaction
Streamline	verb	to make efficient
Strive	verb	try, attempt, work hard
Stuff	verb	put papers in envelopes
Stumble	verb	walk unsteadily, without balance; trip over something
Stuttering	noun	speech that is greatly slowed by elongation or repetition of sounds
Subpoena	noun	an order to speak or be present in a court
Substantial	adjective	large
Surrogate	noun	replacement for a person or thing
Surveillance	noun	continuous watch on something or someone
Suture	noun	stitch
Suture	adjective	used in sewing
Suture	verb	close a wound by sewing
Tact	noun	politeness, consideration of others' feelings

Term	Part of Speech	Meaning
Tailored	adjective	made to fit something or someone specific
Tally	verb	to add up, to figure, to total
Tally	noun	a record, a summary, a total
Tamper	verb	to interfere harmfully
Target	verb	focus on, aim at
Terminate (employment)	verb	fire, tell a person he or she can no longer work for you
Threat	noun	danger or warning of danger
Threshold	noun	starting place
Tickler	noun	reminder
Time consuming	phrase	taking a lot of time
Time frame	noun	the time for doing something
Tone (of voice)	noun	feeling, mood, loudness, or nature of the voice
Track	verb	check progress, record changes
Trend	verb	make a pattern
Trend	noun	pattern
Trigger	noun	something that causes something else to happen
Utmost	adjective	the greatest
Vague	adjective	not clear, not specific
Vehicle	noun	method, carrier
Veteran	adjective	having much experience
Wail	verb	cry loudly
Wand	noun	hand-held electronic scanner; reads information such as bar codes
Welfare	noun	condition
Whirr	noun	sound of something spinning quickly
Willfully	adverb	deliberately, on purpose
Woe	noun	problem, trouble
Wringing hands	phrase	moving hands as if washing them; sign of worry or tension

INDEX

Page numbers in *italics* denote figures, those followed by a "t" indicate tables, those followed by a "b" indicate boxes, those followed by a "p" indicate procedures.